Oxford

Practical Psychiatry

POCKET MEDICAL REFERENCE SERIES

Practical Psychiatry

TIM BETTS

Neuropsychiatry Clinic
Department of Psychiatry
Queen Elizabeth Psychiatric Hospital
Birmingham

and

CLAIRE KENWOOD

Registrar, All-Birmingham
Rotational Scheme

Oxford New York Tokyo
OXFORD UNIVERSITY PRESS
1992

Oxford University Press, Walton Street, Oxford OX2 6DP

Oxford   New York   Toronto
Delhi Bombay Calcutta Madras Karachi
Petaling Jaya Singapore Hong Kong Tokyo
Nairobi Dar es Salaam Cape Town
Melbourne Auckland

and associated companies in
Berlin Ibadan

Oxford is a trade mark of Oxford University Press

Published in the United States
by Oxford University Press, New York

A catalogue record for this book is available from the British Library

Library of Congress Cataloging in Publication Data

Betts, T. A. (Timothy Arnold)
Practical psychiatry / Tim Betts and Claire Kenwood.
p.   cm.—(Pocket medical reference series)
Includes index.
1. Psychiatry—Handbooks, manuals, etc. I. Kenwood, Claire.
II. Title. III. Series.
[DNLM: 1. Mental Disorders— diagnosis—handbooks. 2. Mental
Disorders—therapy—handbooks. WM 34 B565p]
RC456.B47   1992   616.89— dc20   92-8372
ISBN 0 19 263027 X
ISBN 0 19 263010 5 (pbk)

Set by Graphicraft Typesetters Ltd, Hong Kong
Printed and bound in Great Britain by
Bookcraft (Bath) Ltd, Midsomer Norton, Avon

Introduction

A young doctor starting a post in psychiatry (whether as a career trainee or for six months' experience as part of general practice training) faces a stressful and potentially bewildering few months. The transition from a busy medical or surgical job to the slower paced, less physically demanding (but more emotionally searching) world of psychiatry can be difficult.

This is particularly so because psychiatry is a less scientifically rigorous subject than those the trainee has been used to. Psychiatrists have to live with uncertainty and imprecision. Many clinical judgements are necessarily based on intuition and experience: the illness model is occasionally appropriate and useful, but usually the behaviour, feelings, and experiences which have brought the patient to clinical notice are the result of several influences—medical, developmental, cultural, psychological, social, environmental, personal, and others that can only be guessed at. Elucidation and understanding of these influences takes time and often requires a personal input from the psychiatrist. Treatment requires a knowledge of all these factors, and also often makes a personal emotional demand on the therapist. In no other branch of medicine, except perhaps general practice, does the personal interaction between doctor and patient become so important.

Faced with this challenge some doctors retreat into organic certainties, refuse to acknowledge factors other than medical ones, and use a totally illness-related model: others abandon medical principles altogether and adopt models of understanding psychiatric patients which deny illness and embrace political and historical interpretations of behaviour which rely heavily on anti-authoritarian beliefs and theories of collusion and persecution. Both approaches may be right occasionally, but cannot be right all the time: both reflect the turmoil induced by trying to live comfortably with the demands of psychiatry.

Many young doctors feel that in these crucial formative first few months in psychiatry they lack guidance. Nothing teaches like experience and we have a lot of sympathy with the view that it is better to be thrown in at the deep end, as it were, accumulate experience, and then begin to make sense of it. But, valuable as experience is, it can be a poor teacher if it is not structured, and experience is useless without at least some feedback.

Experience of psychiatry as an undergraduate can be particularly misleading, as the acquisition of facts in order to do well in MCQ examinations is a poor preparation for the experiences of the real world and the demands of patient care and assessment.

We have long felt that the trainee, in the early months of psychiatry, needs some kind of practical pocket book into which he or she can dip as the need arises in the first few months of training so that, when faced with a particular problem for the first time, a structured account of what to do is available, to enrich experience, and provide some light in the darkness. As experience develops, such a guide will be consulted less and less, but there is a need for a bridge between undergraduate texts and extensive postgraduate tomes. Such a book will be necessarily didactic and authoritarian and can serve as no more than a preliminary guide.

This then is our attempt at such a book. It is not a textbook of psychiatry and you should not treat it as such. It is unashamedly meant as a crib, as a practical guide for those first perplexing weeks in psychiatry, to help you through unfamiliar situations and emergencies that you are unprepared for, to give you some confidence, and to build up your ability to rely on your own skills. It is not a substitute for practical experience, and can provide only limited feedback of your performance (if you have just had to cope with an unfamiliar emergency using your natural wit, it will be useful to consult the relevant section of this book and see how you did, and whether you had left anything undone). But real feedback can only come from your teachers and your peers (and is often very hard to obtain).

There are four main sections to this book. The first (designed to be read before you see your first patient) is about the basic tools of the psychiatric trade—the interview, mental state assessment, physical assessment, and ancillary assessments.

The next section, meant to be consulted at time of need, presents you with common ways in which mental illness may present, and common problems with which you may have to deal without much prior instruction. It is meant to be a practical guide rather than an exhaustive text, and is meant to do no more than to suggest how you might react to, assess, and behave in certain situations, and to outline what your professional duties and responsibilities are.

There next follows a section on management that is aimed at helping you to choose the correct treatment for a particular condition, be aware of pitfalls and difficulties, and to try to understand the principles underlying what you are attempting to do.

Finally, there is a section containing brief descriptions of the common psychiatric syndromes and illnesses that is meant for no more than a quick revision of the things that you should already know, but may have forgotten. In particular, it may help you to give information and explanations to your patients.

We hope that this book will be useful to those of you embarking on your first psychiatric job (whether for experience as a GP or as a definite career move), and will also help house officers in general hospitals encountering unexpected psychiatric conditions, students starting practical experience in psychiatry, and general practitioners who need a short practical book on psychiatry. It may help you to pass practically orientated exams, but its main purpose is to get you out of a few scrapes and make your early days in psychiatry more enjoyable and interesting: who knows, it may inspire some of you to take up a career in this most fascinating and rewarding branch of whole-person medicine.

To save unnecessary repetition of personal pronouns and in accordance with customary English usage you should assume throughout this book that 'he' embraces 'she' unless the context makes this impossible (e.g. erectile difficulties): in other words we have used 'he' and 'him' also to mean 'she' and 'her'. We have used the feminine gender when the problem being discussed is much more common in women than in men (e.g. anorexia nervosa).

We have chosen to begin the book using the traditional nomenclature and classification that a trainee is likely to encounter in the early days of experience from his teachers, and have then gradually introduced modern concepts, particularly DSM III R so that Chapter 6 is almost entirely based upon it. This, we think, is how most trainees learn to use a scientific classification such as DSM III R.

We have a debt of gratitude to many people, particularly former students and trainees, without whom this book would never have got off the ground, but we are particularly grateful to Gillian Dalby for her endless, cheerful, sweating over a hot Macintosh computer, to Sarah Lawson for her initial reading of the manuscript, helpful suggestions, and encouragement, and to Sarah Boden for her continuing interest, for assessing the manuscript from a nursing viewpoint, and for her help with Chapter 5, based on her joint contribution to counselling training for the undergraduate course in psychiatry at Birmingham University. We also thank Alex Allwood and Alison Beardall for their final helpful reading of the manuscript, and Ann Cartmill who has given so much of her time to checking the manuscript, preparing an index, and providing her warm enthusiasm for the project.

Finally, we acknowledge gratefully the support of our respective spouses and children through trying times (Pam, Hannah, Victoria, George, Florence, and Tim; Adam and James). They have put up with our exacting task without complaint.

Contents

An introduction to classification

You may feel that the classification of psychiatric disorders is arbitrary, nit picking, obscure, and useless. Discussions about the right classificatory niche into which a patient's exotic symptoms should be placed can resemble nothing so much as medieval scholars' debates about how many angels could dance on the head of a pin. You may feel terminally exasperated by the need, when doing a discharge summary, to codify a patient's rich experience of both life and insanity into a single constipating category.

But there is an obvious need to study disease processes, make observations, communicate these to others, and then make sure that these observations are reliable (in the sense that others will make the same observations faced with the same behaviour and that you can replicate your own observations). Once it can be shown that the observations are reliable and valid then some weight can be put upon them and you can begin to classify them into similar groups and clusters. How you do this depends, of course, on the clutter of ideas and concepts already in your mind relating to mental illness and its causes. A Victorian psychiatrist faced with a psychotic patient would have spent much time observing whether the patient excessively masturbated, was bald, and had characteristic bumps on his head (because these observations fitted the current theories of the causes of insanity) and would not, as we do, have explored the patient's delusions or hallucinatory experiences to look for first rank symptoms (although our Victorian colleague did have a comprehensive catalogue of different types of psychotic laughter).

Perhaps our twenty-second century colleagues will be equally amazed at our predilection for classifying delusions as they measure subatomic particle densities in the caudate nucleus—'How quaint,' they will say, 'and the answer was in front of their noses all the time.'

There is also an obvious need to communicate the results of our treatment strategies to each other and to check whether the incidence and prevalence of mental disorders is changing (what impact, for instance, is AIDS making on psychiatric referrals?). Such communication is hampered if we cannot agree on what diseases we are treating or observing. Why, for instance, is drug X getting better results in treating schizophrenia in the United States than in the United Kingdom? The answer may be that drug X is much better at treating hypomania than schizophrenia and American psychiatrists are much more likely than British ones to label hypomania as schizophrenia.

So, some classification is unavoidable and necessary. Apart from the ordinary imprecise clinical classification hallowed by tradition that you and your colleagues will use without thinking much about it, there are presently two competing systems—ICD 9 (shortly to be ICD 10) and DSM III R (eventually to be DSM IV).

The ICD system—International Classification of Disease Revision 9—is basically a single axis **descriptive** or 'glossary' classification that gives a clinical outline of each category. A patient may correspond to only parts of the category in which he is placed, but this does have the advantage of allowing sufficient flexibility to catalogue a large proportion of patients and is useful for coping with statistics when complete accuracy is needed. You will use ICD 9 when compiling statistical returns of patients seen and treated, but probably by the time this book is published you will be using the next revision ICD 10. This has been much changed (and now has research guidelines), and manuals of instructions about how to use it will be available in your hospital with which you will need to be familiar. Do take the chore of filling in statistical return forms seriously: to do this properly you will have to have studied the manual.

DSM III R (Diagnostic and Statistical Manual III (revised)) is an **operational** classification—that is, it employs strict criteria for classification such that one can be sure that patients placed in a particular classification have certain symptoms in common. It is a more precise kind of classification, which is obviously an advantage in research work. It ensures that different studies can be directly compared, knowing that the categories mean the same thing in each. The disadvantage of the system is that sometimes a patient will fall outside any category and cannot be put into the 'nearest' one as in ICD 10.

DSM is a **multiaxial** classification, that is it allows for information in different areas to be recorded simultaneously, which is its other main advantage for research purposes. Axes I, II, and III are used in clinical practice, whereas IV and V are research categories.

Axis I   mental disorder

    II   personality and developmental disorder

    III   physical conditions

    IV   severity of psychosocial stressors

    V   global assessment of functioning

In formal teaching sessions, such as journal clubs, and in literature, you will be more likely to use and encounter DSM III R (it is uncertain when DSM IV will be available). In your examinations you can use either (although you must indicate which one you want to use). Until you gain experience you will tend to use the broader clinical classifications that you will encounter in the first five chapters of this book (and which your clinical teachers will use in their day-to-day discussions with you). After a few months in practice you should, however, be trying to use one of the two classification systems consistently. Chapter 6 (p. 453) in this book is therefore based on DSM III R, partly because it is the classification system that we tend to favour and partly because your academic teachers will be likely to use it. It is a useful exercise to get one of the readily available short manuals for DSM III R early in your training and to try to determine an appropriate classification for every patient that you encounter. This will teach you how to use the system and will help shape up your observation and recording of data. Another useful exercise is to compare the diagnostic categories in the two systems when you are coding statistical information to help learn both the strengths and weaknesses of each.

CHAPTER 1

Principles of the psychiatric interview

A   Interviewing techniques

Start of the interview

- Introduce yourself.
- Indicate amount of time available.
- Use open-ended questions.
- Establish presenting topics.
- Anything else you need to talk about?
- Listen and plan: how much control?
- Plan pacing and amount of passivity.

Middle of the interview

- Introduce each new topic.
- Start each topic with open-ended questions.
- Used closed questions at end of topic.
- Use recapping if direction lost.
- Pay attention to information.
- Deal with distortions to communication by:
    1. using positive facilitation, verbal and non-verbal
    2. using negative facilitation, verbal and non-verbal
    3. avoiding jargon
    4. using confrontation
    5. using supportive empathic statements

6. avoiding diminishing words and statements
7. using directive intervention.

End of the interview

- Anything to add?
- Recap.
- Discuss next step.
- Give information.
- Firm concluding statement.

It is extremely important to get formal training in interviewing techniques, if you have not already had it, as quickly as possible, otherwise you will tend to perpetuate your mistakes and weaknesses and they will become too entrenched to change. Doctors untrained in interviewing skills tend particularly to fail to elicit easily available information (perhaps getting only a third of what they could obtain), to fail to make appropriate rapport with the patient, and to narrow prematurely the focus of their enquiry.

Formal training consists of learning the technical language of interviewing so that you can understand the process of the interview and can begin to analyse your own and other trainees' interviews in a logical and structured way; and to have demonstrated to you models of interviewing skills and to then practise these skills, obtaining feedback of your performance, preferably by means of videotape replay. It is best to undertake this training with a small peer group and with a teacher who uses techniques of positive reinforcement rather than negative destruction. Initially the group may develop a uniform style of interviewing, and providing it is a good style this is no bad thing, but as training develops so individual trainees will shape the style to fit comfortably with their own personalities and preferred methods of working.

Good interviewing skills, important in all areas of medicine, are especially so in psychiatry because assessment of the patient and his management is almost totally dependent on them. The most esoteric knowledge of psychiatry is useless if you cannot communicate with and understand the person in front of you.

In an interview you are attempting to elicit accurate information as completely as possible, and to remain uncluttered by misinformation and misunderstandings derived from failure to understand the language and emotions of the patient. Subsequent management depends on a good rapport or therapeutic alliance developing between doctor and patient as well as a clear understanding of the patient's problems. Good rapport is not just a sycophantic acceptance of the patient's view, it implies the development of a trusting relationship so that views can be challenged if necessary.

The start of the interview

Introduce yourself and establish the identity of your patient. Indicate the nature of the interview and how long it is likely to take. Remember that the patient may have some initial reluctance in talking to a psychiatrist and have a natural reluctance to talk about intimate things, and he must be given enough time to bring up the topics that he feels to be relevant.

Begin with *open-ended questions* (which cannot be answered by 'yes' or 'no') to draw the patient out. Make sure that you have elicited all the main complaints of the patient and have asked 'is there anything else you feel you need to talk about?' before you begin to analyse and dissect the presenting complaints. Recapping these complaints may be helpful before you start the rest of the interview.

In these first few very important minutes of drawing the patient out you should be listening and planning your strategy for the rest of the interview, particularly in terms of the degree of *control* you will need to exert over the interview process (for example, strategies for containing the over-talkative, or drawing out the shy and defensive), and in terms of *pacing*—the relative amount of time you will need to spend, in the time available, on different topics and tasks. For example, the middle-aged man who tells you about his irritability, his indigestion, and his early morning waking with anxiety and the shakes, will need a careful assessment of his drinking history; the young lady who complains of a policeman's voice coming from her wardrobe addressing her familiarly as 'you old shit bag' will need a careful examination of her mental state.

In the first few minutes, therefore, you should be as passive as possible.

The middle of the interview

Here you are more active, but exerting the minimum of control, as you elicit the information you need and examine each topic in turn (always starting a new topic with open-ended questions and finishing with closed questions that can be answered by a 'yes' or 'no') as you *clarify* responses to your initial questions. *Introduce* new topics to the patient so that he can understand where the interview is going, 'You mentioned some rows you had with your mother. I would like to turn now to discuss your family and any problems you have had with them. Perhaps we can start with your mother—can you tell me a little about her?'

From time to time brief *recapping* is useful (particularly if you get stuck!). Do not be afraid of pauses, however, and feel you have to rush in and fill them. During pauses patients feel that you are thinking about their problem, or will themselves volunteer new information. It is useful at these natural break points to review what you have learnt and pause to plan your next move.

When you are pursuing a particular line of enquiry and a fresh item of information emerges, important but unrelated to the present topic, make a note of it in your mind but make sure you finish the present topic before turning to it. For example, 'When we were talking about your feelings for your husband just now, you mentioned the death of your mother and that seemed very important to you. Can you tell me more about it?' This is called *paying attention to information*. Do not, however, be distracted by the new and exciting item of information so that you charge after it and never return to complete your first line of enquiry. This is a common fault and leads to a confused and unsure grasp of the patient's problems.

During this busy part of the interview *distortions to communication* may occur, either because of the emotional state of the patient, because of language difficulties, or because of reticence or over-talkativeness. There are various useful techniques that help to prevent these distortions that you need to become familiar with. Remember that the distortion may not lie with the patient: it may be your own feelings or misconceptions that are getting in the way.

Learn to use *positive facilitation*—both verbal and non-verbal. The phrases 'yes, go on', 'tell me more about that', or just feeding back what the patient has just said ('you felt very upset') may seem banal when written down, but, used in the right context and at the right time, draw the patient out and encourage him to talk about even painful things. Video feedback will teach you the importance of facilitating body language (nods, smiles, relaxed posture). *Negative facilitation* is only rarely needed, but is often inadvertently shown. Here video feedback will help you to look critically at yourself and remove those little quirks of posture and gesture that have effects opposite to those intended, as can your tone of voice.

Avoid *jargon* and *clarify* words and phrases that you do not understand or which may have one meaning for you and another for the patient ('You say you have never been the same since an attack of 'flu'—what was it actually like?'; 'You say you have been depressed. Can you tell me in your own words how that feels?'). Always clarify other doctors' diagnoses: 'known epileptics' for instance often turn out not to have the condition.

Confront displays of emotion rather than politely (or uncomfortably) ignoring them. ('I notice that when we were talking about your wife you looked upset. Can you tell me more about your feelings?' 'I've noticed that whilst we have been talking you've seemed quite angry at times. Can you tell me what is troubling you?').

Supportive empathic statements are also useful with displays of emotion ('You must have been very upset at that time.' 'That must have been very difficult for you.'). Like confrontation, empathic statements are often facilitating and indicate to the patient that, unlike most people (and many doctors), you are able to talk about feelings. This develops rapport. Make sure you show empathy rather than sympathy. 'I can see it still upsets you to talk about it,' or 'You must have wondered how you were going to cope,' is empathy. 'Poor you!' or 'Gosh, what a situation, I don't know how you coped' is sympathy. The problem with sympathy is that it puts the patient into a submissive role and may be irritatingly patronizing: empathy indicates the concern of one human being for another and an acknowledgement of feelings, providing it is not just an unconsidered, unfeeling 'knee-jerk' reaction to what the patient is saying.

Try to avoid diminutive words that thoughtlessly qualify feelings in a belittling way. Many doctors say, 'So you've been feeling *quite* depressed,' or 'So you are *pretty* sad,' because this is a style of speech that the medical profession unconsciously uses without recognizing how patronizing and denigrating of the patient's experience it may sound. This habit of speech is common and is possibly used to protect the doctor's own feelings. Videotape feedback will show you what patients feel about it!

Do not be afraid to exert *control*—beginners are often reluctant to, but patients do not mind being interrupted providing that it is done politely, ('I realize this is important to you, but can we please go back to something else you said earlier about your problems with your work. Can you tell me more about that?'). This is called **directive intervention**.

An important question is how many notes you should make. Accurate recording of information is essential, but rapport is unlikely to be gained with a doctor who keeps his eyes firmly on his notepad. Our own view is that note taking, particularly in the first interview, should be avoided. If essential (to record details of a complicated history for instance) you should break off, say 'Do you mind if I just write down these details as they are important and I do not want to forget them', record them, and then deliberately lay down your pen, turn back into the interview, and indicate both verbally and non-verbally that the face-to-face interview has resumed. The end of the interview, when the patient has gone, is the time to record notes, even verbatim examples of the patient's speech. You will find that your memory will stretch to this. Very unusual speech might need to be recorded at the time.

The end of the interview

It is important to keep to the time allotted. Sometimes, if important material is emerging or there has been an emotional abreaction, you might have to break this rule. Allow yourself at least five minutes for *recapping*. This includes a brief but accurate summarizing of what the patient has said, your own impressions of the interview, and an enquiry about whether he has anything to add. Your own summary will often prompt you to ask further questions or to make further clarifications, which is why you must leave enough time for it.

You should finish with a firm *concluding statement* and end the interview with a statement such as, 'It has been very useful talking to you, but we must close now although I should be glad of the opportunity of talking with you again if you agree.' Many trainees find it difficult to end an interview.

Interview training should also include learning how to *give information* to patients. Remember that very few pieces of information are retained by the patient unless repeated and reiterated, and hardly any is retained if the patient is disturbed or upset.

Do get feedback of your developing skills: even though it is often painful at first, you will eventually find that encounters even with 'difficult' patients become a challenge to those skills, rather than self-defeating. You may begin to realize the truth in the adage 'psychiatrists are doctors who have time to take a proper history.'

B Interviewing people who are mentally ill

- Be natural and unafraid.
- Do not be patronizing.
- Cultivate a sense of perspective.
- Pay attention to your own feelings.
- Acknowledge the patient's reality—but do not confirm it.
- Do not humour the patient.
- Acknowledge and maintain personal space—yours and the patient's.

- Avoid sudden moves or a loud voice. Avoid intrusive eye contact.
- Be cool and polite. Know how to get out of a room or confrontation—or how to let the patient 'escape' if necessary.
- Set, and keep, firm limits on behaviour.
- Ensure quietness and confidentiality.

Although 'How do I talk to people who have a mental illness?' must be one of the commonest questions to occur to the newcomer to psychiatry, most conventional textbooks are rather coy about answering it. There is also no substitute for experience so the sooner you get as much practice as possible the better.

Perhaps the most important thing is to be *natural and unafraid*. Take a genuine interest in the person rather than his symptoms (however bizarre and alarming), and *avoid being patronizing* and making the patient feel wary or afraid himself. Many beginners feel that it is dangerous to show a caring attitude, that if they do the patient will take advantage of it and exploit what is regarded as a weakness. Caring for the patient, as a fellow human being, even when he is being difficult or is very disturbed, is however, very important. Allow yourself to show natural warmth, but avoid any ingratiating greasy 'chumminess'.

For the majority of patients you encounter who are suffering from stress disorders or long-standing adjustment-to-life problems, the general principles of the psychiatric interview are the same as for a medical interview with patients with physical disorders. The difference is that you are much more concerned with placing the patient's present symptoms and complaints into a historical perspective and understanding the influences—biological, social, and psychological—that have shaped the personality and ways of adapting to stress of the person in front of you. You are also much more concerned with confronting and drawing out the feelings and emotions of the person in front of you and acknowledging them. Many British patients and doctors are unused to doing this and find it uncomfortable at first.

Your own relationship with the patient is also more important than in conventional medical interviewing. So much of psychiatry depends on the personal inter-action between patient and doctor that you, your own knowledge and personality, your own beliefs and culture, are part of the assessment process. The first few months in psychiatry are often a little disturbing as your own feelings and values come under scrutiny. As you question the life experiences, behaviour, and quirks of your patients so you tend to question your own and you may not entirely like what you learn about your-self. If you are sensitive (and if you are not then what are you doing in psychiatry—or medicine for that matter?) you will occasionally feel that you are drown-ing in a sea of human misery about which you can do so little. You do need *to cultivate a sense of perspect-ive* and to learn to recognize that very few problems are without remedy and that your main job is to help people to learn how to overcome their own difficulties (rather than you solving them for them), or to learn to live with and adjust to those difficulties that cannot be overcome.

Human resource and human adaptability are more infinite than you may initially realize. In addition, what you do has more of an effect than you may initially realize, thus taking a history, helping someone to take a structured, detailed look at their problems and their life circumstances, is more therapeutic than it may seem at first, and in itself helps many people. In psychiatry you also need to pay more attention to your own feelings and reactions towards the person in front of you. If the patient brings out feelings of hostility and anger in you, it is important to acknowledge those feelings (but not, of course, to act on them), and to ask yourself where your feelings are coming from and what behaviours or attitudes in the patient are releasing them. If the patient is doing this to you, he is probably doing it to others and may need to modify his behaviour or to learn of the effect he has on others.

Your own emotional feelings may also be diagnostic. In the interview it is important to remember that you represent reality and sanity. If, towards the end of an interview, you feel baffled and confused and feel that you have failed to grasp the patient's problems, the patient may be thought disordered or have organic impairment. If, however, the world seems suddenly a wonderful place and you feel uncommonly cheerful and optimistic then maybe the patient is elated, or conversely, if you feel plunged into gloom and despair about the overwhelming problems of the person in front of you, you might have merely picked up his depressed mood. There is no doubt that affect is infective and that your emotional reaction can be diagnostic. *Learn to monitor your emotional reactions*, but learn not to let them mislead you and do not overreact to them. In depression, for instance, empathy is valuable: sympathy is not.

A minority of the patients you interview will be psychotic and removed from your reality. It is important to acknowledge the reality of the experience for the patient without yourself agreeing with it. It is wrong to 'humour' patients by agreeing with their hallucinations or deluded beliefs. You need to keep them in touch with reality, but in a pleasant, supportive way. 'I accept that you have this very strong feeling that people are spying on you, but they are not: it is part of your illness.' 'It must be very frightening seeing green Alsatians running up and down the ward, but they are not there and if you take this medicine the visions will soon stop.'

Even in the most disturbed or psychotic patient there is usually still an island of sanity that you can reach, and no matter how mad a person appears that part of him may still be listening to you and understanding you. So, be cool, be polite, keep the person in touch with reality, do not humour him but acknowledge the intensity of his experiences and empathize with how disturbing or frightening it must be.

Patients who are disturbed are frightening (and also frightened themselves) and you may fear aggression or unprovoked attack. See Section 4J (p. 288) for advice about known aggressive patients, but you have to assume that all patients with a psychosis or with organic brain impairment or confusion might behave unpredictably. Most of them will be frightened; some will be misinterpreting their symptoms or your motives; a few may have hallucinatory experiences urging them to perform aggressive acts. Most psychotic patients, we would emphasize, are in no way dangerous, but until you have gained experience it may be difficult to distinguish the few that might be.

Thus, until you know the patient well *do not frighten him by sudden movements or shouting, and give him enough distance* so that his personal space is not intruded upon. *Do not have too intrusive an eye contact*, and do not tower over the patient if he is sitting or lying. Try to unobtrusively make sure that you are nearer the door than the patient, and know where the alarms are, and that they work. *Let the patient have space* so that he feels that he is not trapped and can break off the interview if necessary and 'escape'. If you see growing signs of tension in the psychotic patient be prepared to break off the interview yourself, particularly if confrontation of the tension suggests that the patient is struggling with aggressive impulses. If you adopt these common-sense precautions (without making it obvious that you are) you will feel safer, will be less afraid, and will therefore be less threatening to the patient.

If the patient is disinhibited, be prepared to *set firm limits in terms of encroachment* on your own personal or emotional space ('John, stop that now: that's out of order. Sit down or I will have to stop trying to help you'). Likewise, firm limits have to be set for patients with manipulative or attention-seeking behaviour (see Section 4N, p. 347).

The setting of the interview is obviously very important, although it might be outside your control. If possible, try to make sure that there is *privacy and quietness* and that the patient understands the *confidential nature of your interview*. Sometimes patients want complete confidentiality and you will then have to indicate that you can only offer a *qualified* confidentiality, in the sense that you can give them an assurance that particularly sensitive information will not be committed to paper or put in the patient's records, but will have to be shared with the patient's consultant or with your trainer or supervisor.

When you are a trainee it is only in extremely unusual circumstances that you should be sole repository of a confidence. Remember that 'secrets' is a game that many manipulative people play. When glowing with the warmth of being the only person that Miss 'X' trusts with the startling nature of her sexual fantasies, it may be disconcerting to discover that no less than four other members of the ward team share that dubious distinction! It is also important to keep to the practice of never making promises that you cannot keep (see Section 4N (p. 347) on the manipulative patient).

Psychiatric interviews often have to be carried out in less than ideal circumstances. Even when stuck in an inadequately curtained cubicle, between a child having her sinuses washed out and a deaf old lady having a proctoscopy, it is often surprising how much people will say and reveal—but can the interviewer pay full attention to what they are saying? Occasionally interviews are carried out in very unusual situations, like jogging around a race track with a manic student, or in a smelly garden shed—'it's the only place in the house which isn't bugged, doctor.'

You also need to think about your dress. For most of us, being able to shed the white coat is a relief, particularly if we can shed white coat attitudes with it. Others will, for a long time, feel naked without it. A sensible compromise in dress is best, which strikes the right note of comforting informality without being insultingly casual. Do not dress like someone in the City, but also do not look like a refugee from a hippy commune. Later, when you know yourself better and are confident in your skills, you can dress how you like. However you dress, be clean and tidy and look as though you wash occasionally. You are still a doctor, so keep your nails short and clean, and wash your hands before and after taking blood or examining patients. If you like the present fashion for facial stubble, make sure it looks as though it is there by design and not mere forgetfulness.

C Interviewing the mentally impaired/confused

- Maintain clear speech: do not 'talk down'.
- Avoid innuendo, jargon, euphemism, and complexity.
- Get advice—study role models.
- Is the patient deaf? Sign language interpretation may be needed.
- Do not shout, face the patient, let him see your lips, and 'read' his face.
- Do not tire him or rush him, allow pauses, use ancillary aids if necessary.

- Do not finish his sentences.

- Interpret, but contain, 'acting out'.

- Keep the patient in touch with reality—be prepared for endless repetition of information and reassurance.

- Interview the carer *after* the patient.

- What is the carer's 'hidden agenda?'

- Is the carer burnt out or over-stressed?

People who have grown up with a limited capacity to comprehend the world as we see it, or with a different conceptual framework to our own, need special care, as do those who, originally endowed with the same intellectual framework as ourselves, have lost it through disease or accident or who still have that framework but have lost the ability to communicate it or to understand your communication. It is important to *maintain clear speech* and a calm manner, and to avoid frustration in both you and the patient. Do not take difficulty in communication personally.

You will need to try to communicate on the same level as your patient, but this does not mean talking down to him or being patronizing, and it most certainly does not mean adopting a childish language. It does mean using simple plain speech, avoiding innuendo and jargon, euphemism, and complexity. If your work takes you often into the world of the intellectually impaired or deprived, or into the world of those who have communicative or receptive difficulty, try to spend some time with experienced speech therapists who provide excellent role models of how to communicate with people with severe communication difficulties.

If you have a patient with a severe receptive or expressive dysphasia, communication is still possible, although if you are inexperienced in this area you will certainly need professional guidance. Occasionally it is difficult to tell the difference between a severe jargon dysphasia and a schizophrenic thought disorder, and advice from a colleague in speech therapy can sometimes be very helpful. Dysarthria is often a problem in those patients with neurological handicap, mental handicap, or indeed in those patients who mutter or grimace because of mental illness. In any patient with a speech disorder, particularly dysarthria, it is important to ensure that he is not deaf. If he is not deaf, then there is no need to shout, although you will find yourself unconsciously tempted to do so. Do take your time and be patient, do not alter your own mode of speaking, and do not try to finish sentences for the patient if, half way through a slow laborious sentence, you guess his meaning. If the patient is profoundly deaf you may need the help of someone adept in sign language. Check that hearing aids are working and make sure the patient can always see your face and lips when you are talking.

If the patient is dysarthric, do encourage him to rest if he is having to make a great effort to speak, and do not encourage elaborate answers but use simple and short speech. Make sure that you are facing the patient so that he can watch your lips and you can watch the patient's face and lips (as facial expression may be very important), and make sure that the room you are communicating in is quiet. If you indicate that you are prepared to be patient, the patient himself may actually slow down his speech (which is often very helpful, particularly for the dysarthric), and writing aids such as paper and a pencil may also be very helpful. Even just a chart with the letters of the alphabet written on it to which the patient can point if he has difficulty in articulating particular letters can be very useful. Patience, quietness, and non-embarrassment on your part helps communication for the speech impaired enormously.

The intellectually impaired, or those who have lost the ability to communicate verbally, are prone to 'act out' their feelings or thoughts and much is communicated through behaviour. States of anger, affection, or despair may therefore be seen as destructive behaviour, as inappropriate touching, or as self-destructive acts. Often such acting out behaviour needs to be contained or channelled into socially acceptable forms, but the underlying communication needs to be understood.

Much of the handicap of the mentally impaired lies in the attitudes and behaviours of those around them. Like people with epilepsy, the mentally impaired have to live with stigma and with overprotection and under-achievement. These can be more disabling than the actual impairment itself. Part of the assessment of the mentally impaired is therefore an enquiry into the attitudes of those who live with them or care for them. Well-meant, but stifling overprotection, which does not allow the person to take risks or learn by experience, is the most damaging of all.

For people who are confused, familiar objects, scenes, and situations may have taken on new meanings, and the person who is confused will often try to explain his altered perceptions. Do not mistake these explanations for delusions, or interpret the altered perception necessarily as an hallucination. Many people with organic brain disease are misdiagnosed as psychotic because the underlying brain disease is not recognized.

Try to keep the confused person in touch with reality (even though this will mean repetition piled upon repetition), and, as with the psychotic, do not try to be kind by agreeing with the patient's distorted or fading memory, but point out when they are wrong. If the patient has some awareness of failing powers and shows distress at this, you might have to modify this reality testing and shaping to avoid causing too much distress.

The confused need to be talked to gently and calmly; distracting or potentially misinterpretable sounds and sights need to be kept to a minimum (as does medication), and someone must be detailed to be with the patient continually, answering their questions, reminding them where they are and what is happening.

It will obviously be necessary, when assessing the mentally impaired or the confused, to talk with someone who cares for the person whether it be in the community or in a hostel. Unless there are compelling reasons not to, it is important to see the person who is impaired first, even if it is only for a fairly brief time. You should avoid the situation in which you end up talking with the carers and never communicate with the person that they are caring for. It is important to recognize two things. Many carers have a *hidden agenda* when they consult you about the impaired person they are looking after, and the interests of the impaired person must come first. You must not let anxiety about your own inability to communicate with the impaired person prevent you from trying to communicate, and must not let it force you into spending a lot of time talking about the affected person with the carer in the affected person's presence, 'over his head'.

You should also remember that many carers of mentally impaired people within the community, particularly if they come from that person's family, will have invaluable information to give you. They themselves might be very stressed and overwhelmed and enquiry into their own stress symptoms and health is necessary. Many carers feel unsupported, unappreciated, and are demoralized and 'burnt out'. This, of course, may well be having an effect on the person they are caring for and will need to be brought out by facilitating remarks such as, 'It must be very difficult coping with this behaviour 24 hours a day,' or just even, 'How do you feel about all this?'

D Interviewing people who speak another tongue

- The patient's culture needs interpreting as well as his language.
- Avoid 'medicalizing' normal cultural expressions of grief and distress.
- Make allowance for your prejudices—do not try to pretend they are not there.
- Use an interpreter who is professional and outside the family if you can. Try to ensure you are being interpreted properly and are actually getting what the patient is saying.
- Brief the interpreter fully.
- Interpreted interviews take a long time—plan them carefully.
- Are there cultural barriers to normal medical practice? If so, can you adapt to them or will they have to adapt to you?
- In an 'ossified' culture, a liberal colleague from the same culture can be helpful.

Language and culture are inextricably mixed. When we encounter someone who does not speak our native tongue as fluently as we do, we make assumptions about his intelligence, his education, and his culture that are totally unwarranted. Having his speech interpreted by someone fluent in both his language and yours only half solves the problem if you do not understand the cultural beliefs, values, and assumptions that lie behind the translation, and do not realize that the interpreter's own value system may be interposed between you and the patient.

You also have to learn to respect (even if you privately disagree with) hallowed cultural and religious beliefs. Although most *clinical* delusions, delusional

interpretations, and hallucinatory experiences lie outside culture, not all do. Where does culturally acceptable strong religious belief and practice end and insanity
begin? If, like us, you have no religious belief you will
need to enquire from an adherent of the particular
religion in question whether his colleague's beliefs and
behaviours are compatible with that religion or whether
they are obsessive or have become clinical. The local
leaders of most sects (unless they have become politicized) can make this distinction for you and should be
consulted. If you do have your own religious belief, do
not let it blind you to the beliefs of others or compromise your tolerance of different cultural practices.

Different cultures and different societies have different levels of tolerance of abnormal behaviour. They also
have different explanations of its cause and markedly
different ways of showing distress, and you have to
learn what these different modes of expression are so
that you can avoid 'medicalizing' normal expressions
of grief or anger and, if the person is clinically ill,
learning to modify your actual treatment and management so that it does not unnecessarily clash with
community values and expectations. A 'native healer'
is likely to be much more effective than you in helping
neurotic illness within his community. You are more
likely to be effective in treating psychotic illness, but
will still need to mobilize community support.

Some communities and individuals may be suspicious of, or even hostile to, Western medicine, particularly psychiatry, and may see it as an expression of
racial discrimination or repression. You also have to
learn that however 'liberal' you think you are, you will
have your unconscious blind spots and prejudices and
you will have to become aware of these so that they do
not influence your own behaviour and judgements.
Nobody is without prejudice, but the majority of us
can make allowances for our prejudice even if we

cannot change it. What we intellectually believe and emotionally feel may not be the same thing, and emotions can, quite unnoticed, powerfully influence our thinking.

When seeking an interpreter it is best to choose one who has the same professional training as you (and therefore understands the descriptive and clinical criteria you are using), who speaks both your language and the language of the patient fluently, and who understands and can explain the culture from which the patient comes. The interpreter may have to explain that certain phrases or modes of thinking do not exist in the other language, which may not have words to express what you are trying to convey.

For instance, the questions 'How often do you have sexual intercourse?' or 'How often do you make love?' convey certain different connotations of meaning (the one clinical and scientific, the other more warm and personal), but they are both fairly neutral and not particularly disturbing or embarrassing. If, however, the only possible translation of either phrase into the other language is 'How often do you fuck?', you may not understand the patient's startled reaction to the question unless your interpreter tells you why.

Professional interpretation should be available (in a hospital or district with many patients from other cultures it *must* be made available and you should complain loud and long if it is not). A register of medical and nursing staff who are fluent in other languages and who have intimate knowledge of other cultures should be kept and if necessary paid interpreters employed. But if this is not available, what is the best alternative? The answer is probably an educated speaker of the particular language who is also fluent in your language. Someone outside the immediate family is preferable as relatives may have their own axe to grind—husbands interpreting for wives, or children for their parents, can be extremely misleading. Although an educated interpreter is best, remember that class distinctions occur in other cultures as well as our own, and hostilities may exist between subcultures within the main culture.

An interpreted interview will take perhaps three times as long as an ordinary one, and since it is expensive in terms of your time and your patient's it should be rehearsed and thought through beforehand. If the interpreter is not used to psychiatry you must explain the kind of questions you will be asking and why you are asking them. If you do not, you may either get the interpreter's own views and opinions rather than what the patient is actually saying, or the interpreter may think you are as crazy as the patient. Pay particular attention to the way the interpreter puts the questions that you have asked. English is a fairly economical language, so if you find that the interpreter's questions seem a lot shorter than yours or the translation seems longer than what the patient has said in return, this may be because the interpreter is not faithfully translating what is being said.

Another reason for the length of an interpreted interview is that you will need to spend a lot of time explaining what is happening to the patient, and discuss topics such as the roles of the various staff on the ward. You will also have to explain what is going to happen and what you think is wrong.

It is helpful on many occasions to have a chaperone of the same sex and culture as the patient available, particularly during physical examinations, if a doctor of the same sex is not available. In some cultures, if the patient is a woman and a female doctor is not available for a physical examination, the woman's husband must be with her. The interpreter should be able to guide you on this. Some cultures that have clearly defined roles for men and women find it difficult to accept the authority and competence of female doctors—attitudes that perhaps even wake faint echoes in Western culture; many elderly Englishmen still call women doctors 'nurse'. A willingness to understand the cultural values and beliefs of the patient should become a two way process and you may need to help the patient adapt to your ways as much as you adapt to his. By all means adapt or modify the rules of good medical practice in the interest of cultural understanding, but do not break them!

Admission to hospital may also be a problem either because it is to a mixed sex ward, because of dietary or religious reasons, or because the whole family wants to come into hospital with the patient. Although admission is sometimes unavoidable, often sensible compromises can be made and intensive care carried out at home with the family's cooperation. Many cultures do not reject mental illness as the Western culture does and see it as their duty to care for the afflicted person. Occasionally, of course, even in an accepting culture the patient's behaviour (for example, promiscuous behaviour in a teenage girl) may bring such social shame on the patient's family that they can no longer cope with it.

It is also worth noting here a curious characteristic of expatriate communities that their memories of traditions and customs in their own country become ossified and often extreme (like that of the British Raj in India) and bear little relation to what the current practice actually is in the previous country. Here the help of a professional colleague from the same culture to persuade the family that standards are changing back in their own country can be very helpful.

Particular distress can occur in people caught between the conflicting demands of two cultures—for instance, the girl from a strict Muslim or Sikh background who hankers after the apparent liberties and freedom of her

English school friends, and who finds the differences between her home life and her outside social life impossible to reconcile. You may be tempted to help her escape into a hostel or refuge via the network set up by social services for such problems, but if you do this without thinking about it very carefully and consulting with some professional from her original culture first, you may unwittingly make her problems worse. Despite the conflict, she would almost certainly be drawing much strength and support from her home life, which she would lose forever at a time when she would be trying to grapple with the problems of her new life.

E Interviewing couples

- Interview each member of a partnership separately and then together.
- Keep individual confidences, although the partners must have an uncontaminated commitment to each other before you can treat them.
- Offer a variety of seating arrangements.
- How do they react with each other and with you?
- Who is the spokesman? Do the partners support each other? Does the silent partner listen?
- Address your first question *between* them.
- Encourage feeling statements and truthful statements.
- Specify behaviours.
- Always look at the positive aspects of the relationship.
- Do not take sides.
- Work with a partner if you can.

In working with people's sexual problems and with marital difficulties, interviewing the couple as a couple and then treating them as a couple is very necessary.

Even though you will probably not start your psychiatric career by doing work like this, it is useful to see many other patients with their spouses or partners to get an idea of how their relationship and partnership actually works. A little knowledge of what to do when you are talking with a couple is therefore useful and educational.

You should make time to ensure that you interview each member of the partnership on their own to start with. This will tell you particular areas of the relationship to look at and examine when you are seeing the couple together, and may also tell you of sensitive spots in the relationship that you should approach with caution.

Individual members of the partnership may give you pieces of information that they do not want the other member of the partnership to know. A classical example of this occurs when one of the partners is having an affair. Confidences like this obviously have to be respected (although the partner having the affair may be surprised to learn that most partners in this situation already have some idea about what is going on). Although you have to keep confidences given to you, it is impossible for either marital or sexual therapy to work for a couple if one of the partners is straying elsewhere. This is for the practical reason that the errant partner is hardly likely to put much energy into restoring relationships with the regular partner if he (or she) is enjoying himself (or herself) elsewhere. If you are given the confidence that one of the partners is having a relationship with someone other than the partner you are attempting to treat, you have to say something to the effect that although you will not reveal the information you will be unable to treat them unless he or she is willing to give up that other relationship and concentrate on improving the present one.

In your first interview with the couple you are mainly

concerned with assessing how well they get on together, whether they have been able to talk over the problem that they are presenting to you (most couples *say* they have, but then demonstrate that they have not), and assessing the strengths and weaknesses of the relationship. You will have to remember that how the couple behave with you in the artificial constraints of an interview and how they behave at home will be different, but you may be able to get some idea of who the dominant partner is and how well they can actually cope together, as a couple, with an external stress.

Try to see the couple in a room where you can offer them a variety of seating positions, and when they come in see where they sit. Do they sit close together, or far apart? Do they have a supportive posture with each other? Do they hold hands or touch? Do they look at each other when they are speaking? When one of them is speaking does the other listen? A very useful exercise when one of them has been speaking for a short while about their mutual problem is to say, looking at the other one, 'Just a minute, I wonder if you can tell me what your husband/wife/partner has just been saying.' You will be surprised just how often the partner was not actually listening and it can be a very useful demonstration.

It is useful to aim your first question, which will of course be of an open-ended nature like 'Perhaps you can tell me something about the problem?', between the two so that you actually learn who the spokesman is. It is also important to give each partner a chance of speaking and also to invite comments from the silent partner about what the other partner has just said. You will also often need to reflect back on how the couple appear to you and will often find yourself acting as a kind of referee, particularly if strong arguments break out. Although arguments are useful, and even rows can occasionally be therapeutic, if they just become an exchange of insults and of negative statements then it is best to stop them. You will usually have to encourage couples to be honest with each other and to say what they are really feeling and thinking. Many couples with a dysfunctional relationship will go to great lengths to protect each other from the truth on the grounds that the truth hurts, and so they will actively prevent the other person from knowing their true feelings.

You will often need to get partners to specify behaviours and not to make general statements. If one of them says that they want the other one to show them more affection you will need to say 'Tell him (or her) what he (or she) has to do to show you that he (or she) is actually trying to give you more affection.' It is important to specify behaviours that can be carried out without too much effort on the partner's part. A small change in behaviour that the partner is willing to make must be supported by some other complementary change in the other partner.

If you are talking with a couple about their relationship, it is all too easy to encourage them to present you with a catalogue of dissatisfactions with the relationship itself and with each other. It is most important not only to look at the weaknesses of a relationship but also at its strengths. What is it that is actually keeping the couple together despite their difficulties? What positive aspects of the relationship do they both see? It is surprising how often couples have become so immersed in the problems of the relationship that they fail to ever rehearse and draw comfort from the things that still bind them together. If you only concentrate on the negative aspects of the relationship, you may, as you rehearse them with the couple, help to drive them further apart. Finding a balance between these two factors is not easy.

One of the most useful things about seeing couples together is to realize the importance of not taking sides in a marital or domestic dispute, and to recognize that there are always two sides to an argument. One partner's behaviour may seem to be completely outrageous, but you always need to ask yourself whether there may be factors in the other partner that are driving the erring partner towards that behaviour. One cannot excuse, under any circumstances, a partner who uses violence against another, but it may be usful to look at the provocative behaviour in the victim, which may be consciously or unconsciously pushing the other partner into losing control. You also need to learn to become tolerant of other people's views and behaviours and accept that couples may be able to live in peace with standards very different from your own.

If you are going to do a lot of marital or sexual work with couples (and it is excellent experience) you may find it best to work with a co-therapist, since marital therapy is particularly tiring and very exacting and is probably one of the more stressful forms of therapy you can engage in.

F   Interviewing children and adolescents

- Interview the child on his own, then the parents, then the family together.
- Understand the child's world. Be as informal as possible.
- Observe very young children at play.
- Be even handed and non-judgemental.
- If you uncover sexual/physical abuse, discuss it with a colleague before acting.
- Assume the child is telling you the truth.

It would be surprising if you started your psychiatric career in the specialist worlds of child or adolescent psychiatry, but in the world of adult psychiatry it is sometimes necessary to interview children and you will certainly encounter adolescence and its problems. Children are often interviewed with their parents, although it is important, if at all possible, that you interview them on their own as well. Adolescent patients must be seen on their own, and except in exceptional circumstances, if the adolescent is the patient, seen first (even if he says nothing to you). You should then talk with one or both parents on their own and then have a family conference in which you see both parents and the child or adolescent together. The principles of this interview are rather similar to those of interviewing a couple, particularly getting people to reflect on what the others have said, giving everybody a chance of speaking, seeing who is the spokesman, and making sure that the positive aspects of the relationship as well as the negative ones are looked at.

As with the mentally impaired, it is important with children to use simple language that they will understand, but not to talk down to them, and to remember that they will have little concept of illness or of abnormality and may have their own misconceptions of and fantasies about psychiatry. It is important to get an understanding of the child's world and how he or she sees it before beginning to enquire about symptoms. A talk about the child's enthusiams, hobbies, likes and dislikes at school, is therefore important before beginning to go through a symptom checklist. Children tend to be afraid of doctors and therefore as informal a setting as possible is important, as is an explanation of who you are and what you are going to do. With very young children formal interviews are hardly appropriate at all, and you will often learn more about the child by observing him at play or with other children of the same age. This specialist kind of assessment is outside the scope of this book.

Adolescents tend to be somewhat hostile to authority

figures and they will tend to see doctors in this light. It is most important that you are seen to be even handed, not an agent of parental authority or control, and that, although you know adolescence is a time of turmoil, you do not wade in with a rather heavy handed 'sympathetic' approach that can set adolescent teeth on edge. Some adolescents are very sensitive about giving personal information to adults and so enquiries about such things as sexual relationships will have to be couched with more than usual tact and care, and you will need to give (and keep) firm reassurances about confidentiality. It is important to remember that some adolescents can, in the middle of adolescent turmoil, look and sound very disturbed indeed, particularly if they are frank with you, but are not actually suffering from a formal mental illness. It is very easy to mislabel and misidentify an intense identity crisis as a psychotic illness or as a severe personality disorder when it is nothing of the sort.

If you uncover evidence of either physical or sexual abuse occurring within the family, discuss this fully with your consultant before taking any action except in an extreme emergency. There should be a local policy of how to deal with this of which you may be unaware. You should, however, assume the child or adolescent is telling you the truth and not dismiss it as fantasy.

In the United Kingdom people aged 16 and above have the legal right to make their own decisions about medical treatment and this means that they have a right to confidentiality. Below that age your own conscience must guide you about whether important information that the child has given to you should be revealed to the parents. The child's best interest must be your guide: in general terms *be very certain* that you are right before breaking confidence, and seek the advice of your consultant (or even your defence union) before you do. Remember that other disciplines do not have (for what they regard as good reasons) the medical profession's scruples about confidentiality. Your first duty is to your patient and not to the parents.

G Interviewing the distressed patient

See also 4G (p. 197); 5C (p. 394); and 6E (p. 489).

- The distressed make us feel uncomfortable and inadequate.
- Raw emotion is unpleasant to be with—we often feel pressured to do something to control it.
- Distress has different cultural guises, and different cultural tolerances.
- It also takes different forms depending on the different stages of recovery the patient has reached and his own personality and upbringing.
- There are several phases of distress and grief:
  1. 'stunned' phase
  2. acute fear and distress phase
  3. denial phase
  4. intrusive or struggle phase
  5. anger phase
  6. depression and despair phase
  7. acceptance phase.
- By and large distress and grief should be acknowledged and confronted, allowed expression, talked through, and supported. Touch and explanation are important. Victims of distress and grief often need permission and explanation to be able to grieve properly, and sufficient time to do it. The frightened must be helped to face their fear and not run away from it.

There are several problems attached to interviewing patients who are severely distressed. There is a natural reluctance to intrude on grief. This relates both to our own feelings, a cultural belief in what is right, and a primitive protective reflex. Other people's distress is also upsetting and makes us feel uncomfortable, inadequate, and insecure, and may remind us of previously harrowing events in our own lives. We do not know whether we should control ourselves and not show the empathic distress that the victim brings out in us, or whether it is acceptable to show, by our emotional reaction, that we are human too. Raw emotion is uncomfortable to be with, and there is a pressure on us as professionals to do something about it—to be put in a parental role of 'making it better'. Because distress is upsetting to be with, others around you will want you to suppress it, but you are not treating them and you must respond to the needs of the person in front of you. Without experience, however, most of us are unsure how to do this and our professional role may seem to conflict with our natural human response to the distressed.

There is, in our particular culture, an injunction and taboo against overt displays of emotion. People who 'give way' to tears or have dramatic emotional outbursts are often seen (by onlookers *and* by themselves) as not playing the game, not showing the fortitude expected of them, and as being 'weak' or 'womanly'. 'Big boys don't cry', we tell our male children. So what do our big boys do? Hold their distress and grief into themselves all their lives until it rots their insides away and they are totally unable to express their inner feelings. As psychiatrists we are not immune to this concept—tears in a man are seen as pathological, but not in a woman (see the Hamilton rating scale for depression). Our professionalism also makes us doubt too much the validity of distress that we see. If we can call overt distress 'acting out' or 'attention seeking', it diminishes the impact it might otherwise have on us.

Another problem that distress causes is that often our interviewing will apparently increase the patient's distress. If the patient is so distressed by it, ought we to be encouraging him to talk about the very things that upset him? Should we facilitate the expression of emotion or should we help the patient to regain composure and shut Pandora's box?

We may not always be able to recognize distress if it presents in unfamiliar guises, is denied by the patient, or is cloaked by a different culture. If we do not know enough about the process and phenomena of distress and grief, how can we expect the patient to? Since we live in a society that shields people from the experience of grief, we will often need to explain its phenomena to those experiencing it. As professionals we need to be able to distinguish between the natural normal process of distress or grieving and when it has become pathological. There are many ways that distress and grief can present. What you see depends on the cause of the distress, and on the culture, education, and constitution of the patient (although we all have our breaking point), and on the phase that the grief has reached. There are several stages to the grief process, but they intermingle and blur into each other, and the earlier stages can be reawakened by memories or by particular stimuli, but they all tend to eventually resolve.

Stages of grief

1. Stunned phase

The individual appears dazed and stunned by the traumatic event and is totally unable to comprehend what has happened. At this stage the victim needs comfort, support, care, and gentle attempts to help him understand what has happened.

2. Fear and distress phase

The individual will be frightened and anxious, sweating, shaking, talking incoherently about the experience (occasionally mute), and sleepless. He needs comfort, reassurance, and the opportunity to talk. He may be feeling out of control and ashamed of showing fear and may need explanation.

3. Denial phase

Denial is partly a psychological mechanism—a deliberate blotting out of the experience to preserve equanimity —and partly a physiological phenomenon related to production of an endogenous tranquillizer that locks into the benzodiazepine receptors in the brain thus producing a dream-like feeling of unreality. Denial is protective and helpful up to a point, but if maintained for too long it prevents resolution of the grieving process, and in denial you may be misled as to how much the patient is actually distressed. The patient needs support and comfort, even though he may not look as though he needs it, and denial may need to be gently punctured by reminders of reality. Denial may be seen in the recovery phase from loss (as in mastectomy) and may then be protective.

4. Intrusive or struggle phase

Anxiety symptoms are prominent. 'Flashback' memories of the traumatic event occur and may be very distressing, and nightmares of the event are common. There is morbid rumination about the event, about its meaning (or lack of meaning), and the futility of existence ('Why should a dog, a horse, a rat have life And thou no breath at all?'). The patient needs to talk, to be comforted, to know that what he is experiencing is normal and will pass. Patients (and relatives) may go to elaborate lengths to prevent being reminded of their trauma or their loss. Try to help them face it and not to run away from reminders.

5. Anger phase

Angry feelings directed at fate, or at possible perpetrators of the event (real or imagined), or at the patient himself for allowing the event to happen and not to control it, are common in distress and grief. They need to be acknowledged, confronted, and talked through. Suicidal or homicidal feelings must be looked for and prevented from being put into action.

6. Depression and despair phase

There is a permeating mood of sadness, unhappy rumination, and despair. Tears are frequent, often arising unbidden, touched off by some triggered memory or evocative experience (many people are distressed at being sometimes too depressed for tears). Somatic symptoms related to grief (such as repeated dry swallowing, sighing, or an abdominal ache) are common and need to be explained to the patient. It is important to let the patient cry and to use triggers like photographs to facilitate this expression of emotion. Do not shy away from the patient's tears or verbal expressions of grief. Support and encourage them and remember that such emotion will be felt and expressed for months after the traumatic event or bereavement, or loss, even when the patient has apparently recovered completely. Do not make the patient feel guilty that he is 'giving way' if he is moved to tears whilst you are interviewing him: what he is doing is normal. Do not medicalize grief.

7. Acceptance phase

Although after severe distress, loss, or grief the person is never quite the same again, eventually the anxiety, anger, and sadness are 'worked through' and the person comes out to a calm acceptance that the event or the bereavement happened, that they have completed grieving, or that their emotional reaction is over. Even so, they can still be reminded of it and are still capable, years after, of showing an emotional response to the memory, particularly during vulnerable times.

Distress and grief in the patient you are interviewing should therefore be acknowledged and confronted. You are doing good and it is not harmful. If you suspect it is there behind the patient's words, use the skills of facilitation to help it emerge. Talk the feelings and the experience through, however painful; allow the patient to show emotion (you may have to suspend the interview temporarily to allow this), and show him empathy. If the patient is distressed, show non-verbal as well as verbal support by touching him or holding his hand. You can also support him by telling him what is happening (as many people are frightened by the intensity of their feelings or by the strange phenomena of grief and distress—like the tingling limbs and lips of hyperventilation). If the patient is terrified of something, help him to face his fear and confront the situation, and not to run away from it. Every time he retreats from fear, he is reinforcing it.

Although severe distress and grief makes you feel helpless, you will find that just being there, listening, ventilating, explaining, and showing support, is all you need to do. In retrospect you will realize that you are helping the recovery process. Do not be discouraged if the next time you see the patient his distress seems as bad or worse: recovery is a slow process that cannot be hurried.

Finally, acknowledge your own distress—you are a human being, not a robot. The patient's experiences may mirror your own, may awaken your past griefs, or be overwhelmingly sad or upsetting. It is no bad thing to let the patient see that you have been moved by his experience (parents of children who die on a ward, for instance, gain much support from the knowledge that the nurses, too, are distressed by their child's death). You do not have to be 'patience on a monument' and can let the patient see that you are affected by what he has said—and yet can remain in support. If you are overwhelmed by distress at what the patient has experienced (perhaps it was too close to your own raw wounds) avoid using the patient as a confidante or therapist (he has his own grieving to do) but do talk it through with a close friend or colleague.

CHAPTER 2

Information to be obtained in the psychiatric interview

A Psychiatric history—general principles

- Be systematic in your approach, even when tempted not to be.
- Delineate the presenting problems.
- From what kind of background does the patient come?
- When was the patient last well?
- Are the symptoms of sudden onset or has there been an insidious change or exaggeration of previous characteristics?
- Have there been any changes in symptoms or the intensity of symptoms since the illness started? Are there any precipitants of the symptoms or change in intensity?
- What effect have the symptoms had on the patient, his lifestyle and relationships?
- What advice and treatment is he already getting and from whom?
- Do not leap to conclusions about cause and effect.

There will be times when you are interviewing patients that it will be impossible to follow the scheme of history taking that is outlined below, particularly if the patient is very disturbed or very forgetful. There will also be times when much of the information will seem irrelevant to the presenting problem. Although in the heat and excitement of an emergency admission of an excited or grossly deluded patient careful recording of such things as his family history and previous personality may seem irrelevant or may be impossible, it should be remembered that it has not been done. When the patient is calm, or when an informant is available, this information must be obtained and recorded.

It is impossible to understand a patient with a psychiatric illness, even with a psychotic illness, unless you know a great deal about him, his present circumstances, his previous life circumstances, and the kind of experiences that have shaped him into the person that he is now. Psychiatrists who try to manage patients purely on the basis of the mental state of the patient at the time of presentation (although this may be a tempting thing to do and may, in emergencies, be the only thing that can be done) will often make mistakes. Psychiatry is about understanding the meaning of symptoms as well as managing them.

In your psychiatric history you are attempting to delineate the patient's presenting problems, obtaining the technical information that you need to formulate a working diagnosis or plan of management, and are trying to understand the background from which the patient comes as this may be shaping or even causing the symptoms that the patient is presenting to you. You need to establish as clearly as you can when the patient was last well in terms of the symptoms that are troubling him. Were they of sudden onset, with a clear break from the patient's normal state of functioning? Was there a slow insidious change? Are you merely seeing an exaggeration of characteristics that the patient has always had? Can you recognize precipitating events, such as bereavement or other forms of loss, change in lifestyle, occupation, etc.? What sort of effect are the symptoms having on the patient, on his relationships, on his occupation, or on his daily living? If changes have taken place in the symptoms since they started, or in their intensity, are there any precipitants or reasons for these changes? What advice or treatment is the patient already getting, and from whom?

When you are talking to the patient about his life and symptoms it may be the first time that he has taken a structured look at his life. Although it may be very obvious to you that the patient has stress symptoms, the patient himself may not recognize it and may not initially see his life as being particularly stressful (but may do so after he has actually reviewed it with you). So, sometimes general enquiries about any problems or any particular stresses that a patient has in his life may meet with a negative response even though such problems or stresses are actually there.

It is also true that all human beings like to try to find the cause of their symptoms. Everyone living in the real world has day-to-day problems. During a period of stress or depression these day-to-day problems, which we can normally cope with satisfactorily, appear to become more prominent and will therefore often be blamed as the cause of the stress symptoms or depression when in fact they have nothing to do with it. A very good example of this is the patient who, when well, is perfectly able to cope with the stresses of his particular job. When depressed he cannot cope, blames his depression on the failure, and therefore feels that the correct treatment for his depression is to leave his job. On recovering from the depression he realizes that the everyday occupational dissatisfactions that he had were totally irrelevant to his depression and he now feels well enough to cope with them. He may, however, find it difficult to get his job back. It is most important that you encourage people who are depressed not to make rapid changes in their lifestyle, in the hope that this will alleviate the depression, until they are significantly less depressed and can make a more rational judgement about whether a particular aspect of their life was actually contributing to their depression or not, and until you know them a lot better. It is important that you do not make snap value judgements about everyday stresses causing the patient's symptoms.

Having therefore taken a full history of the presenting complaints and a structured account of them and other information you need, you should then turn to taking a structured account of the patient's previous development and present life circumstances. Traditionally this is done under the following headings and is usually done in this order.

B Family history

- Find a neutral informant, if you can.
- Construct a family tree back to grandparents.
- Any significant non-nuclear family relationships?
- Nature of relationships with close family members—father, mother, siblings, significant others.
- Assess the family's general function (cohesion, occupation, education, religion, culture).
- Any history of mental illness within the family—any genetic illnesses?
- Any history of attempted or completed suicide within the family?
- Any history of recidivism, violence, or excess drinking within the family?
- Any history of physical or sexual abuse within the family?

A carefully taken family history can tell you a great deal about the patient in terms of the kind of atmosphere he grew up in, the kind of models he had in terms of making relationships, the way he learnt to handle stress and was comforted, and, of course, the genetic endowment of the family. This, of course, is particularly important in child and adolescent psychiatry, but may be very important in adult psychiatry, particularly for patients needing psychotherapy or behaviour therapy.

The family history is therefore worth doing well, but in our experience seldom is done well, and in the patient's notes usually has a few sketchy references like, 'did not get on with father,' or 'three siblings'. There may be occasions when a family history is hardly relevant to the task in front of you, but in most situations the family history is important and it is worth spending a little time on eliciting good information and recording it properly in the patient's notes. It is important to remember that the patient's account of his family life may be distorted by his illness, or by a wish to blame his family life for all his present ills, and so it is necessary to have evidence from an informant who knows the patient and his family well, if at all possible. This informant will usually be another family member, but (as with most of the personal history of the patient) it is often better to have a family member who is not too closely involved with any family dynamics, and therefore have someone who stands a little way outside the immediate family and can look at it objectively and dispassionately.

We would recommend that initially you construct a family tree going back at least as far as grandparents on both maternal and paternal sides, and noting any significant physical or mental illnesses in these family members and whether they are alive or dead. A note should be made of any other significant family relationships that lie outside this family tree but which influenced the patient as a child or adolescent. Sometimes the child will have been brought up by aunts or grandparents rather than by the nuclear family members, or by 'courtesy aunts', because of loss, through death or separation, of the mother or father. Sometimes the significant rearing parent may have been an elder sister or brother. In recording details of siblings it is helpful to include their forename as well as their place in the family.

Then enquire about close relationships with other family members, initially in an open general way by saying something like, 'Tell me about your father, what kind of person is he?' rather than by just saying, 'How do you get on with your father?' To some extent you will be dealing with the patient's own value judgements and you, consciously or not, will also be making your own value judgement about the quality of family life that the patient has experienced. Normal family life can be very difficult to define and, of course, is very much dependent on the general culture from which the patient is drawn, and indeed on the morals and values of any subculture within that culture. Another very useful question to ask the patient is which of his parents he most closely resembles in terms of temperament and other characteristics, and which, if any, of his siblings is he most like.

Early death of a parent or a sibling may have been a very significant event in the patient's life, and therefore enquiry about how the patient felt at the time, whether he was able to grieve for the parent or lost sibling, or whether he feels in some way to blame, is important. It is becoming clear that incestuous relationships within the family are commoner than was once thought and often account for the psychopathology of the victim in later life. It is unlikely that you will initially obtain a history of incestuous contact between family members, and a direct enquiry at this stage, when you do not know the patient very well, will almost certainly be met with a negative answer and may have to be reviewed later. A general enquiry about

'Was there anything in your family relationships that you did not like, or disturbed you?' is a useful general enquiry to make. The patient's general feeling about family discipline, whether it was consistent or not, and whether there is a history of violence, or excessive drinking, or of overt criminal behaviour should be enquired about, as should religious practice within the family.

The family's general function regarding occupation and education, both in the parents and in the siblings, is a necessary part of your enquiry to discover whether there were particular educational pressures or expectations that your patient was not able to meet. Do not expect siblings to necessarily get on, although sometimes you will find that within the siblingship there are close, confiding relationships. The calm, protective elder brother or the warm, supportive elder sister may have been very important in the patient's life and may reflect the patient's present relationships with others. As you gain experience you will realize how often our adult relationships are patterned on our early relationships with parents or with siblings. It is surprising, for instance, how often a woman with an aggressive, drunken father will often choose a similar man as a mate in later life.

There is good evidence that a history of completed suicide in a family is of prognostic importance if your patient is depressed. There is also no doubt that there is a genetic influence to major affective illnesses and to schizophrenia, and you may encounter other genetic illnesses such as Huntington's chorea. There is a familial and possible genetic basis to alcoholism. If your patient is mentally impaired then information about other impaired family members may be very important, as may be enquiry about the rare familial forms of epilepsy. Be careful not to ask 'genetic' questions in such a way that you imply the condition is inherited when it is not. Many people with epilepsy mistakenly think that it is hereditary because they are always asked 'Is there anyone else with epilepsy in the family?' It is better to ask 'Do you know of anyone else with epilepsy?' Even if a condition is not genetically acquired, another family member with it means that the family will already have previously acquired myths and attitudes about your patient's illness.

At the end of your family history you should have a clear impression of any genetic influences that may be running through the family, of any obvious family psychopathology (such as alcoholism, violence, long periods of separation from parents or siblings, loss of a parent or other significant family member), and, although it is hard to define, of the general family atmosphere, which almost certainly will have had a marked formative effect on the way the patient conducts his relationships in adult life.

C Personal development

- Any significant birth events or injury?
- Any significant deviation in milestones (walking, talking, continence, etc.)?
- Any obvious cause for such deviation?
- Any persistent early character traits?

Next follows a chronological account of the patient's development from birth up until the present day. The patient himself may know certain details of his birth and development, particularly if there was something unusual about it. He may be able to give you an account of it even though he has already told you that he arrived on earth in a silver spaceship from the planet Epsilon Minor in the year 1066, if his psychotic ideas are encapsulated enough. Psychotic logic being what it is, he may then give you a perfectly ordinary account of his birth and early development, but say 'That of course was my other life, doctor'.

Prospective developmental studies have suggested that the importance that used to be given to the circumstances of birth and early development was perhaps overrated. The infant brain is plastic and so even quite severe brain damage may merely result in other areas of brain taking over the usual function of the damaged part. Occasionally, however, an exact account of birth events and of subsequent milestones is important, particularly in the mentally impaired, and here an independent witness or even the hospital notes (if they are available) is very necessary. Families develop their own mythology about birth events and even quite mundane events surrounding the birth can acquire an almost mystical significance.

Milestones, that is, the ages at which the child was first able to perform certain developmental skills such as sitting unsupported, crawling, walking, using words, attaining continence during the day and becoming dry at night, may be important providing that somebody has accurately recorded them in the past. Although developmental delay is usually organically determined, sometimes delay in becoming continent, in talking or being dry at night may have psychological causes. Some children appear mute until the age of 4 or 5 years, especially if there has been some emotionally traumatic event, and then begin to speak perfectly normally. Clearly they have understood speech but have chosen not to speak. If there is a developmental delay, and particularly if it is a patchy one, some enquiry should therefore be made about emotional events occurring around the time that the delay probably occurred.

Even at a very early age persistent character traits may be identifiable, particularly in patients with severe personality disorders. When formulating a diagnosis of a personality disorder, it is helpful to know the earliest age at which the child displayed traits such as aggression, failure to respond to punishment, impulsiveness, and whether he had poor relationships with other people.

D Educational, occupational, and social history

- School history: types, dates of attendance.
- Educational attainments and difficulties.
- Any problems with discipline or bullying?
- Relationships with peers and authority figures.
- Higher education or not? Attainments and difficulties.
- Occupational record. Type and number of jobs: unemployment.
- Attainments and difficulties at work.
- Any problems with work/authority relationships?
- How does patient cope with job stress (boredom or too exacting requirements)?
- Any toxic hazard?
- If retired, how is he (and partner) coping?
- Present (and past, if relevant) financial and social circumstances.
- Who supports him?

A history of the patient's schooling should next be obtained. You will need to look at the type of school the patient went to, what educational attainments he was able to reach, any special difficulties he had with particular subjects, what sort of relationships he was able to develop with his peer group at school, whether he had any particular problems with discipline or bullying, and what kind of relationships he was able to form with his teachers. What you are really trying to obtain in this part of the history is an indication of the patient's intellectual ability and whether it became arrested or distorted in any way, and also an account of his developing personality in terms of his relationships with authority figures and also his peer group. A list of educational achievements, including exams passed, will give you a rough idea about his intellectual attainment, but not necessarily about his intellectual potential as the school system has many casualities.

You are obviously looking at, in terms of where the patient is now, what he might have achieved. It is characteristic of some conditions, especially organic ones and schizophrenia, that there is a slow progressive fall in apparent intellectual and academic ability after leaving school. The brilliant sixth former with three grade A, 'A' level passes who a few years later is stacking boxes in the local supermarket may be demonstrating the slow downward social drift of schizophrenia (or he may have a politicized, prolonged identity crisis, or may just be lazy, or maybe, as Thoreau put it, 'marching to a different drum').

The patient's behaviour and experience at school, particularly in terms of relationships, will also, of course, tell you a lot about his developing personality (and any aberrations in it) and again you may see a pattern of disruptive behaviour going back a long way. This would tend to point towards a personality disorder or an insidious psychotic process. Alternatively, you may see that the patient's present illness or difficulties are very different from what you would expect of the kind of person who was developing at school a few years ago. It is often very useful to look at how well the patient coped with stressful events, such as examinations, and also how he dealt with friendships and developing intimate relationships.

The patient may, of course, have gone on to higher education at university or college. Here again you can test out how well he coped with the relative freedom of university life, whether he could continue working in a more unstructured environment, or whether there was unexpected academic failure and a discrepancy in what he was eventually able to achieve.

An occupational record should then be made looking at the kind of jobs the patient has been able to obtain (and whether they are compatible with his academic achievements), how he has coped with the stresses of jobs (whether the stress is one of boredom or exacting time schedules or a difficult boss), and how he has coped with the stress of unemployment if he has had any. What are his relationships like with his work mates? How does he relate to and cope with authority figures at work? Frequent changes of job, whether due to frequent sackings or frequent changes of mind on the part of the patient, may be no more than a reflection of our troubled economic times, but may tell you something about the psychopathology of the patient. Our society currently assumes that people will gradually rise in status, income, and responsibility at work, and it may be illuminating if the patient does not. Job satisfaction should be assessed as should the patient's style of coping with work stress and the attitudes that he has to his work. Is the patient meticulous in attention to small detail at work or slapdash and bored? Is he perhaps over-involved in work to such an extent that he is a kind of workaholic who shows gross obsessional attention to detail, cannot delegate responsibility to others, and finds it difficult to take holidays?

Enquire if the patient is exposed to any particularly hazardous or toxic process at work.

If the patient has reached retirement age look at how he prepared for retirement, how he is coping with retirement, and how he is now spending his time. Assess whether he is coping with the loss of income that retirement usually brings. If the patient is the only one of a partnership that has been working, look at the effect that his sudden arrival at home has had on his partner, as this is a common stress point for even long-term relationships.

General enquiry about the patient's present financial and social circumstances is also needed. In what kind of circumstances and with whom does he live? What tensions exist in his relationships (partner and any children)? Does he have supportive relationships? Is there anyone he can confide in?

E Sexual/marital history

- Sexual adjustment and preferences.
- History of development of intimate/physical relationships.
- Description of present main relationship. Any physical or emotional difficulties? Any other present significant relationships?
- Any previous important relationships?
- Relationship with children or other dependants?

Enquiry into sexual adjustment, sexual preferences, the development of relationships, and the history of marital relationships, comes next in the personal history. Taking a detailed sexual history is outlined elsewhere in this book (see p. 28 and p. 314). In taking this part of the history you are very much intruding into what is often the most intimate part of the patient's life, and tact and patience is very necessary. You certainly should not be too intrusive, and ask only those questions that you need an answer to in order to have an understanding of the patient and of his problems. Some of this questioning can be left to a later time when you know the patient better, providing that you *do* come back to it.

It is best to start with open-ended questions about relationships and friendships and then go on to a chronological account of the more important relationships in the patient's life. Thumbnail sketches of the more prominent relationships should be obtained, and the patient asked whether he has any special friends or confidantes in addition to his main relationship. A general enquiry about the physical aspects of the relationship should be made if this is appropriate. Having delineated the main relationships (both historical and present) in the patient's life, ask a question like 'Have you had any difficulty or worries with the physical side of relationships?', or 'Has the sexual side of relationships been important to you?' Depending on the verbal (and non-verbal) responses to these questions you can go on to gently explore problems, difficulties, and attitudes in an open-ended way so that, having gained the patient's confidence, you can come to an understanding of the part sexuality plays in his life with regard to both its positive and negative aspects.

This scheme of history taking, of course, applies as much to homosexual relationships as it does to heterosexual. Remember, however, that heterosexual men and women can have significant relationships with their own sex and homosexual men and women with their opposite sex. This is why the general question 'Do you have a special friend? Tell me about him or her?' is so useful.

The patient's emotional reaction to the development of secondary sexual characteristics may be important, for example, a woman may not have been prepared for menstruation and have been distressed by it.

F Personality assessment

- Independent informant needed.
- Thumbnail sketch from patient.
- Hobbies, habits, religious or political interests?

- Relationships with others? Gregarious or solitary? Easy mixer?

- Unduly suspicious or aggressive?

- Mood stable or not?

- Obsessional or the reverse?

- Centre of attention? Overly emotional?

- How does he cope with stress and authority figures?

- Forensic history.

Perhaps the most difficult part of taking the psychiatric history is to try to assess the patient's previous personality, but this is a very useful exercise in terms of the prognosis of psychotic illness (and to some extent neurotic illness), the diagnosis of personality disorders, and also understanding the person in front of you, why he is behaving in the way that he is, or reacting to events in the way that he does.

You will obviously record the patient's own assessment of his personality ('Give me a thumbnail sketch of yourself, what kind of person are you?'). Many people can give such an account of themselves and are often tolerably honest. The patient in the grip of a psychosis, particularly if he has personal delusions, will not be able to do so and a patient who is severely depressed will give a negative and misleading account of himself as, of course, will someone who is manic, although his account is likely to be colourful and flamboyant. The severely personality disordered are unlikely to see themselves as others see them.

An account of the patient's personality given by a relative or friend of the patient will be invaluable, but even here caution is necessary because close relatives and friends may be over-involved with the patient, or have their own axe to grind or particular point of view to give.

Assessing a patient's personality can therefore be very difficult. It is useful to have a picture of the patient's normal habits and hobbies, of interests, of religious persuasion, of political views, and of clashes with authority and with the law. If you have not done so already this is a convenient place to take a formal drinking history and to make enquiries about the use of other illegal substances.

You will, however, need to do more than this and will need to look for evidence of a formal personality disorder using the modern descriptive analyses of personality disorders that are now enshrined in classifications of psychiatric disorders (see p. 1).

Can the patient get on with other people? Is he unduly suspicious and oversensitive? Is his mood stable or does it fluctuate? For example, does he have sustained periods of low mood not amounting to depression, or does he have sustained periods of being rather high but not amounting to hypomania, or is his mood more volatile than this? Is he unduly optimistic? Does he make friends easily, mix easily, or does he prefer his own company and have difficulty in mixing with and making relationships with other people?

Is his temper easily provoked? Has he had attacks of rage and aggression that transcend those usual for the circumstances and culture in which he lives? Is he somewhat obsessional? Does he have to follow a set routine, or be perhaps overly neat and tidy, or over-punctual, or is he the reverse?

Does he like being the centre of attention? Is he too easily moved to tears or other displays of emotion? Does he tend to find it difficult to distinguish role playing from reality? Is he somewhat listless and tired all the time? Does he give up easily when attempting tasks that should be within his competence? Does he find the tasks of everyday life difficult to complete? How does he cope with authority figures and with the necessary checks and disciplines of everyday life? Does he find it difficult to take instruction and correction? Is he over-compliant?

You will probably have already determined much of the above from the patient's account of his personal history. Many patients, of course, will have little insight into these aspects of their personality and you will have to gain the information from others.

As a result of your history taking and the answers to your questions, you may feel that you would be justified in placing the patient into one of the ICD 9 or DSM III R categories of personality disorder. It is important to remember that if you do you will need good evidence that the personality traits that you have put together to categorize the patient into a particular personality type are more prominent than those of ordinary people. They must also be durable (i.e., it must be clear that the traits have existed in the patient from an early age, do not fluctuate, and do not merely occur when the patient is perhaps tired, drunk, or under stress). Even if you can place the patient into a personality type, remember that you are using a kind of convenient shorthand to summarize only part of the complexities of the behaviours that go to make up a human being. Most of us who read through the ICD 9 or DSM III R categories and the diagnostic criteria used to formulate them, will often have the feeling that we recognize something of ourselves in all of them and it is important that you do not over-categorize the patient until you know him very well and can see him in perspective.

A separate forensic history is valuable and it may be important to accurately record not only offences for which a patient has been charged and convicted but also those that he has got away with (he may be quite frank in telling you about this). Include juvenile offences and others that may have just resulted in a 'caution'.

G Drinking/drug abuse assessment

- Age at which drinking started?
- Present weekly unit consumption?
- Does it fluctuate? Any binges?
- Previous heavy drinking if not now?
- What company does he drink in and what is his motivation for drinking?
- Is drinking a problem (do others think so)?
- Can he control his drinking? Has he tried to cut down (or have others suggested he does)?
- Any periods of abstinence (and why)?
- Does he conceal his drinking or keep private supplies?
- Any blackouts, next-morning symptoms, craving, or alcohol-related physical symptoms?
- Ever in trouble with the law about drinking?
- Ever lost jobs or had time off work because of drink?
- Other recreational/illicit drugs? How are they taken and how often?
- Motivation for use and drug effects?
- Any drug-related symptoms?
- How are supplies secured?
- Is patient dependent?
- Smoking history.

A formal drinking history, which should be taken from every patient, includes the age at which the patient began to drink and his average weekly consumption (expressed in units—one unit being equivalent to half a pint of beer, one normal sized glass of wine, or a single measure of spirits). Enquire if this intake fluctuates a great deal and if the patient has episodes of binge drinking. Try to discover the kind of company the patient drinks in, whether he drinks for solace or to relieve tension, and whether he regards his drinking as a problem (or whether other people do). Do *not* assume, if your patient comes from a culture that eschews alcohol, that he himself does not drink.

Men with an alcohol consumption of over 21 units a week (14 in women) are drinking above the recognized safe limit. Consumption of over 40 units a week will almost certainly be associated with a drink-related problem, either physical or psychological (or both), but problems can occur well below that level. Episodic drinking ('binges') can also lead to alcohol-related problems even though the weekly average intake is spuriously low. Many people conceal the truth about how much they are drinking even from themselves, and they certainly will from you.

You should enquire whether the patient can control his drinking and whether he has ever felt (or others have suggested) that he should cut down his consumption. Has he had periods of abstinence and, if so, why? Does he conceal his drinking from others by sucking mints or using mouth fresheners, and by keeping secret supplies of alcohol in his office drawer or elsewhere? How many times has he woken in the morning with no idea of where he was the night before? (This is the alcoholic palimpsest or blackout—one of the earliest indications of alcoholic brain damage.) Does he use alcohol to cure a hangover ('the eye-opener')? Does he have morning shakes? If he does not drink for a day or two, does he get a craving for alcohol—can he resist it?

Has alcohol ever got him into trouble with the law (drunk and disorderly or alcohol-related offences like breach of the peace, assault, or drunken driving)? Has he lost jobs through drinking or had alcohol-related accidents? Has drinking led to financial or family problems? Has he ever had withdrawal phenomena like delirium tremens or had the physical symptoms of gastritis or peripheral neuropathy that are the sequelae of drinking?

How much detail you go into will depend on how much the patient drinks (or others tell you that he drinks), but do be careful to err on the side of caution. Use the skills you have acquired in confronting and probing to try to penetrate denial and the fog of self-deceit. Replies to the question 'How much do you drink?' of 'About the usual, doctor', or 'Oh, a couple of sherries' depend a great deal on the patient's concept of what 'the usual' is (and what he thinks yours is!) and on an elastic concept of volume. A 'couple of sherries' might mean a couple of *bottles* of cooking sherry a day to some patients! To those in a hard drinking crowd such as a rugby club, 'the usual' can be very pathological.

Enquiries about exposure to other drugs of recreation or potential addiction need to be made and you will need to confront street names and slang words to be sure you know what they mean. Do not assume that you know what they mean as drug users' language changes rapidly. Questions about drug use and abuse flow naturally from questions about drinking—'So, you have told me about alcohol, what about other things? Ever tried or been offered drugs?' You can assume that most people know of drugs or have been offered them, even if they have not used them. If they have used them, try to discover their motivation for doing so and what effects they have had and whether the patient, if a regular drug user, has had to resort to illegal means to get supplies. Knowledge that the patient uses drugs or abuses alcohol will alert you to make a careful health check during your physical history taking and examination.

Recreational use of some drugs like cannabis is

common in some cultures and is not necessarily indicative of abnormal psychopathology. Experimental 'one off' use of even quite powerful illicit drugs is not uncommon. Continued non-recreational use of cannabis, or resorting to frequent 'buzzes' with solvents or 'speed', or physical or emotional dependence on opiates, is, however, abnormal. You will probably have a stereotyped view of the addict as someone with the snuffles, pinpoint pupils, and needle-tracked arms of the heroin addict, or with the ulcerated nose of cocaine abuse or with characteristic sores round the mouth from glue sniffing. Often this stereotype is right, but do remember that some people can hide their addiction very well. The 'middle-class' heroin addict who has maintained his addiction for years but who is still socially competent, is not uncommon and is difficult to detect.

Record present and past smoking habits. Smoking is just as much an addiction as anything else and a history of heavy smoking of cigarettes, for instance, will mean that the patient will need a very careful physical assessment.

H Previous medical history

- Childhood illnesses and complications.
- Other significant illnesses and hospital admissions or operations?
- Any current illnesses and medication (including 'over-the-counter' drugs) and contraception?
- Any periods of significant minor ill health, GP attendance?
- Patient's emotional/psychological response to physical illness.
- Careful enquiry about any brain injury/insult.

- Any alternative therapies/specific cultural remedies?
- Systematic health review (see 3H, p. 113).
- Dates of any previous hospital attendance with name and address at time.

Record details of all illnesses that the patient has had starting with childhood illnesses (and any of their complications). Hospital admissions and the reason for them and their nature, details of any operations, recent medical history, and recent and current medication should all be recorded. Try to find out what the patient was told about any illness, remembering that the patient may not have full details or full knowledge of previous serious or life-threatening illnesses (partly because the truth may have been denied to him or he may be using denial himself) and so you will need to get information from elsewhere. Periods of minor ill health (for which the general practitioner may or may not have been consulted) might be as just as important to record as major illness. It can sometimes be difficult to distinguish between minor physical ill health and minor psychiatric ill health. Also record the patient's emotional and psychological reaction to the illness and make particular enquiry about any insult and injury to the brain. Is he using alternative systems of health care? What cultural remedies has he tried? What are his own (or his family's) explanations for any illness?

Then ask the usual systems review health screening questions that you would normally ask in a medical interview concerning cardiovascular, respiratory, urogenital, gastrointestinal, and central nervous system function (see p. 113). These questions form a very necessary part of a psychiatric interview, particularly as physical illness may be mistaken for psychiatric illness and vice versa, and many people with psychiatric illness have coexisting physical problems. The answers to these questions will also indicate areas that should be particularly thoroughly examined during the physical examination.

Make sure that you clearly record any medication the patient is taking, both prescribed and 'over-the-counter', and record any method of contraception used. The names and dates of hospital attendances (with the patient's address at the time if it is different from his present address) should be documented together with any change in name of the patient. This comparatively minor chore aids the obtaining of essential information about the patient at a later date.

I Previous psychiatric history

- All contacts with hospital, community, and primary psychiatric care.
- Previous episodes of defined illness with description of symptoms and diagnoses?
- Any significant non-treated episodes?
- Medication and other treatment in past?
- Patient's explanation and understanding of past illnesses.
- Name and address during past episodes.
- Nature of any present medication and treatment and where he obtains it from.

As with the previous medical history you will want to record details about all contacts with psychiatric or primary care services, whether in-patient or out-patient, and previous episodes of defined illness (and, if possible, the diagnosis). In addition to trying to discover what the official diagnosis was of previous periods of illness, it is also important to get from the patient a description of how he felt at the time, and what the experience was like for him. It obviously increases rapport between you and the patient if he understands that you are trying to see things from his point of view, and it enables you to compare his present experience with any previous ones in terms of his own subjective feelings. It also allows you to determine whether there have been milder episodes of the illness that were not formally reported or did not come to medical attention.

Include in your psychiatric history contact with general practitioners and episodes that were not formally treated but which perhaps led to some change in lifestyle, like being sent away to some relative by the seaside for a few weeks' 'rest'. Note any other symptom that the patient now recognizes, in its historical context, might have had some relationship to his present illness (like for instance, previous sustained changes in mood, the significance of which was not recognized at the time). Try to discover what medication the patient has had in the past and make sure that you have an accurate record of what he is taking now. Remember to make an enquiry about whether he has had other forms of treatment, like behaviour therapy, psycho-therapy, and electrical treatment, and the patient's perception of whether they helped or not. Many patients do not regard behavioural treatment or psychotherapy as 'treatment' and will not volunteer that they have had it.

Questions like, 'Has anything like this ever happened to you before?', 'Have you ever had trouble with your nerves?', 'Have there been times when perhaps you have not felt quite yourself?', are particularly useful as they are open-ended invitations to discuss past feelings. As with the medical history, you will need to look at the patient's and his family's explanations for his illness and previous illnesses and particularly any cultural interpretations of it and remedies for it.

CHAPTER 3

Assessment

A Mental state examination

- Elaborate on changes in mental state already noticed.
- Formally test for the presence of psychotic ideas/mental impairment.
- Be systematic and cover all areas: ask all the screening questions outlined in Section 3J (p. 120).

Your examination of the patient's mental state has, of course, been going on throughout the entire interview and you may have already elicited changes in mood, alteration in thought form or content, or evidence of memory impairment. If you have, you may wish to clarify and expand on some of the things that the patient has already talked about. If you have not elicited any evidence of psychotic illness or of memory impairment, it is very necessary that you formally test for the presence or absence of it and also look for mood changes. You must ask about suicidal intention in every patient (see Section 3J, p. 120 for *questions that should always be asked*).

Although you will have already made most of the observations you will need, it is important that you spend some time in your interview considering the patient's mental state and going through a systematic review in your mind, using the headings that follow, so that you can be sure that you have left nothing uncovered. You will have made a lot of observations about the patient unconsciously, and this is your chance to clarify these observations and perhaps ask yourself how you came to make them. If you find evidence of an abnormality in one modality of mental state, do not abandon the rest of the examination to pursue a fascinating hare! Make sure that you have covered every area outlined below. Many patients with schizophrenia, for example, have a significant mood disorder, and a not inconsiderable number have, in addition to auditory hallucinations, olfactory hallucinations that will not be recorded unless asked about.

Use the usual method of change of topic statements, open-ended questions, and then closed questions to assess all modalities of the mental state using the screening questions outlined later and also listed on p. 120.

B   Appearance and behaviour

- What is your *immediate* impression (behaviour may change).
- Anything abnormal about his gait, behaviour towards others, dress?
- Gently confront obvious differences from cultural norms.
- Observe motor activity (abnormal movements, retardation, or overactivity)?
- Are behaviour and observed emotional responses appropriate or not?
- Does he look ill?

On first meeting with the patient, even if it is in his own home, it is useful if you can watch him walk into the consulting room or area. You will get an immediate impression of how he is dressed, how he behaves towards others, and of his gait and posture.

Behaviour may, of course, change during the interview and the initially hostile and suspicious patient who sits hunched facing away from you may eventually relax and have normal non-verbal contact with you. It is, however, the immediate physical picture that can be so helpful and which, if you do not perceive it straight away, can be missed (like the facies of a patient with myxoedema or the festinant gait of someone with Parkinson's disease).

Bearing in mind that different cultures do have different expectations of dress and behaviour, it is important to gently confront aspects of behaviour, dress, or appearance that seem to clash with the culture to which the patient belongs (or if the patient appears to be adopting aspects of a culture other than his own). It is better to record aspects of the patient's appearance without initially making interpretations of what that appearance means, except to record the patient's explanation. 'John, you are not wearing any clothes at the moment. Is there some reason for that?' 'God told me to take off my clothes and be free.'

You will need to make a note of the patient's motor activity. He may appear underactive and sluggish or retarded, or he may be overactive with restless pacing and endless twisting of the hands or wedding ring (although many psychiatrists describe the 'wedding ring sign' as an indication that the patient has marital problems, it is usually only an indication of general tension). Be particularly on the lookout for tardive dyskinesia and the restless feet of akathisia. The patient with tardive dyskinesia often seems oblivious to the movements, even if his attention is drawn to them, whereas the patient with akathisia will volunteer that he cannot keep his feet still and has an inner feeling of restlessness.

A full description of most of the disorders of movement that you may encounter is given in Section 4O (p. 359). It is important to emphasize that abnormal movements are quite common and that they can often be either subtle (as in the early stages of chorea when they may look just like fidgeting) or look so bizarre that it is assumed that they must be deliberate even though they are not. It is worthwhile reviewing a videotape of movement disorders during the early part of your training, and noting in particular that, until you can recognize them, dystonias can look very 'hysterical'.

The patient's behaviour in the interview may sometimes seem very inappropriate. Remember, however, that many patients on first seeing a psychiatrist are very anxious. Anxiety can make people behave in a very stilted and affected way, or may make them either garrulous or almost mute. It may at times make patients answer at seeming random because they are so keen to escape from what they see as a very threatening situation. Do not mistake this for psychotic behaviour.

One other important observation to make is whether or not the patient looks well. Most of us as doctors develop an instinct for recognizing when a patient is seriously physically ill, and it is worth trying to keep this instinct. Never make the mistake of assuming that just because the patient has presented to a psychiatrist he must therefore be psychiatrically ill, or that there is nothing physically wrong with him (no matter how eminent the authority that has said that there isn't!).

C Cognitive function

- Always test cognitive function.
- Introduce it properly, and ask if he has noticed any difficulty.
- Ask if he can remember your name and function, and his name, address, and date of birth (check).
- Check orientation in time and place (to within an hour). Does he know the function of nurse, doctor, etc?

- Ask dates of first and second world wars, brief test of general knowledge, general information.
- Can he register information and remember it (name and address)?
- Digits forward (up to seven). Digits backwards (up to six).
- Serial sevens test.
- Abstract thinking (proverbs).
- Go on to fuller tests (Section 4F, p. 173) if any apparent abnormality is present and not explained by the patient's mental state or educational abilities.

In conventional textbooks it is usual to put assessment of cognitive function at the end of the mental state examination and you may sometimes feel that this is the most appropriate place for it. We are putting it near to the front of the examination to remind you of its importance and to encourage you to make this assessment in every patient you encounter, whether or not it is likely that the patient has a cognitive disturbance. The reasons for this are firstly, that unless you look for it, and look for it early, subtle cognitive impairment may easily be missed (but will, of course, have a profound effect upon the diagnosis you are trying to reach and will modify the rest of your examination). Secondly, you may otherwise forget to do it in the excitement, for instance, of uncovering a delusional system. Thirdly, it is important to do it in every patient you see so that you will learn the kind of responses to your questions that the non-cognitively impaired give (so that you can recognize real impairment more easily and have more confidence in your diagnosis).

Life and mental state examination is full of surprises. Although you may have already begun to suspect that a patient has a memory impairment from the history you take, it will not always be so. You may be misled by facile social speech that is full of empty stock phrases, or even by confabulation, only to discover later, with some surprise, that the patient has practically no recent memory and cannot retain new information.

When testing cognitive function, doctors often preface the tests with an apologetic remark to the effect 'Do you mind answering some silly questions?' because they feel faintly ridiculous asking what seem to be questions with very obvious answers. Do not be tempted to do this, because you are diminishing the importance of what you are doing, both for yourself and for the patient, and 'silly' questions beget 'silly' answers. Preface your cognitive testing instead by saying something like '*I am going to ask you some questions now that we ask everybody. Tell me if you have particular difficulty with any or if you are not sure what the question means.*' 'Before we begin perhaps you can tell me if you have noticed whether you have had any particular difficulties with your memory recently, getting the right change for the shop, or in finding your way?' Make sure you have already introduced yourself clearly and that you have asked the patient for his name, address, and date of birth (and have checked his accuracy). 'First of all can you tell me what the date is today? And the year? And what day of the week is it? What time is it? Where are we at the moment? And the name of this place? And (for example, pointing to a nurse) what does that person do?' In this way you have tested **orientation in time, place, and person**.

Remind the patient that you introduced yourself at the beginning of the examination, and then ask him if he can remember your name and what you do, and ask him to tell you roughly how long the interview has already taken. Patients who have been in hospital for a long time become confused about dates without necessarily being organically impaired, but everybody should be able to estimate the time of day to within an hour. They should be able to appreciate where they are, the function of the place in which they are (for example, a hospital ward, police station), and the function of the people they encounter (i.e., they should know the role of a nurse or of a policeman).

The facility and accuracy with which the patient can recall details from his past will often give you a clue to the integrity of his **long-term memory**. (To be sure you will need confirmation of his accuracy from someone else. It may also be checked by asking about such things as the dates of the first and second world wars, if the patient is old enough to have lived through them. If the patient is younger then ask him a few questions of general historical knowledge.)

You should then estimate the patient's ability to **register information** and assess his **short-term memory**. The most usual way is to initially check for concentration and immediate recall by testing **digit span**. You offer the patient a series of random single-digit numbers, given with an even intonation and spacing (such as, 5 . . . 4 . . . 3 . . . 6 . . . 9 . . . 1). Avoid an obvious sequence like 1 . . . 2 . . . 3 . . . or 3 . . . 5 . . . 7. Then ask the patient to recall them in the order in which they were given. Start with two or three digit sequences and add a digit each time the patient succeeds in repeating them back correctly. Three attempts should be made at the highest level the patient has reached before deciding that he has failed to reach this digit span. The exercise should then be repeated with the patient repeating the digit sequence he was given backwards (i.e., 4 . . . 2 . . . 7 becomes 7 . . . 2 . . . 4. Always give the patient an example before starting). The average person can recall seven digits forwards and four backwards. Many things, apart from organic impairment, can effect concentration (anxiety, preoccupation with hallucinations, worries, etc.). It is therefore important to test concentration before short-term memory and other cognitive functions.

The usual way to test short-term memory is to give the patient a name and address to retain and ask him to recall it after five minutes (make sure the number of elements in the name and address do not exceed the patient's own digit span). Give him the name and address (for example, Frank Robinson, 23, Chesterfield Road, Derby—if his correct digit span is six) and get him to repeat it once (so that you can check that he has retained it). Then ask him to repeat it after five minutes. All the elements should be remembered if his short-term memory is intact, but make sure that he knows beforehand that he has to remember the address for five minutes.

It is usual to ask a few questions about general information and current affairs (even old chestnuts like asking the name of the sovereign or prime minister). Make enquiries about topics of the day in newspapers and on television. If the patient has been in hospital or ill for a long time he may have little interest or knowledge of current affairs. You should make a *general assessment of the patient's intelligence*. It is not always obvious that a patient is of limited intelligence, but enquiry about whether he can read or write is often helpful, as well as that about whether he can cope with everyday things like shopping, getting the right change, travelling on buses, etc.

Abstract thinking is tested for by asking patients to give you the symbolic as opposed to the literal meaning of proverbs (for example, 'people who live in glass houses should not throw stones'). Concrete thinking is suggested when a patient of sufficient educational or intellectual background to understand the abstract meaning of the proverb, can only give you the literal answer.

These tests do not take too long to do and are merely screening tests, but they should give you some idea of whether or not the patient has cognitive impairment.

They should also give you a rough idea of whether the patient's present apparent intelligence is commensurate with his educational background or whether there may have been some decline. If there is evidence of possible impairment, the fuller tests outlined in Section 4F (p. 173) should be used. The patient's educational level, his limited intellectual capacity, or his mental state (for example, severe retardation) may produce 'false positives'.

It is important to remember that cognitive function often fluctuates in organic conditions and all you can do is record the patient's cognitive function as it appears to you at interview. You will need to gather evidence of the patient's behaviour over several days, either at home or in the ward setting, to really know whether sustained cognitive impairment is present or not.

D Mood

- Is there an obvious change in mood (depression, elation, anxiety)?
- Is it sustained or does it fluctuate?
- Is behaviour consistent with verbally expressed mood?
- Always ask about suicidal ideas, feelings, and intent. *Be blunt.*
- Explore suicidal ideas, feelings, and intent *thoroughly* (Section 4H, p. 215).
- Look also at reasons for staying alive.
- Any evidence of anhedonia and morbid thoughts?
- Any ruminations or overvalued ideas? Depressive delusions or hallucinations?
- Record pattern of sleep and any change in it.
- Changes in appetite, weight, concentration, memory, and sexual desire?

- Does he blame himself or anyone else for his depression? Any feelings of guilt, self-blame, unworthiness, or poverty? Does he feel that he may be ill?

- What does he think is the reason for any mood change?

You need to try to make an assessment of the patient's prevailing mood during the interview. Is there sustained lowering of spirits and depression? Is there obvious retardation or agitation? Is there sustained euphoria, or pathologically high spirits, or sustained tension and anxiety? Does the patient's mood fluctuate markedly during the interview, perhaps from euphoria to tears and back again, or do you see lowering of mood only when perhaps painful or difficult subjects are touched upon? You are recording the patient's mood as it appears to you at the interview, rather than as judged by what he says it is. People can be feeling very anxious or depressed, however, without it being reflected in their overt behaviour, and the reverse is also true.

Look critically at how the patient appears to you and listen to his verbal tone, as well as to what he is actually saying. There may be obvious incongruities between expressed and observed emotion—seen, for example, in the patient who is full of gloomy talk but who smiles (often an empty, chilling smile), or the patient who denies anxiety but who sits shifting on the edge of his seat with his legs and arms crossed fiddling incessantly with his wedding ring.

Learn to look critically, therefore, at the patient's posture, mannerisms, facial expression, gestures, and eye contact, and record them. Video feedback of your interviews will teach you the importance of this and what to look for, and how, when necessary, to confront incongruity of expressed and apparent mood—'I understand how low you feel, but I notice that you are smiling. Why is that?' 'You say that you feel quite calm at the moment, but let me show you how you are sitting. Now, what do you think that is telling me?'

The overall mood of a patient in an interview may therefore be congruent or incongruent with his normal mood, or depressed or elevated, or tense and anxious, or a fluctuating mixture of them. Alternatively, it may be one of perplexity. Perplexity is the physical expression of a mood of puzzlement and uncertainty. Record mood as it appears to you during the interview. You will also need to obtain information about how the patient's mood has appeared to others, either at home or on the ward, over the past few days or weeks.

It is most important that you enquire about suicidal ideation in every patient and, if present, find out how sustained and how strong any such feelings and thoughts are and whether the patient is likely to act upon them. A full assessment of the suicidal patient is described in Section 4H (p. 215). Even if you do not suspect it, it is important to ask, no matter what appears to be wrong with the patient. Vague suicidal ideas or fantasies about personal demise and its effect on others ('Will I be missed?') are, of course, extremely common, particularly in adolescence (most of us have had them) and should be distinguished from more sustained and deeply felt ideas of self-harm.

Some beginners in psychiatry fear that if they raise the topic of suicide they may put it into the patient's mind, but you can assume that the idea is already there. Anyone who is depressed will have thought about suicide even if only to dismiss it, and almost everybody who has suicidal feelings will be glad of the chance of discussing them and realizing they are perhaps not as abnormal as they thought. In discussing the topic do not use so many euphemisms that you and the patient end up with a rather unclear idea of what you are discussing. Be blunt and direct in your questions.

('I can see that you have been feeling low for some time. Many people who feel like this are so despairing that they think seriously about harming themselves. I wonder if you have ever thought of killing yourself?')

Always make sure that you record the answer to the question in the notes. If you get a positive reply, as you often will, then you will need to discover how pervasive the thought is, how strongly it is felt, what the patient himself feels about it, whether he had planned to act on it (or whether he has already tried to act on it and not told anybody), and, most important of all, what prevents him from carrying it out. This may be religious reasons, the fear of upsetting relatives, or the effect that it will have on his children. The reasons for staying alive, despite the patient's present bad situation, should be explored. The patient who denies any suicidal thought, if he is depressed, should be treated with grave suspicion, as should the *smiling depressive* mentioned above. Sometimes such patients will have already made the decision to kill themselves and are merely waiting for the opportunity. Making the decision to die often has a cathartic effect on mood.

Although you are assessing mood as it appears to you and are concentrating on the patient's behaviour and verbal and emotional tone, you will, of course, also be influenced by what the patient says and will be alert to descriptions of loss of pleasure in normal pursuits (**anhedonia**) and to **morbid thoughts**. These are over-gloomy and pessimistic thoughts that the patient has about his life and his situation that tend to be ruminative and, although not delusional, are difficult to alter. Sometimes, of course, the patient, if elated, may have an overly rosy view of the world and its pleasures that is out of keeping with cynical reality.

You will occasionally also discover, either in your initial history taking or by asking screening questions, that the patient has affect-laden delusions, either hypochondriacal, or of guilt, self-blame, unworthiness, or poverty. Rarely **nihilistic** or **grandiose delusions** may be expressed. The patient may also have mood congruent hallucinations or illusions.

As part of your routine questioning you will have also enquired about sleep, appetite, sexual desire, concentration, and memory, which are often characteristically altered during changes in mood (see Section 4G, p. 197).

E Form of speech (thought form)

- Is there a speech disorder present? Is it of form or content? Is it organic? Does it affect writing as well as speech?
- Assess rate and quality, volume and tone. Are there sudden shifts in topic or sudden long pauses?
- Can he stick to the point or does he wander off, and if so, why?
- Is there non-social speech or poverty of ideation?
- Record any very unusual speech immediately.

You will need to judge the patient's speech. When you do this you will also be rating his thinking since the only way we can really judge what and how the patient is thinking is by what he says. With experience you may be able to make intuitive guesses about his thinking (and the patient's behaviour may tell you that he is hallucinating even though he denies it). A great deal of your formal examination of a patient's mental state will therefore be spent listening to and analysing what the patient says (and, if necessary, recording verbatim samples of his speech). You will not often have to record speech immediately during the interview, but if a patient is particularly thought disordered, or is using neologisms, then it is important to record it at the time because its very uniqueness will make it difficult to remember and recall. 'Has anything unusual or strange ever happened to you?' 'Such as death, do you mean doctor? Yes, I've been dead several times—dead of the Germans mainly, but I've always been restored to life by psychogalvanic electromagnetism.'

It may initially be difficult to recognize that you are dealing with somebody who is speech disordered and you will have to develop the critical faculties needed to recognize whether a speech disorder is present (always remember to check if it is also a *writing* disorder), and you will also have to develop the skills to recognize whether you are dealing with an organic or *functional* speech disorder. The distinction is not always easy to make and it is best, if you are unsure, to let the patient talk without interruption for a while and to let his words wash over you. Simultaneously ask yourself the question whether you can understand what the patient is saying and if you cannot, is it because of the *way* that he is saying it (**thought form disorder**) or because of *what* he is saying (**thought content disorder**). You have to be able to recognize that unusual forms of speech may not in themselves be pathological and may indeed just be indicative of the patient's educational background. You need to know your culture well, and also your language, its grammar and literature, otherwise in your ignorance you may see a disorder when it does not exist.

Why for instance, although very hard to understand, is some of the work of James Joyce or the poetry of Dylan Thomas not considered to be thought disordered? Why is Mrs Malaprop's 'allegory on the banks of the Nile' a malapropism and not a neologism? The answer is that Joyce's stream of consciousness, although difficult to understand at first, is very like our own. Were our own stream of consciousness to be written down in such painful and intimate details as Joyce's, it would read very much the same (in terms of its form, although perhaps not in terms of its content!). In the same way the words of Thomas's poetry seem incomprehensible at first, but the sound of the words makes sense and awakens echoes in our minds that indicate that we and the poet have a shared experience and a shared understanding. We all know what Mrs Malaprop meant. Her misuse of 'allegory' when she clearly meant 'alligator' just tells us that she has intellectual pretentions above her educational level. We can also guess, from the context in which the sentence occurred, that the word alligator was the one really intended.

When we speak we all make allusions to things within our memory and our experience that may not be immediately understood by other people, and we all have in our language a common store of stock phrases and expressions, the context of which we understand but which people from another culture may not. A doctor from abroad who does not know the phrase 'butterflies in the stomach' for instance, may make the assumption that a patient describing such an experience has somatic hallucinations. When a patient calls his toe 'the finger on my foot', we might think he has a nominal dysphasia not realizing that it is a literal translation from his own language.

The difference between such normal (even if difficult to understand) thinking and writing and psychotic thinking and writing is that the shared bond, the common experience, is no longer there, and the symbolizations, assumptions, and allusions of psychotic thought become so private and so disordered as to no longer make sense. This is not to say, of course, that the more you get to know the patient and his previous life and experiences, the more you will not actually understand what he is trying to convey to you. It is important to learn early on in psychiatry that, although psychotic behaviour, speech, and ideas probably have physical bases to them (of some postulated change in brain transmitter chemistry and genetic predisposition), the patient is still trying to explain his alien experience to you and it is important to try to make some sense of what he is saying.

As you listen to the patient's speech you are assessing its rate, quantity, volume, and tone. Can the patient stick to the point or does he seem to go round and round it and never quite get to it? Is he showing obsessional attention to detail? Are there unexpected shifts in topic, and if there are, can you follow them or do they seem incomprehensible? Is he talking to you or just muttering to himself (**non-social speech**)? In addition to sudden changes in direction, is his speech full of rhyming and clang associations, puns and assonance?

The rate of speech might be slow, as in retardation, or might cease altogether, as in mutism (see Section 4P, p. 370). It might be very fast, and there might be great pressure of speech (as is seen in mania and in some excited people with schizophrenia). Shifts in topic occur, sometimes very rapidly. These shifts are sometimes understandable, as in mania, even if they leave you intellectually breathless, but sometimes, as in schizophrenia, the shifts occur without any obvious logic or your understanding (**derailment**). Shifts in topic may be so rapid in schizophrenia as to present you with what is called a 'word salad' or **verbigeration**. Speech becomes almost incomprehensible because of the rapid, often allusive, changes in topic. In a word salad almost all sense is lost because words follow each other without any connection (it can sometimes be difficult to distinguish this from jargon dysphasia —severe expressive dysphasia—but most dysphasic patients can still make themselves understood. Testing for nominal dysphasia, dyspraxia, dyslexia, or an expressive or a receptive dysphasia will usually help you to tell the difference). Word salad is now rare.

It is usually possible to tell the difference between manic speech, which flows and makes sense (although it can sometimes be hard to keep up with a patient's elated ideas and fantasies), and schizophrenic speech, which, although often rapid, does not seem to flow and makes little sense. Internal rhyming, clang associations, punning, and assonance can be found in both manic and schizophrenic speech, but in manic speech such phenomena are usually easier to understand and may even occasionally be witty, whereas it is unlikely that this will be so in schizophrenia.

Even the most psychotic patient, or even one with an organic disorder, may have very little wrong with his speech. In some patients who are psychotic, however, it will gradually become clear as you listen that there is a **poverty of ideation**. There is very little meaningful content in what the patient is saying, his speech is vague and woolly and there is a **loss of determining tendency** so that the patient never actually arrives at the point. This is to be contrasted with the patient who shows obsessional attention to detail, who also takes a long time to get to the point, but *is* actually getting there and has got some idea of where and what the point is. As an example, when asked 'How are you today?', the patient who is showing obsessional attention to detail may say something like 'Well, to answer that question properly we have to go back 13 years. Now at that time . . .' and will eventually end up, ten minutes later, saying 'Not too bad today, thank you'. The patient who shows poverty of ideation will wander on for several minutes about the world, his mind, and 'reality' until after a few minutes both you and he will have forgotten the original question you asked and it will never be answered, and you will be in despair at never being able to get to grips with what he is saying. Contrast this with what we might term 'politicians' speech', which *deliberately* sets out to be obscure!

When describing or rating the patient's speech you should try to avoid making a diagnosis, but rather make a *description* of what you have heard. Leave the diagnosis until later. You will be lucky if you can resist the temptation to diagnose, but try not to. Doctors in the future may not agree with your diagnosis and curse you if this is all you have recorded, but bless you if you have written a clear description of what the patient actually said and how he said it.

F Content of speech (thought content)

- Confront any obvious abnormalities.
- Use systematic screening questions (see Section 3J, p. 120) on everyone.
- Any preoccupations, ruminations, overvalued ideas, obsessional acts, obsessional thinking, phobias, or delusions?
- Has the patient insight into any abnormal thoughts?
- Any paranoid ideas or delusions?
- Any ideas or delusions of guilt, unworthiness, poverty, or self-blame?
- Any hypochondriacal ideas or delusions, dysmorphophobia, monosymptomatic delusions, or nihilistic delusions?
- Any grandiose ideas or delusions?
- Any sexual ideas or delusions?
- Any first rank schizophrenic delusions? For example, passivity/control, thought withdrawal or blocking, thought echo, thoughts heard out loud, thought broadcasting, delusional mood, delusional perception.

Although we classically distinguish between disorders of thought form and disorders of thought content, it is sometimes difficult to be certain which one you are dealing with. For instance, you observe that the patient suddenly stops in the middle of explaining something to you, does not speak for perhaps 20 or 30 seconds, and then suddenly starts with an entirely unrelated topic. This is clearly an abnormality of thought form, but there may be an underlying abnormality of thought content as well, and it is important that you confront the patient with this behaviour so that you discover the true underlying abnormality. The patient may, for instance, have experienced thought blocking (thought form disorder) or thought withdrawal (thought content disorder). Likewise, you may notice that your patient adopts a listening posture from time to time, or begins to look intently around the room as though he can see something that you cannot. It is important to confront this abnormality of behaviour so that you discover the underlying perceptual disorder. For example, 'I notice when we were talking just now that you seemed to be listening to something that I could not hear. Can you tell me what it was?' If you are sure he is hallucinating you can say, 'John, what are the voices saying at the moment?'

In your examination of the patient's thought content you will obviously often pick up points that the patient has already made and elaborate on them. If, however, the patient has given you no indication that he might have a disorder of thought content, you will need to ask several screening questions, no matter what you think might be wrong with the patient, to make sure that he is not harbouring some kind of delusional system or other disorder of thought content. It is very important that you do this. One benefit of doing this is that you will learn to distinguish the normal negative replies to your questions from people who do not have the experience from the more evasive replies of patients who actually do have the experience, but who do not want you to know that they have.

It is important to remember that disorders of thought content include other things apart from delusions, and that abnormal beliefs may not always carry the strength of a delusion but nevertheless it is still important to record them. Thus you will be recording any **preoccupations** the patient has (with symptoms of illness, for instance, or with particular ideas), and **ruminations**, in which the patient is not only preoccupied with an idea or a feeling but either constantly ruminates about it or has recurrent, difficult to shake off, often panic-laden thoughts about a particular topic or topics. Both these phenomena will tend to present themselves to you during your history taking, but it may not always be apparent just how much time the patient spends ruminating about his problems unless you enquire.

It is important to also enquire about **obsessions and compulsions** and **phobias**. Obsessions are ritualized pieces of behaviour or thinking that the patient knows to be silly or unnecessary, but which he feels compelled to carry out because of a feeling that if he does not some evil or unpleasant consequence will befall him. The compulsion relates to the fear of consequences rather than to any feeling that the patient is being externally directed to behave in a particular way or think a particular thought. Do remember to check for obsessional *thinking* as well as behaviour as the patient may know full well that his obsessional thoughts are abnormal and may not volunteer them unless asked.

Although you will already have touched on this, recheck to see if the patient has *anxiety symptoms* or *panic attacks*. Ask if he has learnt if any particular situation seems to bring on the panic attacks, and whether he has actually learned to avoid certain situations that are particularly likely to make him feel anxious. **Phobic anxiety** (often, but not necessarily, accompanied by panic) is precipitated by certain situations but not others (such as anxiety in crowds or travelling on buses, etc.). Some phobias are so common as to be normal (for example a fear of insects), but even with these you should distinguish between a normal level of phobic feeling about, say, spiders in the bath and a phobia that has become so pathological that the affected person can no longer enter the bathroom.

In this part of your examination of the patient's thought content you will also be trying to establish the patient's judgement about what he thinks is wrong with him and the degree of **insight** he has into the fact that he is ill or that he has a problem. Some people who have a psychotic illness will have no insight at all whereas others with the same illness will recognize that they are ill. In addition, you will be assessing whether the patient has any **hypochrondriacal ideas** and will also see if the patient has a **dysmorphophobia**. At its minimum, hypochondriasis is either a preoccupation with symptoms that have no organic basis, or is being overly concerned with health and having a fear of disease. At its maximum, however, it becomes delusional. Dysmorphobia is a belief which like hypochondriasis can be held with delusional force, that the patient is misshapen or unattractive, and characteristically fastens on one feature of the patient (nose, ears, or breasts, for instance). These ideas may exist on their own or may be part of other delusional systems, such as paranoia, and may sometimes be associated with significant depression.

You should also check to see if the patient has **overvalued ideas**. This is usually fairly obvious from what the patient tells you during your history taking. Overvalued ideas are thoughts or ideas that tend to dominate the patient's conscious life, are often affect-laden, and are understandable in terms of the patient's past experience and his personality. Although unduly prominent and taking up too much of the patient's thinking time, they are not held with delusional force.

Finally, you will need to be sure that the patient has no abnormal beliefs (**delusional ideas**). The patient with delusions may not see them as being abnormal and may therefore not volunteer them, since they are so much part of his life, unless you specifically ask about them. A delusion may be defined as an unshakable belief or conviction that is out of keeping with the patient's culture and which cannot be altered or dispelled by any proof to the contrary. Some psychiatric classifications identify **partial delusions** (that is, those delusions that can be modified or those about which the patient has some insight), and **full delusions** when the belief is totally unchangeable.

Different cultures have different acceptable beliefs. A particular acceptable cultural belief might still be an overvalued idea, or a patient may be preoccupied with it or be ruminating about it, but if it is an idea that is compatible with the patient's culture then it is not a delusion. If you can find a sufficient number of people who share a particular belief, no matter how odd it may appear, then again the belief is not a delusion. Patients with delusional ideas may, of course, find themselves attracted to sects that have similar beliefs.

It is possible for two (sometimes three or four) people to share a common delusional system. Usually this is because the more powerful member of the pair, or group, imposes his delusional system on to the weaker brethren. If you remove the dominant member, the delusional beliefs of the others usually collapse very rapidly. This is known as **folie imposée**, or **folie à deux**. When it does occur it is usually seen in families or in pathological relationships.

The possession of a delusional system almost invariably implies that the patient has a psychotic illness. Luckily for psychiatrists the delusions that occur in psychotic illnesses tend to run to a pattern, although their content may change over the years as human knowledge and experience advances. For instance, delusional belief about being influenced by witches is declining whilst belief in control or interference by alien spacemen is increasing. The major forms and types are outlined below.

Sometimes the patient will be bursting to tell you of his delusions, whereas at other times he may try to conceal them, although will often confide them to you if your question makes it clear that you already have an intuitive understanding that he has a delusional system. (In the same way a patient with hallucinatory experiences will often be much more likely to tell you about them if your questions indicate that you already have a shrewd idea that he has them.) It is therefore important that you ask everybody some screening questions about the presence of delusions.

A good general screening question to start with is '*I wonder if you can tell me if you have any particularly strong thoughts or feelings that you tend to think a lot about—about yourself perhaps or about the world we live in*?' If you get a negative reply then ask a supplementary question, '*I wonder if you feel that you are special in some way, or if you are being got at or persecuted in some way*?' If you still get a negative reply you may well feel that it is worthwhile going on to ask the screening questions outlined below to try to be as sure as possible that the patient does not have a delusional system. At this point you should ask a screening question about perceptual experiences, the usual one being '*Has anything strange or unusual happened to you, which perhaps has puzzled you or you are not quite sure about*?'

Paranoid delusions

The word paranoid, unfortunately, has come to have different meanings for the different schools of psychiatry, but we are using it here to mean an idea of persecution or intended harm, or of being spied upon. The patient may just be preoccupied with, or ruminating about, paranoid ideas, and his sense of persecution may be either an overvalued idea (and clearly related either to his mood or to his sensitive and suspicious personality) or it may be a true delusion. Certain cultures are much more paranoid than others, and people in such cultures will often interpret inner feelings (such as depression or even elation) as being the result of some outside agency trying to harm them or influence them.

Paranoid delusions may be fairly diffuse and unfocused, or may be part of a very elaborate delusional system in which the original idea of an outside agency wishing to cause the patient harm has become systematized and complex. The elaboration and systemization of the paranoid delusion may in itself not be psychotic although the original idea is. It is also important to be really certain that the patient *is* deluded that people are out to get him. We can cite several examples of patients who were thought to have the delusion that their families were trying to dispossess them of their dwelling place only to find that this was actually true. Another example was an Iranian student who was thought to be deluded in his belief that the Iranian secret police were after him, which was subsequently found to be true. Do not believe that every idea of persecution is necessarily delusional without checking first (a sad reflection perhaps of the society in which we live).

Because they are so common, it is usual to always ask a screening question about paranoid delusions '*Do you ever feel or think that somebody or something is trying to harm you or get at you in some way?*' If the patient says 'Yes', then use open-ended questions and your skills in probing to try to get a complete picture of what the patient actually believes. The patient will have the delusional belief that he is being poisoned, spied on, or harassed either by some identifiable person (who may be a relative), by some body of people (such as the police or the Jehovah's Witnesses), or by some less identifiable organization, such as the government, the communists, or people from outer space. The patient often cannot tell you why he has been particularly chosen in this way for persecution, but occasionally he will see it in a rather grandiose way in terms of being a special person or sometimes in a much more negative way in terms of being punished for past crimes. Both these interpretations should make you think in terms of an affective illness.

Paranoid delusions are common. They may exist on their own as a separate syndrome, may occur as part of a schizophrenic illness, may occur both in mania and depression, and are not uncommon in patients with organic brain disease. The possession of paranoid delusions is therefore not particularly diagnostic and is certainly not indicative of schizophrenia, and so further careful examination of the patient's mental state is necessary before you can come to any diagnostic conclusion.

Delusions of reference

These may or may not occur in association with paranoid delusions. The ideas may again be held with delusional force, may be preoccupations, or may be overvalued. Essentially the patient experiences references to himself in communications that a reasonable person would not think were about him. The communication may be verbal or non-verbal and, as with paranoid delusions, may be affect-laden so that the patient may experience the delusion as pleasant, unpleasant, or neutral. As with paranoid delusions, the patient may have the idea but not have formulated it very much, or the idea may have become extremely systematized.

Screening questions, which should always be asked, include '*Do you ever have feelings that people are talking about you, or are referring to you?*' and '*Do you ever think that things you read in the papers or see on television have a special meaning for you?*'

Common delusions of reference include people talking about the patient in the street (this is not an auditory hallucination—inanimate objects may be the source of auditory hallucinations but rarely people that the patient can actually see), or people may be making gestures of special significance to the patient, or the patient may see hidden messages referring to himself in the way people are dressed, the way objects are arranged in shop windows, or in announcements on the television or the radio. Sometimes it is hard to tell when a delusion of reference ends and delusional misinterpretation begins (see below).

As with paranoid delusions, delusions of reference are not particularly diagnostic and can occur in all psychotic illnesses and in organic brain disease.

Delusions of guilt, unworthiness, and self-blame

Many people who are depressed entertain negative ideas about themselves, feel that they are being punished for past misdeeds, and have a very poor valuation of themselves. At times these ideas become of delusional intensity. Ideas of guilt, unworthiness, and self-blame therefore span the whole spectrum from preoccupations, ruminations, and overvalued ideas, to full delusional beliefs. To some extent the possession of delusions of guilt and unworthiness reflect the culture from which the patient comes and are particularly likely to occur in those who are religious or at least come from a culture in which the religious ethos tends to be one of encouraging feelings of guilt and ideas of punishment.

In delusions of guilt, the patient characteristically remembers some innocent pecadillo of youth (such as kissing a girl behind the school bicycle sheds at the age of 16), invests this innocent act with the majesty of a mortal sin, and then feels that his present depressive feelings are a true and just punishment for such a crime against the Almighty. Such an idea is held with unshakeable force and when dealing with such patients you must be very careful not to accidentally reinforce it. One of us saw such a patient, who had guilty delusions related to a harmless act of masturbation, cut his throat from ear to ear five minutes after the visit of a Catholic priest who had foolishly tried to offer the man absolution, not realizing the delusional nature of the man's beliefs. The man himself felt that he could never be forgiven for such a terrible sin and the priest's response was, of course, confirming his delusional idea. 'These are the excesses to which religion can lead,' Lucretius remarked about somewhat similar circumstances. Such delusions are a reflection on any religion that tries to make mankind feel guilty about harmless and normal activity.

Delusions of poverty, unworthiness, and self-blame are also common in patients with depression. The patient believes, against all efforts to persuade him otherwise, that he is ruined, that he has lost all his money, and that he has reduced his family to pauperdom. Even if you go to the length of showing him his bank statements he will tell you that this is merely the bank trying to be kind and protecting him from the enormity of his loss. Patients with delusions of unworthiness will tell you that they have disgraced their families or disgraced their country, and patients with delusions of self-blame tend to take the evils of the world on to themselves. They will believe, for instance, that the present troubles in Northern Ireland or any recently occurring natural catastrophe is actually due to them and that in some way they have caused it. People with these delusions will often confess to being the perpetrators of some infamous crime currently having the attention of the community.

There are several important practical points about the management of a patient with such delusions. Having heard them, be careful not to reinforce them and make sure that the patient realizes that your interpretation of his delusion is that he is ill. Once you have elicited the phenomenon do not dwell upon it and do not let the patient do so. Neither you nor those looking after the patient should endlessly rehearse the patient's catalogue of guilt and blame. Also, make sure that when the patient has recovered from his depression he has also recovered from his delusions and that he sees that they were a reflection of his illness. It is quite likely that your patient will become depressed again and he may be able to learn to recognize that when he is depressed he develops these abnormal beliefs. You will therefore be helping him to cope with the next episode of illness better.

Patients with delusions of guilt, poverty, unworthiness, or self-blame are usually actively suicidal (and may, if they feel that they have involved their family in their poverty or guilt, be homicidal as well), and this aspect of their mental state needs very careful assessment. You should assume that they need urgent treatment and active guarding against self-harm until they are clearly better. Screening questions about ideas of guilt, unworthiness, and poverty should therefore always be asked of people who are depressed and include *'Do you ever think you are being punished in some way?'*, *'Are there things you feel particularly bad about?'* and *'Is there anything you are particularly ashamed of?'*

Hypochondriacal delusions

As previously indicated, patients may be preoccupied about their health, ruminate about it, or have overvalued hypochondriacal ideas. Hypochondriacal delusions may occur as an entity on their own, and many psychiatrists regard the patient with an unshakeable hypochondriacal belief or dysmorphophobia as having a monosymptomatic delusion.

People who are depressed are often preoccupied with their health. Possibly depression makes them more aware of the odd twinges, aches and pains, and bodily sensations that we are all prone to and which we ignore when in good health and good spirits, but which we allow to develop an overwhelming significance when depressed. It is important to remember that in patients with hypochondriacal delusions the delusion may be founded on some real, if slight, physical symptom that will need careful evaluation.

Hypochondriacal delusions in depression tend to have a somewhat bizarre quality to them. The patient believes his brain is rotting, his bowels have been blocked for six months, water is rising in his body and when it touches his heart he will die, or he is rotting with venereal disease. Monosymptomatic hypochondriacal delusions tend to be about cancer or infestation.

A depressed patient with hypochondriacal delusions is likely to be prone to suicide. If he has a delusion that he has a venereal disease and has infected his family he may occasionally be a risk to them as well. Try to distinguish between patients who have strange *symptoms* of bodily ill health and patients who have strange *ideas* about bodily health. We have seen several patients with symptoms of neuropathy related to carcinomatosis labelled as hypochondriacal because they were complaining of sensory symptoms and parasthesia that the referring doctor had failed to recognize. Always ask yourself what might have triggered the patient's delusional ideas off in the first place.

It is unlikely that you will actually need a screening question for hypochondriacal delusions because almost invariably they will be part of the way the patient presents to you, but you should always ask how the patient interprets the cause of his depression if he has not mentioned a hypochondriacal idea. The screening questions you ask in terms of general health will often throw up hypochondriacal delusions, if they do not present elsewhere, and you should always ask the question *'Do you feel that you might be physically ill?'*

Nihilistic delusions

True nihilistic delusions are extremely uncommon. The expression comes from the Latin word *nihil* meaning nothing, and to have a nihilistic delusion the patient has to have the fixed and unalterable belief that part of his body is missing ('I have no brain' or 'I have no head'), or have similar feelings about his surroundings. Some patients even feel that the entire world has disappeared and that they are merely sitting in a grey formless void. Such nihilistic delusions may be thought of as the psychotic end of derealization and depersonalization rather than as an extension of hypochondriacal delusions. They usually occur in severe depressive illnesses, but may be encountered in schizophrenia or in organic brain disease. Patients are usually very distressed by the experience and will readily volunteer it during screening questions about bodily perception and about how they view the world. Confronting them with evidence that their idea is false, for example, by showing a woman who believes that her head is missing her own head, either on video or in a mirror, is not effective—'That is not my real head, doctor, it's just a puppet you have put there to try to fool me.'

Grandiose delusions

These are the reverse of the delusional experiences described above. Occasionally, grandiose ideas may merely be a preoccupation or an overvalued idea, but usually they are delusional. They take the form of belief in great wealth, of possessing extraordinary powers, or of being famous, or of having a special relationship with the Almighty, or of having some important religious task to do, like being sent to save the world. These delusional ideas occur most commonly in hypomania and are therefore sometimes likely to be infective and to involve others. They will also leave the patient feeling very foolish when he recovers (like a hypomanic vicar who danced naked on the lawn of his bishop's palace). Belief in new-found powers of being able to walk on water or fly may occasionally lead to unpleasant accidents.

Although grandiose delusions are commonly found in hypomania, they may occasionally be encountered in schizophrenia and in organic mental states as well. Classically, of course, they are supposed to be extremely common in cerebral syphilis, but in fact this condition usually presents with a depression or a simple dementia (see Section 6D, p. 471). It is important to treat grandiose delusions as seriously as one treats a delusion of guilt and to recognize that they can be equally as damaging and need prompt treatment. It is unlikely that you will need to ask a screening question about grandiose delusions as the patient is usually only too ready to press his beliefs upon you, but patients who retain partial insight may not immediately declare their beliefs and therefore you should always ask the question 'Do you ever feel that you have special powers or a special mission or that there is something out of the ordinary about you?'

Grandiose delusions often have a religious theme and it may sometimes be difficult to distinguish a true delusion from a shared cultural belief. If you have any doubts it would be well worthwhile reading Section 1D (p. 23).

Sexual delusions

As with hypochondriacal delusions, delusions of infidelity (morbid jealousy) often occur on their own as a monosymptomatic delusional state. Some people are more jealous than others. Often at times of crisis in their life or during periods of low mood, they will become preoccupied by thoughts of their partner's infidelity or ruminate about it, or develop it as an overvalued idea (some men with potency problems or with other sexual difficulties will project them on to their partner). Sometimes ideas of jealousy will develop delusional strength. In patients with such delusions it does not matter whether the partner has actually strayed or not. Some partners faced with a barrage of questions about their fidelity, or with a partner who is constantly seeking clues to the imagined infidelity by searching the partners clothes and belongings, or spying on them, will sometimes seek peace from the constant strain by making a false confession (or even a real one) in the hope that this will bring peace. It does not. Such morbid jealousy (sometimes called the Othello syndrome) must be taken seriously and treated as an illness, and the partner may need to be temporarily (or sometimes permanently) separated from the sick partner for safety (remember what happened to Desdemona!).

The delusion is commoner in men, but can occur in women and may be symptomatic of a depressive illness or even occasionally occur in hypomania or schizophrenia. If it is occurring as part of a psychotic illness, it is usually much easier to treat than if it is a monosymptomatic delusion.

Erotomania usually, but not invariably, occurs in a woman. She develops the delusional belief that some person (who may not even know her) is in love with her and is giving off secret signals of this love. The woman's waking life becomes preoccupied with the imaginary lover and she constantly pesters and tries to communicate with the object of her desire. This can make his life extremely difficult, particularly if he is meant to be a pillar of respectability in the community, like a clergyman or a doctor. It is important to take this condition seriously, partly because love can often turn to hate, and partly because of the effect that it has both on the victim and also on the deluded. It is usually another form of a monosymptomatic delusion, but it can occur in affective illness or in schizophrenia. Unlike most delusional experiences, however, it may be resolved by confrontation.

Occasionally, patients have delusional sexual experiences, usually as part of schizophrenia. These are usually the patient's explanation of an underlying sexual feeling that may in itself be normal, like a wet dream, or the experience may have an hallucinatory element to it. Sexual delusions and hallucinations are also seen in organic states and in the elderly, as in the old lady who has a delusional belief that the devil enters her bedroom and has intercourse with her every night.

Delusions of jealousy will often be presented to you by the partner rather than by the person who has them, but it is useful to ask the patient screening questions about jealous feelings. Your sexual history will usually have already determined whether the patient has any strange or unusual sexual experiences.

Delusions specially related to schizophrenia

There are certain delusional and perceptual experiences that we recognize as being characteristic of schizophrenia. Since schizophrenia is one of the commoner psychiatric illnesses, and since its diagnosis carries such importance, it is very important to consider schizophrenia in the differential diagnosis of any patient who the examiner thinks may be psychotic or who has puzzling neurotic symptoms. In a clinical examination it is the one thing that a candidate is fearful of missing! As a result, if the interviewing doctor does encounter phenomena that suggest the patient may have schizophrenia, he sniffs the smoke of battle like an old warhorse and gallops off after the first rank symptoms of schizophrenia without ever wondering what is happening on the rest of the battlefield, and he may end up with a very incomplete view of his patient and fail to elicit other evidence of mental illness including affective disturbance. This is why we have put the elicitation of schizophrenic symptoms towards the end of this section on delusions rather than at the beginning. Another reason for having schizophrenia-related delusions at the end of this section is because it is often quite difficult to decide if the patient is describing a delusional experience or a hallucination.

Passivity ideas (delusions of control)

If the patient has already told you of some phenomenon that seems to be imposed on him, like an emotion or a thought, or he has a compulsion to act in a certain way, you should always enquire as to what he feels may be making him feel, think, or behave in this particular way. Often, delusions of control will have already become apparent and will just need to be fully elucidated. Some patients, however, recognizing that their experience is extremely alien and that they are likely to be thought mad if they express it, will be more reluctant to tell you about such experiences, and therefore you should always ask the screening question '*Do you feel that you are always in control of your own thoughts, actions, or feelings*?' Patients with delusions of control experience the belief either that some outside force is directly controlling their behaviour and making them move or behave in a certain way that they are powerless to resist, or that an outside force is making them feel a particular emotion, such as anger, or is directing thoughts into (or taking them from) their heads.

Clinical examples of this include the patient who feels that he is walking like a robot because a radio transmitter on the local police station is beaming movement controls into the back of his head, or the patient who feels that blasphemous thoughts are being inserted into his head by telepathy, or the patient who feels that external forces are putting anger into his head 'to put me in danger'. In all these examples of made acts, made thoughts, and made feelings, the patient has an unshakeable belief that it is happening. This should be contrasted with people who feel that sometimes their acts, thoughts, or feelings are not entirely their own, but this idea is culturally determined and is not held in a delusional way. A vague belief in fate having a hand in one's affairs, for instance, is not a delusion of control, and patients who have hallucinatory voices telling them to do things (which they may or may not resist) are also not suffering from delusions of control. Patients who feel that they are acting directly on the orders of God are not suffering from this particular delusion.

If you think that your patient may be having a true delusional experience, it is important to enquire about *acts*, *thoughts*, and *feelings* being controlled from outside.

In addition to thoughts being put into the patient's head, he may experience the delusion that thoughts have been withdrawn. Clinically you may notice the patient suddenly, often in mid-sentence, stopping, remaining silent for a short while, and then continuing on a different topic. When you enquire about what has happened he may tell you it was just as though his thoughts had *stopped* to be replaced by an absence of thought. The experience is not that his thought stream has suddenly changed direction, but that his thoughts have stopped and for a while his mind is empty. This is **thought blocking**, and is a *first rank* symptom of schizophrenia.

If the patient's thoughts stop, he may also experience the feeling that something has entered his mind to remove them, in other words an external agency has taken his thoughts away and either replaced them with a new thought or with blankness for a while so that eventually he has to start on a completely new train of thinking. This **thought withdrawal** is also a first rank symptom of schizophrenia, and is a passivity experience. The question '*Do you ever have trouble with your thinking*?' should therefore always be asked.

The patient will sometimes have the experience of his thoughts being repeated or echoed in his head. Make sure that this experience is that of the thought repeating itself (sometimes once and sometimes several times) and that this reduplication of thinking is felt as a *thought* and not as a voice. This is another first rank symptom of schizophrenia and is known as **thought echo** or **écho de la pensée**. Thought echo is rare and is not the same thing as hearing one's own thoughts out loud.

If the patient does have the experience of apparently hearing his thoughts spoken out loud *in his mind*, but does not have the conviction that other people can hear these thoughts being spoken out loud, then this is another first rank symptom and is more of a delusion than a hallucination. It is usually referred to by the German expression **gedankenlautwerden**. It is a private internal experience, and the patient knows that other people do not share the experience.

If the patient, however, believes that other people *can* hear his thoughts and that they are spoken out loud outside the patient's head (or through the medium of television, for instance) then this is the delusion of **thought broadcasting** and one could argue as to whether it is a delusion or an hallucination, although it is usually classified as a delusion. It is also another first rank symptom of schizophrenia. Patients who have the delusion of thought broadcasting, as opposed to the internal experience of hearing their thoughts, are much more likely to be distressed by it.

Delusional mood

Often as a precursor to the more entrenched delusional beliefs outlined above, some patients (usually transiently) develop an awareness that the world has changed or is different in some way without being exactly able to say how it has changed or is different. It is a strange, puzzling, and sometimes frightening experience that often presages a more full-blown psychotic experience, although it may exist in its own right. Just as nihilistic delusions can be seen in some ways as the psychotic end of derealization and depersonalization, so in a sense can delusional mood. Most patients who have it (it is not common) are also puzzled and perplexed. A suitable screening question would be '*Do things seem different to you? Have things changed in a way you cannot explain?*'

Delusional perception

This experience, another first rank symptom of schizophrenia, is also rare and often misunderstood by the examiner. In delusional perception the patient perceives something (usually visual) that in itself is normal and *then* develops from this perception a delusional idea that the perception has a particular and personal reference to him. It is important to make sure that the perception comes first and that the delusional misinterpretation takes place subsequently. Many patients who are already deluded will incorporate perceptions into their delusional systems. Thus a patient who observes a traffic light turning red and then develops the strong idea that this is a signal that he is changing sex, has a delusional perception. The patient whose paranoid ideas about communists taking over the world are reinforced by a traffic light changing to red does not have a delusional perception. It is important to make sure that the perception is a real one and is not in itself an hallucination. The patient who sees the Almighty descending in a golden chariot into his hospital ward and then forms the idea that he is the new Son of God is not having a delusional perception (since it is unlikely that the staff and other patients can also see the Almighty descending in his golden chariot).

The experience is usually sudden rather than gradual. Because the experience always has a special quality for the patient, a very suitable screening question is '*Have you ever had the experience that something had a special message or a special meaning for you*?', although you will need to distinguish this from a delusion of reference.

G Disorders of perception

- Always ask screening questions (Section 3J, p. 120) and cover *all* modalities of perception.
- Was it a *true* hallucination or a pseudohallucination?
- Was the patient falling asleep, waking up, or sleep deprived?
- Was it an illusion rather than a hallucination?
- Did it occur in clear consciousness or not? Was the patient confused?
- If it was brief and repetitive, were any other phenomena occurring with it?
- If a visual hallucination, how vivid was it? Did the patient believe it? Any other sensory change with it? Elementary or not?

- If a hallucination of smell, distinguish it from para-nosmia and delusion.

- If a hallucination of taste, distinguish it from a per-version of taste or delusion.

- If a hallucination of touch or other bodily sensa-tion, distinguish it from a pseudohallucination, parasthesia, or a delusion (particularly of control).

- If a hallucination of hearing, was it elementary or not? Distinguish it from a pseudohallucination or a delusion (ideas of reference). If voices, could they be recognized? What did they say? If addressing the patient, second or third person? Was there a run-ning commentary? Were the voices derogatory, ac-cusing, or pleasant?

In addition to abnormal beliefs, the patient may, in response to the screening question '*Has anything strange or unusual happened to you recently*?', reply indicat-ing that he has had some experience of altered percep-tion. He may, of course, have told you about it as part of his own presenting complaints, or it may already have emerged in the history taking, but it is important in every patient you see that you make a general en-quiry about altered perception. If you are at all suspi-cious that the patient has a psychotic or organic process, then in addition to the main screening question men-tioned above you should ask other questions relating to every modality of sensation. It is also important that if you discover a patient with abnormalities of per-ception in one modality, particularly if they are very prominent, that you make sure to check whether he has abnormalities of perception in the other modalities of perception. An example of this is that a substantial minority of people with schizophrenia have olfactory hallucinations and will declare them, but are seldom, if ever, asked about them.

As with abnormal beliefs, there are grey areas in assessing hallucinatory experiences and it is important, particularly if you are going to put a lot of diagnostic weight on the patient's hallucinations, that you are certain that he is having true hallucinatory experiences. Some people have the natural ability to summon vivid and realistic images into their minds, usually visual, but also auditory, olfactory, or tactile. These can be as vivid as reality (although the person knows they are not real and that they do come from his own mind). Although they are usually under voluntary control, they can also appear, apparently spontaneously, if the patient is troubled. They are presumably the explanation for the brief hallucinations of the recently bereaved, who see a realistic image of their loved one sitting at the dinner table or coming home from work, or hear very clearly the loved one's voice (the 'hallucinations of widowhood'). Such a hallucination may be so real that it is believed and is often a comforting experience. Likewise, the very troubled may have comforting hallucinations of, for example, a friendly spirit surrounded by glowing light, or may have unpleasant images of open graves or grinning corpses. Although these experiences are vivid, the patient can usually recognize that they come from within his own mind and are therefore **pseudohallucinations**.

True hallucinations do not have an 'as if' quality and are not perceived as coming from the patient's own imagination or mind, but are perceived as real external events into which the patient has no insight. They occur in psychotic states and may also occur in organic mental illness. In a true hallucination there is no basis for the hallucinated perception. In **illusions** there is a perception that is misinterpreted. For example, a patient might see a clock on the wall (the perception) but reports it as the grinning face of the devil (the illusion), or a patient in a hospital bed might hear the gentle hiss of the piped oxygen supply above his head but reports it as the sound of rain falling. Illusions can occur both in psychotic illness and in organic illness, but are probably commoner in the latter.

True hallucinatory experiences are usually abnormal, but can occur as a normal phenomenon in people on the point of falling asleep (hypnogogic hallucinations) or awakening (hypnopompic) and in those who are extremely sleep-deprived (as some of you who have recently completed house jobs will remember). They also occur in states of sensory deprivation. Hallucinatory experiences also occur in altered mental states related to mind-altering drugs and drug intoxication. It is important to always check if the hallucination occurred in clear consciousness or whether there was an element of confusion.

Elementary hallucinations are brief hallucinatory experiences in which the experience is confined to a fragment of perceptual experience (i.e., a flash of light, coloured spots or knocks, thuds, etc.). They often have an organic import.

Visual hallucinations

Patients who have visual hallucinations, particularly if they are prominent, should be thought of as having organic brain disease until it has been excluded. The experience has to be distinguished from vivid imagery, normal visual hallucinations (hypnogogic and hypnopompic hallucinations), and pseudohallucinations. It is rare, but not impossible, for a patient to have a visual hallucination that he can also hear, smell, or touch. Hamlet's vision of his dead father, which he could not only see but also hear speaking, was a pseudohallucination (assuming you do not believe in ghosts!) as speaking visions, particularly if they have some special message or special memory for the person receiving them, are unlikely to be organic or psychotic in nature and are much more likely to be a powerful pseudo-hallucination. Usually visions are silent.

In assessing the experience of patients who have visual hallucinations, it is important to determine if the patient was just falling asleep or just waking up when he had the experience, whether he was particularly excited or dejected when the experience occurred, and whether the experience seemed to occur in clear consciousness or whether there was evidence that the patient was confused at the time. If the experience was brief and repetitive, it is important to enquire whether anything recognizably epileptic was also happening during the episodes. Elementary visual hallucinations require a careful search for structural disease of the brain or of the visual tract.

Organic visual hallucinations are usually vivid and often frightening, and usually (but not invariably) occur during a period of agitation and confusion, as in delirium tremens, and will often distress the patient considerably. (A man, for instance, running up and down the ward stark naked with his finger stuck up his anus, thought that he was being pursued by red hot pokers that seemed to be aiming themselves at that particular part of his body.)

Most patients with visual hallucinations will either readily admit that they have them, or it will be obvious from their behaviour that they are having them, but you should always ask screening questions about visual experiences, such as '*Do you ever have the experience that you can see things that other people cannot? Do you ever have visions?*'

Hallucinations of smell

It is useful to ask a screening question for olfactory hallucinations as, though common, they are not usually volunteered by the patient. '*Have you been troubled by or noticed any unusual smell or smells lately?*' Pseudoolfactory hallucinations can also occur. Be careful to distinguish hallucinations of smell from paranosmias in which the patient perceives a real smell differently from the way most people experience it.

Smell has a strongly evocative effect on memory and so it should not be surprising that the reverse can happen, presumably the explanation of olfactory pseudo-hallucinations. True olfactory hallucinations can occur in schizophrenia (when they often have a bizarre quality and are accompanied by a delusional explanation), in depression (when they are usually unpleasant, as of rotting flesh), and in organic states involving the temporal lobe (classically the olfactory experience of a simple or complex partial seizure—often the smell experience has an alien bizarre quality to it or may be indescribable). Rarely they occur in hypomania or ecstasy states and then often have a pleasant or mystical quality, like the smell of incense. Patients can also have a *delusion* that they smell or give off an unpleasant odour. This is encountered particularly in depression or as a kind of dysmorphophobia and is not the same as a hallucination. Enquire of the presence of an olfactory aura in anyone with tonic clonic seizures as the patient may not have realized its importance and it can sometimes be used to trigger a behavioural treatment of the epilepsy.

Hallucinations of taste

Both hallucinations and pseudohallucinations of taste can occur. Perversions of taste (due to drugs, a dry mouth, etc.) are also common and should be distinguished from true hallucinations. Since taste is an individual sense not readily shared with others (we all see, smell, and hear the same external percept whatever sense we make of it), it can be very difficult to decide if the patient is having a true gustatory hallucination or if his sense of taste has merely changed.

Hallucinations of smell and taste can also be hard to distinguish from each other. People with bulimia sometimes experience a sweetish taste in the mouth before a binging episode, and an experience of a sweet or sour taste is not uncommon in severe anxiety or during overbreathing. You will need to distinguish those people who have a *delusion* that they are being poisoned or covertly medicated from those having true gustatory hallucinations. Such hallucinations occur in schizophrenia, depression, and organic states and are usually elicited by the screening question *'Have you been troubled by or noticed any peculiar taste in your mouth, or in your food or drink recently?'*

Hallucinations of touch and other bodily sensations

True hallucinations of touch (or other bodily sensations) can be elicited by the screening questions *'Have you had any unusual or strange feelings on or in your body? Have you ever felt that something was touching you when no one was there?'* Pseudohallucinations of touch related to emotional sensitivity to normal physiological skin responses ('goose flesh' and a sensation of the skin crawling) must be distinguished from tactile hallucinations, as must feelings of sudden chilling and warming. Delusions of bodily sensation as in delusions of passivity ('when the transmitter on Digbeth police station controls my muscles it makes a burning, buzzing feeling on the back of my neck') are not hallucinations of touch. Likewise, parasthesia are not an hallucination.

True hallucinations of touch are usually found in schizophrenia, occasionally in organic states, and classically in cocaine intoxication (when the feeling is of formication or ants crawling under the skin). Schizophrenic tactile hallucinations often have a bizarre quality to them. Hallucinations of sexual feeling also occur (distinguish them from misinterpreted normal feelings like spontaneous erections), as do hallucinations of other bodily sensations, like the kinaesthetic sense or internal alimentary feelings, although these are often more delusional.

Hallucinations of hearing

We have put these, the commonest hallucinatory experiences, last mainly to encourage you to look for those in other modalities first. The presence of auditory hallucinations will often have been declared by the patient, or guessed at from the patient's behaviour and then confirmed ('I think you are hearing something I can't'), or revealed by the general screening question 'Has anything strange or unusual happened to you?' If not, always ask the specific screening question 'Have you ever heard anything that you feel other people cannot hear?' If there is a negative response ask directly 'Do you ever hear voices?'

As with visual experiences, auditory pseudohallucinations are common as are hypnogogic and hypnopompic auditory hallucinations. Fatigue and sleep deprivation will also cause them (they are then usually fragmentary and elemental), and they are common in states of altered consciousness. Not all auditory hallucinatory experiences are of voices, but may comprise other noises or music. If voices are heard they may be loud or soft, clear or muttered, recognizable or unknown to the patient, and may be a singular voice or several voices. Sounds are usually heard external to the hearer, but may occasionally be heard coming directly from some part of the body (if so it is important to establish that they do not have an 'as if' quality).

Elemental hallucinations (for example, brief noises or a name being called) are usually of little importance but may reflect organic damage in the left temporal lobe, as may more formal hallucinations of snatches of music or song or even a repetitive vocal phrase. One such patient with a left posterior temporal epileptic discharge would hear and then say 'forty tons of fall out'. This phrase had her much puzzled until some years later it was pointed out to her that it was a line from one of the Liverpool poets and was probably an ictal re-awakening of an otherwise forgotten memory. If auditory hallucinations are brief and repetitive, enquire (as with visual experiences) if something else recognizably epileptic was going on at the same time.

Most auditory hallucinations are vocal. They are extremely common in schizophrenia (when they often have the special qualities outlined below), but also commonly occur in psychotic depression (when they are usually accusatory or derogatory), in hypomania (when they are usually expansive and warm), and in organic states and in alcoholism (not related to delirium). The possession of auditory hallucinations is therefore in itself not diagnostic. Having elicited the fact that the patient has such hallucinations, you will need to check if they have a special schizophrenic quality (and also make sure that they are not really a delusional experience that the patient is describing, as in delusions of reference).

If the voice or voices talk about the patient as *he* or *she* (i.e., refers to the patient *in the third person*) then this is taken to be a first rank symptom of schizophrenia. The experience is usually felt to be unpleasant, except when the voice or voices are saying pleasant things, but that is unusual. The voices may also make a **running commentary** on what the patient is doing—similar to the continued interior monologue that many great writers have (but not as true auditory hallucinations!). George Orwell described such a mechanism in 'Why I Write'. An auditory hallucination of a running commentary is a first rank symptom of schizophrenia.

Voices that address the patient in the second person

are not diagnostic of (but may occur in) schizophrenia, their content often then related to the delusional system that the patient has. They also occur in depression, hypomania, and organic states, their tone and content often giving a clue to the underlying mood disorder. If the patient admits to hearing voices, it is important to ask him if they talk about him, what they say, and how they address him (if they do). It is important to make sure that a running commentary is really describing what the patient is doing ('He gets up—he walks to the door—he goes out') and that the experience is not just a voice making general remarks about the patient ('He's too fat. He's wicked. He shouldn't do that').

H Physical assessment in psychiatry

- Full physical history and screening questions:

  Central nervous system:

  Headache—recent onset or change?
  Vision   —recent deterioration?
  Hearing   —recent deterioration?
  Speech   —any recent difficulty?
  Writing   —any recent difficulty?
  Memory   —recent deterioration?
  Gait   —recent deterioration?
  Dexterity —any recent clumsiness?
  Sensation—any recent change or parasthesia (particularly focal)?
  Strength   —any recent loss or change (particularly focal)?
  Any seizures, loss of consciousness, or abnormal movements?

  Respiratory and cardiovascular systems

  Recent breathlessness or decline in effort tolerance?
  Cough and/or sputum?
  Nocturnal dyspnoea (paroxysmal or not)?
  Orthopnoea?

Ankle swelling?
Chest pain on exertion?
Palpitations?

Abdominal system

Weight? Recent gain or loss?
Any change in bowel habit? Incontinence? Passage of mucus?
Any rectal bleeding or melaena?
Any vomiting?
Any abdominal pain?
Any indigestion/dyspepsia?
Any reflux/waterbrash?

Genito-urinary system

Menstrual history—any change? Is patient pregnant?
Intermenstrual bleeding?
Postmenopausal bleeding?
Postcoital bleeding?
Unusual discharge?
Any dysuria/frequency/retention or other difficulty passing water?
Any erectile change?
Any backache or urinary tract pain?

- Fully and carefully examine all new patients and repeat examination in any uncooperative patient when he is calmer.

- Never assume that a physical symptom is psychogenic no matter how obvious it may seem.

- In disturbed patients, always use a chaperone of the same sex as the patient whether you are male or female and no matter what sex your patient is.

A substantial minority of patients with emotional illness have a significant physical disability as well, which may well modify your diagnosis and complicate your plans for treatment. (A similar proportion of patients with physical disease have a significant emotional disability, but some physicians do not seem too concerned with this!) Physical illness may often present as apparent psychiatric illness (some cerebral tumours, myxoedema, thyrotoxicosis, Addison's disease, carcinomatosis, Huntington's chorea, etc.) and vice versa (depression, anorexia nervosa). There are also several physical contraindications to the treatments you may offer your patient. For all these reasons a thorough physical assessment is part of the mental state examination and should be performed on every new patient and repeated if there is a significant change in the patient's symptoms, no matter who has already examined the patient and pronounced them physically fit. Many patients are worried that their emotional symptoms are due to physical illness and find a thorough physical assessment reassuring.

Thorough physical assessment starts with a careful physical history going through the usual screening questions that are part of the routine physical examination. This is followed by a thorough physical examination, making a particularly careful examination of the skin for bruises, needle marks, etc.), which should be directed particularly at those areas in which screening questions have suggested a possible problem. The central nervous system should be very carefully examined.

Constant practice at performing physical assessments and examinations will prevent the psychiatrist from becoming rusty, and the task should never be relinquished to someone else. If your patient was admitted overnight, repeat the duty doctor's examination. If you stop examining your patients you will have stopped practising whole-person medicine. Very disturbed patients may resist examination or be uncooperative, and it is important to examine them properly when they are calmer. Always examine patients even when they seem to have an 'obvious' psychiatric explanation for their symptoms—you will make mistakes if you do not. A very religious elderly woman became mute when she discovered that her son had left his wife and young children for another woman. The muteness was selective in that she would talk to nurses but not to doctors. She was initially uncooperative and a sketchy physical examination revealed nothing amiss, but a more thorough examination performed later revealed a mild right-sided hemiparesis that was due to a left temporal glioma. Another patient, a girl of 21, was referred for psychotherapy for recurrent and intrusive guilt feelings. It was noted that when she had a guilt feeling she also wet herself. The cause of what were, in fact, simple partial seizures was a right temporal tumour that would not have responded too well to psychotherapy!

During the physical examination of a severely mentally disturbed patient, it is important to have a chaperone of the same sex as the patient—no matter what your sex is. The job of such a chaperone, apart from acting as a witness, is to help reassure and give explanations to the patient. The only exception to the rule of always examining your own patient is if you are engaged in psychotherapy with that patient at the time when the transference relationship may make the examination acquire an unwanted emotional significance, or if you are male and you are asked to examine a female victim of serious sexual abuse, when it would be better for a female colleague to do it.

I Physical investigation in psychiatry

- Routinely screen full blood count, film, indices, and ESR.
- Routinely screen electrolytes, calcium, urea, creatinine, protein, alkaline phosphatase, and other liver-function tests, gamma glutamyl transaminase, blood glucose, and cholesterol.
- Be *selective* about screening other parameters, such as thyroid function, B12, or serum folate levels.

- Serological screening for syphilis in high risk groups, and adopt local policy for HIV.

- Chest X-ray for weight loss, respiratory symptoms, neurological symptoms in alcoholics, and heavy smokers.

- Avoid routine skull X-rays.

- CT of brain and skull only if there are clinical indications.

- EEG (electroencephalogram) for investigation of epilepsy, the mute or apparently unconscious patient, sleep disorders, and undiagnosed attack disorders (sometimes). Visual evoked potentials may be indicated in investigating dementia.

- ECG (electrocardiogram) if symptoms suggest it.

- Consult with radiologist or neurophysiologist before ordering CT or EEG, and provide full information.

Routine (but careful) physical assessment and examination of all new patients is clearly necessary, but should all such patients undergo any further physical investigation? Although the pick-up rate will be low, most psychiatrists feel that routine haematological and biochemical profiles can be justified, particularly as they are cheap and may occasionally reveal treatable illnesses or possible causes of the patient's symptoms. With alcoholism being so prevalent, routine liver-function tests, gamma glutamyl transferase estimation, and red-cell indices are helpful, and in patients who may be about to take lithium the measurement of renal and thyroid function is mandatory.

The problem with routine screening is that it often throws up unexpected or aberrant results, which either lead to unnecessary anxiety or to fruitless further investigation. Normal results do not necessarily mean that there is nothing wrong with the patient and may provide false reassurance. Abnormal results may also have nothing to do with the patient's psychiatric state and may need skilled interpretation outwith the competence of the average psychiatrist. We suggest that, although a routine haematological and biochemical profile in *new* patients can be justified, other *routine* screening of such things as thyroid function, folic acid levels, etc. should not be done and such screening reserved for those patients in high risk groups (such as the elderly or the alcoholic), or for those whose physical assessment or investigation suggests possible abnormalities in this area. This should also apply to serological testing for syphilis, which should be reserved for those with a history of venereal disease, service in the war, or a high risk lifestyle or profession, and for patients with evidence of organic brain impairment or physical signs suggestive of cerebral syphilis. There will be local rules about HIV screening, which you should follow.

At one time routine chest X-rays were expected in psychiatry, particularly because tuberculosis was so common in crowded asylums. Nowadays this is not a recommended practice and chest X-rays should be reserved for those with respiratory or cardiovascular symptoms, weight loss, neurological symptoms, and to heavy smokers or drinkers. Routine skull X-rays are also not recommended because the pick-up rate of abnormalities is very low and the investigation may well provide false reassurance.

Cranial computed tomography (CT) facilities are patchy in the United Kingdom and the investigation is not easily available to most psychiatrists. Our experience suggests that the detection of *treatable* abnormalities in psychiatric patients is low with this investigation, and it should be reserved for those patients whose history or physical examination suggests possible intracranial abnormality. Ordering a CT investigation just because the patient has puzzling psychotic symptoms is unlikely to be productive, but if the patient has episodes of confusion mixed in with his psychosis then you are much more likely to detect a possible treatable lesion. The problem with CT is that it often turns up non-treatable abnormalities (like cerebral atrophy), the significance and meaning of which are uncertain. Some CT-demonstrated atrophy, as in anorexia nervosa or alcoholism, is also reversible. It is too early to suggest what the place of magnetic resonance imaging (MRI) should be in psychiatry.

A much abused investigation is the EEG. This is not a routine screening investigation and its false negative and false positive rate is high. It cannot be used to make psychiatric diagnoses and a normal EEG is no reassurance at all. It is useful in helping to localize epilepsy (but *not* in diagnosing it), in the differential diagnosis of patients who are mute, in detecting some early cases of encephalitis, it has a minor role in investigating dementia, and is an important tool in investigating sleep disorders. Visual evoked responses in the EEG (to flash and pattern stimuli) may turn out to be a useful investigation in helping to distinguish between depression and dementia. Ambulatory EEG investigation (up to 16 channels) is useful in the investigation of attack disorders providing that they are occurring often enough for them to occur whilst the patient is being monitored, a good description of the event can also be recorded and skilled interpretation of the record is available. A sleep-deprived EEG is also useful in diagnosing attack disorders. In some patients monitoring respiration and blood oxygen tension during sleep is helpful, particularly in chronic fatigue states if sleep apnoea is suspected. Discussion with the neurophysiologist in charge of the EEG department is vital to get the best results from EEG investigation (as is the case with neuroradiology). An ECG will sometimes be needed, as might ambulatory ECG monitoring, but this is not a routine investigation.

We would emphasize that the best screening test of all is a careful and considered physical history and examination, which takes time and patience but is worth doing well. There are no routine psychological tests. The use of psychological testing (and its abuses) and the role of the clinical psychologist will be considered in Sections 4F (p. 173) and 5B (p. 387).

There is one other important point about physical investigation. Do it well, do it thoroughly, and then leave it alone if you can. Doubts and uncertainties about the patient, his progress, and his diagnosis should not lead you to repeat physical tests in the vain hope that something organic might turn up one day—it very rarely does and your heroic investigatory efforts may leave you with a puzzled, exhausted, and uncertain patient.

J Questions that should always be asked

We are providing a list of screening questions in the mental state examination (all referred to elsewhere in the relevant sections) that should always be asked after the relevant history of the presenting complaint, family and personal history, personality assessment, and enquiry into previous psychiatric and mental history, if you have picked up hints of possible organic or psychotic illness.

- Has anything strange or unusual happened to you, or have things happened that you have found it difficult to explain?*

- Any problems with your memory or with finding your way or getting change in a shop? (Can you read and write?)*

- How are your spirits? (How have you been feeling lately?)*

- Have you had any particularly strong thoughts or feelings that you think a lot about—about yourself or about the world we live in?*
- Have you felt bad enough to think of killing yourself?*
- Do you feel got at or persecuted in some way?*
- Is someone trying to harm you?
- Do you feel that people are talking about you or that things refer to you? Does the television or radio have special messages or meanings for you?
- Do you feel that you are being punished in some way? Are there things you feel particularly bad about or anything you feel ashamed of?
- Do you think you might be physically ill?*
- Do you feel that you have special powers or have a special mission?
- Is there someting out of the ordinary about you?
- Has there been any difficulty with your thinking recently?*
- Do you feel that you are always in control of your thoughts, actions, and feelings?
- Do things seem different to you—have they changed in a way that you cannot explain?*
- Has anything that has happened had a special meaning or message for you?*
- Have you seen things that you think others cannot see? Have you had any visions?*
- Have you been troubled by or noticed any unusual smells?*
- Have you been troubled by or noticed any peculiar or different tastes in your mouth or food?
- Have you had any strange or unusual feelings in your body? Have you ever felt something was touching you when there was nothing there?

- Have you ever heard anything that you feel other people cannot hear? Do you hear voices?*

  * Every patient should be asked these questions, even if there is no hint of organic or psychotic illness.

CHAPTER 4

Presenting problems

A Psychiatric emergencies—general points

- Whose emergency is it anyway?
- You are often treating other people's anxiety.
- Make sure that you can be found when on duty.
- Respond swiftly and politely to calls for help.
- Give practical advice if you cannot attend at once.
- *Plan* your response—cognitive rehearsal before attending is helpful.
- Remember your role as a psychiatrist—you are not a policeman.
- Ask yourself, what are the best interests of the *patient*?
- Act calm and you will feel calm: look calm and you will calm others.
- Approach the patient 'matter of fact' and do not take sides.
- Obtain as much information as you can.
- Make an accurate record of what took place (including negative information).
- Have a debriefing after the emergency is over.
- Formally 'hand over' the patient to those who are normally responsible for his care.
- If staff are overreacting there may be a hidden agenda.
- Know where you can turn for help and advice, and use it freely at first.

- Above all, do not be stampeded into losing your psychiatric skills and objectivity, and don't be a telephone psychiatrist.

There are probably few absolute emergencies in psychiatry. Most exist in the mind of the person who has called you, or in the patient's mind, and indicate a loss of tolerance of the patient's behaviour or feelings (but are real enough for all that). You are often responding to the anxiety of relatives or attendants rather than to the patient's need, but this anxiety may be making the patient's own behaviour worse, and managing their anxiety is then the best thing that you can do for him.

It is therefore quite appropriate to ask yourself *'Whose emergency is it anyway?'* when summoned to help, but make sure, even if your response is not that which was expected of you, that you do respond *swiftly and politely* to an emergency call. Psychiatrists can all too easily acquire the reputation of being too laid back in the way that they respond to calls for help from general practitioners, casualty staff, or ward staff. When on duty, make sure that you can be contacted easily and even if, for good reasons, you cannot attend the patient straight away you are able to give some practical advice at once. For example, 'I'll be with you in one hour, but meanwhile try your best to contact a relative and ask the duty social worker to meet me. If you can't contain the patient's aggression you are entitled to ask the police to help'.

Try to *plan* your response to an emergency. *Rehearse* in your mind the possible causes of the behaviour you are about to meet and think about the information you will need and your best approach to the patient to try to reach both a diagnosis and a plan of management. Learning to think on your feet will come with experience, particularly if you think over experiences after you have had them.

It is important to remember that your role in an emergency is to act as a psychiatrist and not a removal man, a policeman, or even Rambo. Avoid heroics. Your job is to diagnose psychiatric illness and to suggest a remedy and a prognosis (the remedy *might* include compulsory detention). Dealing with antisocial behaviour, drunkenness, and hooliganism is not part of your remit, but recognizing altered mental states, delirium, psychosis, or severe distress is. Your job is to make decisions in the best interest of the patient and not necessarily to make life comfortable for everyone else. Often the best interests of the patient and, say, his relatives will coincide, but this is not always so. If you cannot agree with the demands of angry or distressed relatives at least listen to them and try to defuse the situation.

In a crisis people often have unrealistic expectations of the psychiatrist. Once frightened they tend to lose both their common sense and the skills they are endowed with, and they tend to wait, passive and inactive, for the miracle worker to arrive. Attempts at communication with the troublesome patient are often suspended so that when you arrive very little is known about him. You are expected, with no information, to instantly calm the patient either using the force of your personality or some magic knockout drop known only to psychiatrists. Unfortunately, it does not always work that way.

It is important that you know as much about the patient as you can before reaching a decision because responding purely to his mental state can lead to mistakes. The better you know the patient the better will be your decisions about diagnosis, management, and disposal. It is worth spending considerable time and trouble finding an informant or relative to talk with either before, during, or after the emergency, although the ward or casualty staff will be unlikely to think that this is important unless you tell them, and they will be pressing you to do something. Your need for information before you see the patient will often seem like a delaying tactic to uninitiated nurses, and you may have to tactfully explain that just as a surgeon, even in an emergency, will not open up a belly until he has a reasonable idea of what he is going to find inside, so you cannot decide what to do for the patient until you have a better picture of what is going on.

Your immediate task is to keep calm, and to calm others, and then to use your skills of listening, observing, and not being provocative, judgemental, or threatening. How do you keep calm? Until emergency situations stop terrifying you (probably the week you retire!) *act calm and you will feel calm, look calm and you will calm others.* Approach the patient in a matter-of-fact way and do not have a panicky crowd of nurses or relatives with you when you first see the patient (as he will pick up their fear), and do not appear to be taking sides. 'John, I'm Dr X and I understand that your parents are very worried because you have shut yourself in your bedroom and won't eat. I've asked them to wait downstairs whilst I talk with you. I'd like to hear your side of it and try to help sort things out. Is there anything troubling you or anything I should know about? I see, that must be very frightening. Have you any idea why the Martians should be looking for you in particular?'

In an emergency it is very necessary to keep your psychiatric head and to take an adequate history, perform a mental state examination as thoroughly as circumstances will allow (plus a physical examination if it is possible and appropriate), and not to act precipitately unless the circumstances really demand it. When you do decide it is time to act then do so decisively and swiftly.

Make sure that you make an accurate record of the

patient's behaviour and of what he said. The patient may recover quickly, either because of the natural history of the condition or because of your treatment. The making of an accurate diagnosis (and therefore prognosis) may well depend on your written record as no one else may have seen the patient disturbed. Your record should include not only positive information but also negative points—what the patient did *not* say or do may be equally important, and a declaration of the absence of certain delusions or perceptual disorders, although enquired for, may be important for making a diagnosis. If you omit to say, for instance, that you enquired about hypochondriacal delusions but none were elicited, the person reading your account will not know if you had just forgotten to ask about them or record them, or whether the patient really did not have them, and his view of the patient will be incomplete and blurred.

Also record your interviews with other people and note how they may be contacted again (for example, the name, rank, and station of any police officer, or the name, district office, and contact phone number of any social worker).

Many emergencies leave a nasty atmosphere behind them. Make sure that you talk through the experience afterwards with those involved (for example, an attempted or actual suicide on a ward). It is natural for staff to feel angry, afraid, and upset after such an incident and they will often feel abandoned and may become victims of scapegoating. Senior nursing and administrative staff in particular may look for someone to blame after such an incident, often to cover up their own inefficiency or lack of resources. It is useful to have an informal 'post-mortem' about the event to learn from it and to plan a better response to the next incident (for example, a disturbance in casualty). Emergencies can be a stimulus to learning, and it might be useful to keep a journal of such events and to have regular meetings to discuss them and how they were handled. Sadly, their educational potential is often wasted. Make sure that you formally hand over the patient to those normally responsible for his care if you have been acting in an emergency capacity (for example, over a weekend).

As a junior doctor, never go on emergency duty or on-call without knowing who is covering you and where you can contact him or her. At the start of a new job you might be unaware of local conditions and rules of procedure, methods, and routes of disposal or community supports, and will need advice. Contact freely the senior psychiatrist covering you, and if you find that you consistently cannot get this support when you need it consider taking a job elsewhere!

One local rule that often causes problems is the existence of a hospital blacklist. If patient X is on a hospital's blacklist, that hospital might not be prepared to readmit him under any circumstances. Such rules are silly. Each request for admission, each crisis in the patient's life, needs to be assessed on its own merits, although the patient's known previous behaviour will need to be taken into account in making a decision about disposal. If a hospital has a policy about not admitting a particular patient, then it must also have a policy about what to do with him when he presents elsewhere and must be prepared to offer community support or to have some agreed alternative means of disposal and not to leave you 'holding the baby'. Do not let the hospital unilaterally abrogate its responsibilites.

Another problem is the well-known patient, presenting as an emergency, who staff will tell you is an 'attention seeker' or time waster. Make up your own mind. People have died of alleged attention seeking! Be wary of staff 'gossip' about well-known patients as such opinions are not always well formulated and there may well be a 'hidden agenda' (see below). If you do not know the patient very well it is best to give him the benefit of the doubt, and if you do know him ask yourself whether or not circumstances have changed or whether the patient may be different this time. Knee-jerk responses have no place in psychiatry, particularly knee-jerk rejections.

There will be times when you will think that the reaction of relatives or nursing staff is out of proportion to the actual degree of disturbance that the patient is showing (for example, the general hospital ward sister who seems terrified of the possibility that a patient might harm himself and is demanding instant removal of the patient who, post-overdose, is still confused and not assessable). In these circumstances there is often some hidden agenda that you are unaware of (such as the crusty old physician, faced with a serious bed shortage, who is demanding that sister 'gets rid of that nutter blocking my bed', or an incident such as a patient recently jumping from the ward's day room to his death making everyone involved feel guilty). Gentle confrontation of what seem to be unreasonable attitudes in staff and relatives may be helpful.

Do remember, however, that doctors have only brief and intermittent contact with patients, and can come and go off the ward. You are not the ward sister who has to cope with difficult behaviour day in and day out, resulting in her reaching the end of her tether because she has three staff off sick and has 'had it up to here' with a crazy, manipulative girl who has taken three overdoses this month—'Why don't you doctors do something?' You may not be able to do something about the girl, but you will be able to help sister abreact and be able to support her.

Your role in an emergency is rather like that of a junior officer of a platoon of young soldiers in a fire fight. *Keep your eye on your objective*, keep your men's morale high by not showing the fear that you feel, concentrate on practising the skills you have learnt, and *lead from the front*. Nelson's adage 'No captain can do much wrong if he lays his ship alongside that of the enemy,' also applies to emergency psychiatry. Psychiatry is actually a very practical discipline. Emergencies are not solved by elegant theories or elaborate tactics, but by getting stuck in, talking and communicating. Do not be a telephone psychiatrist—go and see the patient. Talking to him will solve most problems.

B Patients who are excited

- Try to understand what is causing (or lying behind) the excitement.
- Previous history (developmental, social, and psychiatric) is important.
- Assess mood, hallucinatory experiences, and look for organic impairment.
- Is there evidence of drug abuse?
- Is there risk of violence or self-harm?
- Is the excitement related to the patient's culture or life circumstances?

Differential diagnosis

1. organic mental states
2. psychotic illness
3. affective disorder
4. intoxications
5. acute situational reactions
6. 'neurotic' illness
7. personality disorder.

Management

- Is the excitement self-limiting?
- Can you talk the patient down?
- Will he accept treatment?
- Does he need restraining?
- Use oral medication if you can (liquid), but intravenous medication if not. Use haloperidol or droperidol for rapid calming, chlorpromazine (oral only) for immediate sedation (watch side-effects in the elderly or ill), and thioridazine (oral only) for agitation. Specific therapy (for example antibiotics, fluid replacement, antidepressants) might also be needed.
- Once the patient is calm, help him remain calm with continued medication.
- Talk over the experience with the patient, relatives, and nurses.

Setting the scene

Grossly excited patients will often present as an emergency, although lesser degrees of excitement are more tolerable and for a short while may even be charming (they may be difficult to distinguish from normality and may also be contagious).

Excitement implies a constant pressure or drive towards overactivity both in thought and in action, and may imply an emotional lability between tears and laughter, although many excited people have a consistently elevated mood. There is often irritability (with explosions of anger if the person is crossed or frustrated) and there may well be a paranoid element to the excitement. Seriously excited patients often have little insight into their behaviour. They are usually sleepless, eat little, and often lose weight dramatically. If a state of high excitement is maintained for any length of time, exhaustion occurs (with the attendant risk of intercurrent infection and even cardiac failure or death). Lack of insight will often lead the excited to performing rash acts that would not normally be contemplated (like spending too much money or taking part in unwise sexual adventures).

The excited can be intensely irritating to others if contact with them is maintained for long (in short doses the excited can be invigorating, stimulating, and, because of the infectivity of affect, may temporarily excite others and lead them to perform similar rash acts or adventures). Because they cause irritability, or are irritable themselves, the excited are often assaultive or may themselves be victims of assault. For this and other reasons excited patients need to be carefully managed, and once you have elicited the cause of their excitement they need to be brought back to a normal mood as quickly as possible and may need to be detained for their own sakes, as well as for the sake of others.

Few patients will complain of being excited particularly if, in addition to excitement, there is elevation of mood or feelings of ecstasy. Such patients will often resist treatment because they have never felt so well in their lives, and it may be difficult to persuade inexperienced social workers or relatives that the patient is ill and needs treatment until he has done something extremely foolish. Usually patients with excitement will present to you after such an act or when people have grown weary of them. Patients with recurrent hypomania, however, may eventually gain insight into the hypomania and will often present early for treatment saying that they fear they are having another mood swing.

When you are presented with a patient in a state of excitement, and this is the primary management problem, there is a wide differential diagnosis to consider and, although it may be difficult because of lack of cooperation on the patient's part, you will need to look at all the factors of the patient's mental state very carefully.

Assessing excitement

It is all too easy to react to and to try to control the excitement without understanding the underlying cause. This often happens because of the 'do something doctor' pressure that you will be under. But careful assessment of the patient will pay dividends in terms of his future management and prevention of future episodes of potentially embarrassing and disruptive behaviour.

The previous family history, developmental history, and personal history may all be helpful in reaching a diagnosis. A family history of manic depressive illness, previous antisocial behaviour, or a previous forensic history may aid in formulating the cause and prognosis of the patient's illness. A history of sustained, but untreated, mood swings or of previous drug abuse or experimentation may point to the cause of the present symptoms.

You will also need to assess the mental state of the patient as well as you can. Enquire for and examine any hallucinatory or delusional experiences the patient has as they may point to the diagnosis (but remember that first rank symptoms of schizophrenia cease to be first rank if there is evidence of organic impairment or if there is a mood disorder present—the only patient we have ever seen who possessed all the first rank symptoms of schizophrenia at once was manic). A careful assessment of mood is therefore needed. The patient who is restlessly pacing, singing hymns, and shouting 'make way for Mr Wonderful' probably has an elevated mood, whereas the patient who is restlessly pacing, wringing his hands, and saying 'what have I done, I'm evil' is probably depressed.

You must also try to do some organic mental state testing. This may be extremely difficult particularly in manic patients. For example, 'Why are you asking *me* these silly questions you *stupid little bugger*, don't you know what day it is? Well I do, but I'm not telling you!' You may end up unclear whether the patient is organically intact (but will not cooperate) or whether his non-cooperation is due to organic impairment. Physical examination (both general medical and neurological) is important, but again there may be such little cooperation that it is impossible and you may have to repeat it when the patient is calmer (as is the case with physical investigations like a chest X-ray or an EEG). Try to determine whether the more obvious (and treatable) physical causes for excitement are present, and also look for evidence of drug abuse or ingestion and take a blood and urine sample if you suspect it (i.e., gross sudden excitement in a young person with no other obvious cause).

Excitement is both irritating and contagious and so your assessment may be hampered by either of the these factors being present in those surrounding the patient (for example, outside the room there might be a very excited young lady, dressed in a sheet and tinsel, pacing up and down singing hymns *con brio* and somewhat hoarsely, while inside the room her elderly parents with beatific smiles are saying to the psychiatrist 'We want our daughter treated with the proper respect, doctor. You see, she is pregnant with the infant Jesus').

It is also important to bear in mind that the excited may be seriously aggressive or suicidal and both these risks need careful assessment (see Section 4H (p. 215) and Section 4J (p. 288)). Particularly careful assessment needs to be made in those who are excited and who come from a different culture as they may be erroneously labelled as having a mental illness when in fact they are merely reacting in a way that you do not understand to circumstances that you do not comprehend.

Advice from someone of the same culture may be invaluable.

Differential diagnosis

Organic mental states

1. delirium (acute brain syndrome)

2. dementia (chronic brain syndrome).

Organic mental illness has many different ways of presenting, but excitement, particularly in delirium, must be one of the commonest. Because the interviewer is reacting to the excitement and the perceptual disorders that often occur in delirium, it may be difficult to recognize the sometimes quite subtle accompanying changes in mental state that indicate that the patient has an organic impairment. This is particularly true in patients whose excitement has led to exhaustion. Delirium tremens, for instance, may present as a wildly excited patient pursued by perceptual experiences who often presents a serious management problem. It is difficult to keep the patient still long enough to find out whether he is orientated and whether he still has a retentive memory. The differential diagnosis of delirium is dealt with on p. 180, but all forms of delirium may present as excitement. Remember also that acute medical conditions can give rise to excitement and are particularly likely to be encountered postoperatively, on medical wards, or in casualty. These include:

1. *acute* (or acute on chronic) anoxia due to respiratory disease, CO_2 retention, myocardial infarction, etc.

2. infections—lobar pneumonia, typhoid, etc. (subphrenic abscess postoperatively)

3. acute brain insult (for example, cortical stroke, brain abscess, encephalitis)

4. delirium tremens
5. hypoglycaemia
6. *acute* renal failure
7. *acute* liver failure (portal encephalopathy)
8. unwise sedation of people in pain
9. postictal states, non-convulsive status epilepticus
10. 'myxoedema madness'.

Episodes of delirium may also occur in those who are dementing, and some patients who are dementing also show paradoxical excitement, particularly at night, when they react to the delusional or perceptual experiences that sometimes accompany dementia or react to their awareness of their failing powers by becoming excited. *Catastrophic reactions* (gross overreaction to simple changes in the patient's environment) will often present as states of excitement and once again it may be difficult, unless you look for them, to recognize the underlying intellectual problems.

Psychotic illness

1. schizophrenia (including catatonic excitement)
2. schizophrenia with an affective component
3. brief reactive psychosis
4. paranoid psychosis.

Schizophrenia can present as a state of excitement, often accompanied by florid delusions and hallucinatory experiences. Excitement may be related to the internal distress that a patient feels about his schizophrenic experiences and present as agitation, or may occur because the patient is acting out or acting upon hallucinatory or delusional experiences. Only a careful analysis of the nature of the hallucinatory or delusional experiences will distinguish such states of psychotic excitement from affective or organic disturbance. A particular form of excitement in schizophrenia is seen in **catatonic excitement** (which nowadays is very rare). This usually, but not invariably, follows a period of catatonic stupor. It is a state of wild excitement that starts extremely suddenly and usually terminates spontaneously. Serious aggressive behaviour may occur during such an episode.

Some people with a paranoid psychosis may also be agitated and excited, particularly by the content of their delusions or hallucinations. Patients exposed to extreme emotional stress may break down into a short psychotic episode, often with schizophrenic or affective symptoms, that resolves spontaneously and which may present as excitement. Some people with schizophrenia have a strong affective component to their illness and here again the presentation may be one of excitement.

Affective disorders

1. mania/hypomania
2. agitated depression.

Hypomania (and the rare mania) are, as might be expected, amongst the chief causes of states of excitement. Hypomania is easy to recognize when it presents classically as an excited patient with grandiose ideas, a warm affect, infectious enthusiasm, punning speech, flight of ideas, inexhaustible energy, and irritability if crossed. Even this classical presentation may sometimes be difficult to spot if it has been preceded by a significant life event (because *reactive* hypomania certainly exists), and minor degrees of hypomania (which in retrospect you realize the patient had) can be very difficult to recognize and distinguish from just ordinary high spirits unless you have had previous acquaintance with the patient. You therefore need to maintain a high index of suspicion.

Hypomania does not always present in the classical

way and some patients with hypomania, although they appear excited and inwardly driven by intense energy, may be paranoid and aggressive rather than elated. You may also be confused if their delusional and perceptual disorders are very prominent and you may not recognize the affective nature of their delusions or of their hallucinations and therefore misclassify them as schizophrenic (see Sections 4C (p. 143) and 4D (p. 153)). Many young patients who are given an initial diagnosis of recurrent schizophrenia eventually turn out to be having recurrent affective episodes. This is one of the commonest diagnostic mistakes to be made in psychiatry.

Agitated depression can also present as a state of excitement with restless pacing, projects abandoned half completed, and intense agitation. Many depressed or agitated patients also try to put on a kind of forced cheerfulness and it may be difficult to see behind this hollow mask to assess what the patient is really feeling, although careful assessment of the mental state will tell you.

Intoxication

Intoxication may be a primary cause of the excitement (in which case it usually settles quickly, but not always) or may be superimposed on top of another primary cause (as in the manic patient who is also drunk). Acute, uncontained excitement after an intoxicant is also more likely to occur in those whose previous character predisposes them to it, or in the brain damaged or the physically ill. Drugs acquired on the street are likely to be contaminated so that apparently unexpected reactions can occur.

Common intoxicants

1. alcohol
2. cannabis
3. amphetamine and other 'speed'-like drugs

4. cocaine and its derivatives like 'crack'
5. PCP (fortunately rare in the UK)
6. paradoxical reactions to prescribed drugs (tricyclic antidepressants, benzodiazepines, antiparkinsonian drugs)
7. solvents.

It is important to always think of intoxication, but it is also important to remember that it may not be the sole cause of the patient's symptoms, as in the head-injured drunk. Many mentally ill people also drink, so that merely detecting the smell of beer or spirits on the breath does not mean that the patient is only drunk.

Although cannabis usually produces a wakeful tranquillity, paradoxical reactions can occur. Wild excitement, in the young in particular, may result from ingestion (sometimes unknowingly) of 'speed' or PCP, rare so far in the UK. Characteristically, there is often markedly increased salivation. Sudden excitement in the elderly is often due to an unexpected reaction to a prescribed drug.

Acute situational reaction

People responding to acute environmental or interpersonal stress may become excited, but the excitement will be more understandable than in psychotic illness and in keeping with the situation the patient is facing and will not have any psychotic features to it. Such reactions are probably more common than we realize and are very much part of the differential diagnosis of excitement states, particularly in certain cultures like the Afro-Caribbean one.

'Neurotic' illness

Panic and extreme anxiety can present as excitement. In the severely anxious there may be such a pressure of speech and activity and such little attention paid to the examiner and his questions, that an erroneous impression of hypomania or delirium may be given. Dissociated states of excitement may also occur in hysteria (for example, ecstasy states) and may be mistaken for a psychosis.

Personality disorder

People who are personality disordered may be prone to sudden excitement or transient changes in mood. They are also more likely to suffer acute situational reactions and take intoxicants. The personality disordered may also suffer from psychotic illness or organic mental illness, their personality problems colouring the presentation of the disorder. This is why a multiaxial classification system is so useful (see p. 3).

Management

The principles of management are those of taking as careful a history as you can in the circumstances, and looking particularly at the patient's previous personality and psychiatric (and medical) history. Mental state examination should concentrate on detecting the patient's prevailing mood (searching particularly for masked depression) and the presence of hallucinatory experiences in all modalities, and assessment of any organic impairment and delusional experiences and the degree of risk of violence. Physical examination and investigation should initially, if possible, concentrate on those illnesses outlined above. You should be able to reach a working diagnosis.

Having done so, you will need to try to decide if the condition is self-limiting and will resolve on its own (in which case masterly inactivity and containment is best), or whether, in the interests of the patient's health and safety, you will need to intervene to control the excitement, either as the start of treating the underlying illness (as in mania) or to investigate it further.

Many excited patients can be talked down, at least temporarily, or can be *distracted* and their energy diverted into more productive channels. For example, psychiatrist to a manic student who is imperiously demanding that the entire ward comes on a ten mile run with him, 'OK, but we are not quite ready yet and so how about playing ludo with Nurse Jones for the moment.' 'Right you are, doc.' In this way the young man is kept occupied without overstretching ward resources, until his medication has time to work.

A few patients cannot be talked down or are completely out of control and they will need restraining in the interests of their health and safety (see Section 4J, p. 288 for advice on this). Patients need not be detained under the Mental Health Act to be restrained—you have a common law duty to prevent them or others from coming to harm. If they are not formally detained you will need to make a careful note of the patient's mental state and your reasons for restraint.

Talking down is accomplished by approaching the patient in an open, friendly manner, attempting to confront him with his behaviour and excitement and trying to get him to appreciate the effect he is having on others (remember that he may have a short-term memory deficit so that this may need to be repeated numerous times). Offer to talk through the problems that may underly the behaviour, but do not make promises you cannot keep.

Try to help the patient to see that he is ill (even manic patients will often appreciate this) and in need of help and treatment, and institute it quickly if he agrees. If he does not agree then you have to decide whether to overpower him, apply restraint, and treat him against his will. There will be times when this is the only thing that you can do, but unless there is extreme urgency, discuss it with your consultant first. See p. 301 for advice on restraint.

Physical treatment will be mostly symptomatic (as with the use of haloperidol for mania), or occasionally specific (as with penicillin for treating the delerium of lobar pneumonia). For most excited patients you will be applying chemical restraint until the underlying condition has resolved. Many patients will accept oral medication, given initially in liquid form (for example, haloperidol liquid or chlorpromazine syrup). Absorption of liquid is more rapid and it is easier to assess whether the patient has taken it. Very occasionally you may need to conceal haloperidol liquid in the patient's orange juice, but this subterfuge can only be justified if the only other way of calming the patient is to overpower him, and you must discuss its use with your consultant.

For the delirious patient, droperidol or haloperidol is best and can be given intravenously if needed (see Section 4J, p. 288). Try to avoid intramuscular injections if at all possible as this route can lead to erratic and slow absorption of the drug and an irritated patient. Chlorpromazine is often used, but may cause disabling hypotension in the ill or elderly. It is useful as a 'one-off' sedative in the excited patient who is exhausted and who needs to sleep. Its liquid form is particularly useful for this. Thioridazine orally is useful for agitation. Avoid oral benzodiazepines in the excited, except in delirium tremens. Diazepam intravenously can be useful in an emergency but can sometimes disinhibit the patient further. If using a benzodiazepine such as chlordiazepoxide for delirium tremens, start with a high dose (say 25 mg three times a day) and taper off over seven to ten days.

Future management

Whether you have used chemical restraint or been able to talk the patient down, once he is calmer you will need to make a formal diagnosis and plan of investigation and management. If medication has been needed to calm the patient make sure it continues for a while so that the patient remains calm. If controlling the patient has been particularly difficult and physical force has had to be used, make sure you talk over the need for it with the patient when he is calmer, and talk through the experience with the relatives and the nursing staff, who may well be feeling shocked and guilty.

C The patient who is hallucinating

Also read Section 1B, p. 12 and Section 3G, p. 104.

- Not all hallucinations are abnormal.

- Keep the patient in contact with reality, and do not agree with the experience, although indicate it is real to the patient.

- If the patient is experiencing hallucinations in one modality, check for similar experiences in other modalities.

- Distinguish carefully between perceptual disturbances, illusions, pseudohallucinations, and true hallucinations. Do not mistake delusions for hallucinations (for example, thought broadcasting).

- Careful mental state examination is mandatory, particularly assessing mood, accompanying delusional experiences, and for signs of organic illness.

- Previous life experiences and previous psychiatric disorders may help you to understand the patient's particular hallucinatory experience.

- Visual hallucinations are organic until proved otherwise, as are elemental hallucinations.

- Auditory hallucinations are likely to be related to psychotic illness.

Differential diagnosis

1. organic mental states
2. psychotic illness
3. affective illness
4. intoxication
5. situational reactions
6. neurotic illness-pseudohallucinations
7. personality disorder-pseudohallucinations.

Management

- Manage the underlying disorder.
- Overwhelming or very disturbing hallucinations may need treatment with intravenous medication such as haloperidol.
- Occasionally the patient may need restraining if he is acting on the hallucinations.

Setting the scene

In the lay mind, hallucinations of all kinds are associated with madness. This means that patients who are overtly hallucinated tend to be reported to psychiatric care early (particularly if hallucinations are prominent or the patient is acting upon them), but it also means that many people who suffer hallucinatory experiences, and who retain some insight, will be reluctant to declare them. It may only be when you have the obtained the patient's confidence and trust that you will learn of his perceptual experiences.

Different cultures also have different explanations for hallucinations and may not always agree that the patient's experience is a sign of illness. A patient of ours, for instance, who had temporal lobe epilepsy giving rise to visual hallucinations of the devil, achieved much power and notoriety within her religious community as a result and it took a long time for both her and her companions to accept that she was ill and needed treatment. Psychotic hallucinatory experiences may also, at times, become politicized. A good example of this occurred with Joan of Arc whose hallucinatory experiences were convenient for the French in their struggle against the English but once they had ceased to be useful she was abandoned to her fate.

People who are hallucinating may retain some insight into the unreality of the experience, or may believe it implicitly, although (as stated in Section 1B, p. 12) almost anyone who is having a psychotic experience will retain some island of sanity within him that you can still communicate with. Hallucinations may be the most prominent part of the patient's presenting mental state, or may be clearly occurring as part of some other process (as in patients who are manic or grossly thought disordered).

Not all hallucinatory experiences are abnormal (although, even if they are not, the patient may think that they are). Hypnogogic and hynopompic hallucinations are normal (although may be disturbing for the patient), as are the 'hallucinations of widowhood', even when they are occurring in the middle of a severe grief reaction. It is important not to regard these normal phenomena as indicative of a severe depressive illness.

Your job, as a psychiatrist, is to respond to those hallucinatory experiences that are presented to you, and to diligently seek out those that are not. As was indicated in Section 1B (p. 12), it is important not to agree with the patient's hallucinatory experiences. Acknowledge them and in particular acknowledge their reality for the patient, but also indicate that they are false and, when appropriate, that they are a sign of illness. Your job is to keep the patient in contact with reality. The behaviour of a casualty officer who was recently seen peering at the skin of an agitated patient with a hand lens attempting to identify the green, black, and purple insects that were allegedly crawling over the patient's skin should not be emulated. The casualty officer had lost his objectivity.

Assessment

Hallucinations can occur in all modalities and there are various types of hallucinatory experience. In your history taking be careful to distinguish between distortions of perception, illusions, pseudohallucinations, and true hallucinations (read Section 3G, p. 104) as they have different diagnostic imports. If a patient is hallucinating in one modality always check for hallucinatory experiences in the other modalities. In patients who are hallucinating you will also need to carefully examine the patient for alterations in mood, signs of organic impairment, delusional experiences, and disorders of thinking. Vivid visual or olfactory hallucinations should make you want to rigorously exclude an organic disorder. Auditory hallucinations, although not exclusively psychotic, should make you look hard for evidence of affective or schizophrenic illness.

An understanding of the patient's upbringing, background, and previous life experiences is sometimes necessary to understand the nature of his hallucinatory experiences. Although psychotic hallucinations are often stereotyped and common to all people with hallucinations, the patient's previous experience sometimes colours their nature or their form (and the patient's reaction to them will certainly be coloured by his previous life experiences). In a patient having vivid pseudohallucinations, the nature of the phenomenon will often be very much in keeping with the patient's previous life experiences (for example, a woman repeatedly admitted to a mental hospital because of a persistent visual hallucination of a threatening face was finally relieved both of her hallucination and of her need to be in hospital when she was encouraged to explore the nature of the pseudohallucination, which turned out to be the face of a relative who had previously sexually abused her).

The patient's previous psychiatric history is clearly important in terms of assessing and diagnosing the reason for the patient's hallucinations, although may be misleading, as in the patient who has a previous history of 'schizophrenia' that turns out to be a recurrent affective disorder. The patient's medical history may be relevant, as may his drug history (for example, the patient with hypertension who develops visual hallucinations due to a recent prescription of propranolol).

The patient's reaction to his hallucinations will vary. The vivid hallucinations of delirium are usually frightening and believable, and the patient may react vigorously to them. Hallucinations may sometimes be comforting and the patient react with pleasure, but usually they are disturbing. Some patients react with apology, some greet their hallucinations like old friends, and some will talk about them as though they were still present long after they have gone, especially if the patients have been led to believe by the medical system that their only importance in life is to have hallucinations.

Differential diagnosis
Organic mental states

1. delirium (acute brain syndrome)
2. dementia (chronic brain syndrome).

Hallucinatory experiences are common in organic disease, particularly delirium, are usually easily detectable, and may affect the patient's behaviour a great deal. They are often accompanied by excitement (although occasionally by stupor), and by signs of organic mental impairment (which may vary from the most profound disorientation and complete lack of retentive memory to looking like a very mild confusion).

In delirium, visual hallucinations are usual, often vivid, and often terrifying. Visual illusions are also common. Both illusions and hallucinations occur in other modalities of sensation, particularly olfactory and auditory. They almost invariably lack any special schizophrenic quality, and command hallucinations are rare.

The differential diagnosis of delerium is dealt with in Section 4F (p. 180), but it is important to remember that certain acute medical conditions may present with hallucinations as the principal management problem, and are particularly likely to be encountered post-operatively, on medical wards, or in casualty. These are described in Section 4B, p. 135. Elemental visual hallucinations (and occasionally auditory hallucinations) should also make one think particularly of brain disease.

Some forms of chronic brain impairment may present or be associated with hallucinatory experiences (for example, cerebral syphilis). Hallucinatory experiences, both visual and auditory, may occur in any kind of dementia in response to episodes of delirium (due to an intercurrent chest infection, etc.). In both delirium and dementia, misperception of the environment leading to illusions is common.

Brief and repetitive hallucinations, particularly visual, auditory, or olfactory, may be simple partial seizures. These sometimes present diagnostic difficulty particularly if, during the seizure, nothing else obviously epileptic is going on (like alteration of consciousness, automatism, etc.). Unfortunately, even ambulatory EEG monitoring may sometimes fail to reveal their epileptic nature, since simple partial seizures are confined to a small part of the cortex and may not be reflected in changes in a scalp EEG recording.

Psychotic illness

1. schizophrenia (all types)
2. schizophrenia with an affective component
3. brief reactive psychosis
4. paranoid psychosis.

All types of hallucinations occur in schizophrenia, although they are characteristically auditory and have specific schizophrenic qualities (Section 3G, p. 111). First rank auditory schizophrenic hallucinations can, however, only be said to be schizophrenic if there is no evidence of organic mental impairment and the patient is not significantly hypomanic or depressed. The first rank hallucinatory symptoms of schizophrenia are voices talking about the patient in the third person, and voices that make a running commentary of what the patient is doing. It is important to distinguish between *auditory delusions* (such as thought broadcasting) and *auditory hallucinations*.

Visual hallucinations can occur in schizophrenia (distinguish them from delusional perception). Olfactory hallucinations, usually of an unpleasant nature, are common. Tactile and gustatory hallucinations also occur in schizophrenia and often have a bizarre quality to them.

The hallucinatory experiences of the other psychotic states are usually auditory, but lack the special schizophrenic qualities.

Affective illness

1. mania/hypomania
2. depression.

Hallucinatory experiences are common in both these illnesses and tend to be related to the patient's prevailing mood. Thus people with hypomania tend to have cheerful, comforting auditory hallucinations, and may have visual hallucinations often of a religious and rather grandiose nature. People who are depressed tend to have auditory hallucinations that often have a strong derogatory or accusatory content to them, or which reflect the patient's guilt feelings. The depressed may occasionally have visual hallucinations, but often such hallucinatory experiences are in the nature of pseudo-hallucinations. Olfactory hallucinations, usually unpleasant, are common in depressive illness, but conversely, pleasant olfactory hallucinations only very occasionally occur in mania.

In a patient with depression, it is important to make sure that the patient is actually having an olfactory hallucination and not in fact a delusional experience (as in the patient who thinks he is rotting and therefore giving off a powerful smell).

Intoxication

Hallucinations, particularly visual, are common in drug, but not alcohol, intoxication. It is important to distinguish between intoxication causing an hallucinatory experience and the patient who is mentally ill and also intoxicated. Intoxication can also awaken a previously dormant psychotic illness.

Common intoxicants

1. alcohol
2. cannabis
3. amphetamine and other 'speed'-like drugs
4. cocaine and its derivatives, like crack
5. LSD
6. PCP

7. paradoxical reaction to prescribed drugs (tricyclic antidepressants and other centrally active drugs like propranolol)

8. solvents.

Alcoholics can develop a chronic auditory hallucinatory state that may be difficult to distinguish from schizophrenia. This is not the same condition as acute delirium tremens consequent upon alcohol abuse or the sudden withdrawal of alcohol.

Although visual hallucinations are associated with alcohol in the lay mind, those acutely intoxicated with alcohol very rarely hallucinate. An alcoholic who has visual hallucinations almost certainly has delirium tremens. Cannabis rarely causes hallucinatory experiences (unless the cannabis is contaminated), but may occasionally trigger off a psychosis.

High doses of amphetamines and similar drugs, if taken for some time, can produce a drug induced psychotic state resembling schizophrenia in which hallucinations occur. Auditory and visual hallucinations can occur in abusers of cocaine and its derivatives, and there is a particular tactile hallucination associated with chronic cocaine use (formication). People who take PCP may have vivid hallucinatory experiences that are usually visual, but may be olfactory or auditory. LSD can produce vivid hallucinatory and perceptual experiences, usually visual, into which the person often has insight and from which he can often be talked down.

The elderly and the ill are particularly likely to have hallucinatory and illusory experiences if given certain centrally active drugs like tricyclic antidepressants and antiparkinsonian drugs. These are usually visual hallucinations, but auditory, olfactory, and other experiences may occur.

Solvent abuse usually leads to sudden alteration in mood, but occasionally may give rise to predominantly visual hallucinations.

Situational reactions

People in the grip of strong but normal emotion may hallucinate. Such experiences are usually pseudo-hallucinations and the classical example is the 'hallucination of widowhood' in which the person either sees a clear image of the dead person he is mourning or hears the dead person speak. Pseudohallucinations are more common in some cultures than in others.

Neurotic illness

People under stress, particularly with reactive depression or anxiety, may have pseudohallucinations that are often a reflection of the underlying distress (visions of open graves, etc.). Hallucinatory experiences may also occur in dissociative states. They are usually visual or auditory and are powerful pseudohallucinations, but may be mistaken for true hallucinations and a psychotic experience.

Personality disorder

Some people who are personality disordered are particularly prone to intoxication and to pseudohallucinations.

Management

The management of hallucinations is almost invariably the management of the underlying disorder, which is why a careful mental state examination of the patient is necessary. People who are having normal hallucinations, such as the hallucinations of widowhood or hypnogogic or hypnopompic hallucinations, need reassurance and explanation, and pseudohallucinations may need interpreting. Otherwise the treatment of the underlying disorder, whether it is delirium, schizophrenia, or depression, almost invariably results in the loss of the hallucinatory experiences. If the hallucinatory experiences are particularly vivid and frightening, they may need to be treated in their own right with a powerful neuroleptic or tranquillizer (sometimes given intravenously) to help reduce the intensity of the experience until the other treatment helps. Intravenous haloperidol may be particularly useful for the auditory hallucinated patient, and sometimes intravenous diazepam may also be helpful. Occasionally, the patient who is overwhelmed by his hallucinations and who is acting on them will need restrainting or talking down (Section 4J, p. 301).

D Patients with odd ideas

Also read Sections 1B (p. 12), 3F (p. 84), and 3J (p. 120).

- Odd ideas may be overvalued, ruminative, obsessional, or delusional.

- Not all odd ideas are pathological.

- Do not reinforce delusional beliefs by agreeing with them.

- Indicate to the patient that you acknowledge that they *seem* real to him.

- Check that the idea really is delusional (some may be odd, but true).

- Some deluded people are very persuasive, and folie à deux can occur.

- If the patient has one type of delusional belief, check to see if he has others.

- Full psychiatric and physical assessment is needed to understand the patient and the cause of his illness. Assess for risk of violence.

Diffential diagnosis

1. delirium
2. the dementias
3. other organic brain disease
4. medical disorder (particularly endocrine)
5. the schizophrenias
6. paranoid psychosis
7. reactive psychosis
8. monosymptomatic delusional state
9. hypomania/mania
10. depression
11. intoxications (usually chronic abuse)
12. some medicinal drugs
13. neurotic illness/personality disorder (rare unless associated stress reaction or related to intoxications)
14. simulated psychosis.

Types of delusion

- Paranoid—common to all causes.
- Delusions of reference—common to all causes.
- Delusions of guilt, poverty, unworthiness, and self-blame—usually depressive (check suicidal intent).
- Hypochrondriacal delusions—mainly depression or monosymptomatic, but may occur in schizophrenia.
- Nihilistic deluions—rarely anything else but depressive.
- Grandiose delusions—hypomania, some organic states, may occur in schizophrenia and are then often bizarre.
- Sexual delusions—may be monosymptomatic, occur in depression, and occasionally in schizophrenia.

- Schizophrenic delusions—passivity ideas (delusions of control), thought insertion, thought withdrawal, thought blocking, thought echo, thoughts spoken out loud, thought broadcasting, delusional mood, delusional perception.

Setting the scene

Odd ideas are the stuff of madness, but unfortunately they can also be the stuff of human progress and many new ideas initially labelled 'mad' are now part of orthodoxy. Odd ideas are also the stuff of harmless eccentricity. It is important for the psychiatrist to confine his attention to those odd ideas that are necessarily within his remit and not to become an agent of society or of orthodoxy. He should merely confine himself to recognizing and treating those odd ideas that relate to causation by psychiatric or physical illness.

Delusions may present in a florid way with an excited patient thrusting his strange ideas upon you, but may need to be extracted from a patient who realizes that his ideas will not be acceptable to others. You therefore have to respond to (and recognize) those delusional systems that are presented to you and diligently seek out those that are not. Delusions that relate to psychiatric (or physical) disease tend to run to type, although their content may change as human experience changes. They are therefore usually easy to recognize, and it should be possible to distinguish between those people who just have novel or eccentric ideas and those people whose ideas relate to mental illness. Odd ideas may also be overvalued, obsessional, ruminative, or appear odd because the patient is preoccupied with them (see Section 3F, p. 84).

As with hallucinatory experiences, it is important not to reinforce the patient's delusional belief by agreeing with it, but it is important to acknowledge the reality of a particular belief for the patient. You should indicate clearly that although you accept that the idea is real to the patient, it is false and is a sign of illness. Obviously before you do this you should be certain that the patient is actually describing a delusion. This is particularly important in those patients with paranoid delusions as occasionally their paranoia may turn out to be true. The patient who believes he is being persecuted by his family may occasionally be right. Although rare, there have been instances of people who have claimed that they were being poisoned by others only to have their claims dismissed, but who have belatedly been shown to be right at subsequent post-mortem. So, when assessing a delusion you do need to ask yourself 'Could this person be right?' (If, however, you start wondering this about the patient who claims to have arrived in a silver spaceship from the planet Arcturus then perhaps you need a holiday!) If a patient has one particular idea that he is preoccupied with, check to see if he has others (for example, hypochrondriacal ideas as well as paranoid ones—see Section 3F, p. 84).

It is important to remember that some deluded people can be very persuasive, particularly people who are both paranoid and articulate. Folie à deux is a real possibility, particularly in close-knit families or in small groups that feel threatened themselves by the rest of society. It is in such groups that a Messiah-like figure is particularly like to arise.

Assessment

Since delusional ideas can occur in a wide variety of both physical and mental disease, thorough assessment of the patient who is expressing odd ideas is necessary. Hurried assessment will lead to an incomplete understanding of the patient and where his ideas have come from. If you are to help him lose them (with some dignity), you will not only have to give him medication but will also have to understand him as a person. Often the roots of a delusional system can be seen to originate in the patient's past life or previous experience and so his family history and personal developmental history may be very important in understanding the roots of the patient's present delusional system. His previous physical and psychiatric history may also be important and a very careful examination of his mental state, both of the delusional system itself and whether or not the patient possesses any other odd ideas or any of the first rank symptoms of schizophrenia, is necessary. In addition, a full account of any hallucinatory experiences and an assessment of his mood must be made. Remember to assess the risk of violence and danger to others (see Section 4J, p. 288).

Since delusions also occur in organic mental illness, a full organic mental state testing is necessary (in dementia delusional ideas may occur very early in the dementing process before organic impairment is much apparent). Physical examination is therefore also necessary in patients who are deluded. (A well respected doctor suddenly developed the delusional idea that men were breaking into his house each night and having intercourse with his wife and, believing her to be involved in the conspiracy, he viciously attacked her. His horrified colleagues had him admitted into psychiatric care without performing a full assessment and ascribed his weight loss to his mental state. A proper physical examination would have revealed the carcinoma of lung with hepatic and cerebral metastases that were to kill him two weeks later.)

Differential diagnosis
Organic brain disease

1. delirium
2. dementia.

Apparent delusional ideas can occur because of the patient's misidentification or misinterpretation of his surroundings induced by his perceptual disorders. This is particularly so in delirium. If the perceptual disorder can be relieved, then the delusional beliefs, which are often transient, will usually disappear with it. Any type of delirium may present with these fleeting delusions, and if the organic impairment is only mild the underlying organic basis for the apparent 'psychosis' may be missed (see Sections 4C (p. 143) and 4F (p. 173)).

Delusional ideas occur in dementia, often at the beginning of the illness, and can sometimes be understood as the patient's explanation of his failing intellectual powers. Paranoid delusions are common and bizarre hypochondriacal ideas may also occur. Brain abscesses, viral encephalitis, or Creutzfeldt–Jakob disease may all start with a delusional state (usually paranoid) that may be misdiagnosed until cerebral degeneration becomes obvious.

Because the dementing patient usually loses some control over his impulses, the patient with delusions related to his dementia may be particularly likely to act on them. Dementia, like depression, may also reveal for the first time ideas or impulses that the patient has had for many years but which he has struggled to control because he appreciates that they would be socially unacceptable. The respectable middle-aged man who suddenly starts molesting little children may be dementing (or depressed). 'A nice man is a man with nasty ideas' as Oscar Wilde said.

Sustained delusional ideas, usually of a paranoid nature and not related to hallucinatory experiences, are particularly likely to occur in certain chronic medical conditions (most commonly endocrine disorders). Severe myxoedema sometimes leads to 'myxoedema madness', which is a paranoid delusional system often with auditory hallucinations and occasional visual hallucinations accompanied by signs of organic mental disturbance and paradoxical excitation. Thyrotoxicosis, much more rarely, can cause a patient to have paranoid delusions, sometimes in the setting of a depression and sometimes on their own, and without obvious organic mental impairment.

A delusional psychosis may also occur in hyperparathyroidism when it is usually, but not invariably, accompanied by marked depression. With very high blood concentrations of calcium, frank delirium may occur. The characteristic symptoms of muscle weakness, anorexia, vomiting, and generalized fatigue should alert one to the possibility of raised calcium being the cause of the patient's symptoms. Hypoparathyroidism may also occasionally cause a delusional illness, particularly following surgery on the neck. There has been some discussion about whether the low calcium level in the blood, the high phosphate level, or hypermagnesemia, causes this syndrome, which is also usually accompanied by signs of acute calcium deficiency (tetany, carpopedal spasms, etc.). Chronic water intoxication is commonly associated with a paranoid state, and it can be difficult to determine which is the cause and which is the effect as some patients with paranoid schizophrenia are compulsive water drinkers.

Both Cushing's syndrome and Addison's disease may also cause delusional states, usually of a persecutory nature. In Cushing's syndrome the disorder is usually secondary to severe affective change, which may be either depression or mania.

Pernicious anaemia may occasionally present as a paranoid delusional state in which there may also be affective change, usually of a depressive nature, plus signs of organic mental impairment. Mental changes may occasionally appear early in the condition before subacute combined degeneration of the cord is apparent. The condition will almost always be picked up on haematological screening, which will show characteristic changes in the red cell indices. Whether folic acid deficiency on its own can cause a similar syndrome is open to dispute (and some doubt). Nicotinic acid deficiency (pellagra), which is occasionally seen in alcoholics and vagrants, classically presents with diarrhoea, dermatitis, and delusions.

Delusional states may also occur as a result of brain disease itself. Cerebral tumours may be associated with the development of delusional ideas, particularly if they are situated in the temporal lobes. Presenile dementias, particularly Pick's disease and Huntington's chorea, are often preceded by a delusional state, especially of a paranoid persecutory nature. Cerebral syphilis (which still occurs) may be accompanied by a delusional state with or without affective change. Occasionally, multiple sclerosis may be associated with a psychotic illness in which delusions are prominent. This may be due to affective change, but is not always so. Organic mental impairment or neurological signs will usually also be present. Vasculitis, particularly cerebral lupus erythematosis, may also initially present as a delusional state.

Partial epilepsy whether or not secondarily generalized (particularly if the focus is in the temporal lobes) may be associated with a paranoid delusional state that resembles schizophrenia. The epilepsy may come first followed by the psychosis or vice versa. Presumably both are a reflection of some underlying disturbance in the temporal lobe which causes both the psychotic and the epileptic symptoms. Some epileptic twilight states (partial or subconvulsive generalized status) may be accompanied by delusions and hallucinations.

Dialysis dementia, although usually presenting as an acute organic mental impairment or delirium, sometimes with focal neurological signs and seizures, may occasionally be preceded by a short period of delusional experience, again usually persecutory. This condition is thought to be associated with aluminium toxicity. Uraemia may also result in a delusional state, sometimes accompanied by hallucinations, as can liver failure. The more rapid the kidney or hepatic failure the more likely that the patient will have mental symptoms.

Wilson's disease (hepatolenticular degeneration), due to increased copper levels in the blood with increased serum ceruloplasmin, is often associated with a psychotic state in which paranoid delusions are common. Acute intermittent porphyria may also present as a paranoid delusional state with auditory hallucinations. Characteristically, of course, this occurs in bouts with intervening normality. Abdominal pain and neurological symptoms will also be present and vomiting is common.

Some patients with narcolepsy show a late paranoid change with delusional ideas, and this may not just be secondary to the amphetamine that the patient may be taking. Postoperative delusions (again usually paranoid) may relate to infection or to any of the causes outlined above. It may also be a true reactive psychosis to the stress of the operation itself, and in some cases signs of organic brain impairment will be absent.

Psychotic illness

1. the schizophrenias

2. paranoid psychosis

3. reactive psychosis

4. monosymptomatic delusional state.

Delusional ideas are part of the presenting symptoms of schizophrenia and part of your mental state examination of the deluded patient will be aimed at determining whether the diagnostic first rank delusions of schizophrenia are present or not (Section 3F, p. 84). If they are, then they are only diagnostic of schizophrenia if they are occurring in clear consciousness and in the absence of both organic brain disease and marked affective change (either hypomania or depression). These delusions are of passivity or control, thought withdrawal or blocking, thought echo, thoughts heard out loud, thought broadcasting, delusional mood, and delusional perception. In patients presenting for the first time with apparent schizophrenia over the age of 40, look particularly carefully for an underlying organic basis for the symptoms and remember in both older and younger patients to look critically for a primary mood disturbance.

Patients with paranoid delusions that do not have the special schizophrenic qualities (and who do not have any diagnostic schizophrenic hallucinations) may have a paranoid psychosis. Again look carefully for any underlying affective or organic cause. In older patients sensory deprivation, such as severe deafness, may be an important factor.

Overwhelming stress in the patient's life, usually acute, may give rise to a brief delusional psychosis, (sometimes with schizophrenic features) which arises quickly and settles rapidly, particularly if the stress is removed, the patient returning to his previous personality and with no residual symptoms. Recognizing that a psychosis is reactive requires knowledge of the patient's present life circumstances and previous personality, which is why a full psychiatric history is so important.

Some patients have a single delusional idea, usually hypochondriacal but occasionally paranoid, which does not become systematized and elaborated but remains in its original form. The condition is sometimes accompanied by a secondary depression. Delusions of bodily infestation are common, as are delusions of jealousy (Section 3F, p. 84).

Affective illness

1. hypomania/mania
2. depression.

Delusional ideas are common in both hypomania and depression. Such ideas are grandiose or paranoid in hypomania, and paranoid, guilty, hypochondriacal, or nihilistic in depression. The affect-laden nature of the delusion is usually obvious, but paranoid delusions occurring in both mental states may be diagnosed as belonging to something else unless the underlying mood disturbance is recognized. They will not be relieved unless the underlying mood disturbance is treated.

Intoxication

Intoxicants causing odd ideas:

1. alcohol
2. cannabis
3. amphetamines
4. cocaine
5. LSD
6. anticholinergic drugs
7. tricyclic antidepressants
8. corticosteroids
9. ethosuximide
10. dopamine agonists: bromocriptine.

Most intoxications are acute with obvious mental impairment, excitement, and hallucinations, but in which any delusional symptoms are usually not prominent. Chronic misuse or intoxication can, however, sometimes lead to a chronic mental state in which delusions, usually paranoid, are more prominent and may be the presenting symptoms. A chronic paranoid state occurs in alcoholism and can also occur with chronic heavy cannabis ingestion, both without signs of organic impairment. Chronic amphetamine abuse can lead to a psychotic state resembling paranoid schizophrenia, and chronic cocaine abuse may lead to a psychosis. A few people who use LSD may develop a prolonged psychotic experience in which delusions may occur.

Similarly, with some medically prescribed drugs (common examples listed above) chronic use may be associated not with an obvious delirium but with a chronic psychotic state in which hallucinations and delusions may occur. It may take some time to recognize that the condition is iatrogenic.

Neurotic illness

Overvalued ideas, preoccupations, ruminations, and obsessional thinking are, of course, common in people with neurotic disorders. True delusions do not, however, occur except, rarely, during acute psychotic reactions or intoxications.

Personality disorder

Likewise, the personality disordered are prone to adverse reactions to both stress and intoxication and may therefore have brief delusional states and entertain overvalued ideas etc. *Sustained* delusional ideas are uncommon in the personality disordered, although one can often see a personality disorder presenting in an increasingly bizarre and extreme way until the person involved clearly crosses the psychotic borderline and his former ideas, originally merely overvalued, eventually become delusional. This is particularly so with paranoid ideas.

Some patients may pretend to have psychiatric disability, and some may recount their delusions as a piece of learned behaviour helping to perpetuate the 'sick role'. Recognition of this is difficult and the prognosis is poor.

Management

The management of odd ideas, particularly delusions, involves the recognition, removal, or treatment of the underlying cause or disorder, whether medical or psychiatric. In the case of psychiatric illness this will usually be with the appropriate medication. Patients who are not psychotic but who have overvalued ideas, ruminations, etc., need counselling, psychotherapy, and cognitive behavioural techniques to help them break out of their entrenched thought patterns, if they are disabling enough to be treated.

E Patients with difficulty in thinking, expression, or communication

Also read Sections 1C (p. 18), 1D (p. 23), and 3E (p. 79).

- Disorders of articulation (whispering or muttering).
- Speech too fast and/or too loud.
- Words cannot be understood.
- Words can be understood but do not make sense.
- Always be patient and listen politely.
- Seek advice (i.e. speech therapist).
- Record speech (audio or video) if persistent difficulty.
- Confront the patient with your difficulty.
- Can he communicate in writing?
- Make sure he is not deaf.
- Make sure he can see you as well as hear you—touch may help and comfort.
- Does he realize you cannot comprehend him—does he care?

166 | Practical Psychiatry

- Does he expect you to understand him?
- Neurological assessment of cranial nerves IX, XI, and XII, swallowing, phonation, and cortical function often needed.
- Is he using patois or dialect?
- Is it a private language?
- If rapid or loud is it organic speech, psychotic, or manic?
- If words incomprehensible is it patois, psychotic, or organic speech?
- If words comprehensible but sense not, is it a psychotic, organic, or demented speech?
- Is the patient anxious or 'talking in tongues', or preoccupied with an overvalued idea?
- Do not mistake organic speech for the excitement of delirium or for psychotic speech.
- Disordered speech (thought) can occur in organic brain disease, psychosis, affective illness, intoxication, and rarely in neurotic and personality disorders.

Setting the scene

Since we largely express our thoughts through speech, and since the medium of speech is our main method of communication, problems in understanding the words, expressions, and continuity of a patient's speech can make for particular difficulty in determining what is wrong with the patient. Beginners in psychiatry can find this particularly unnerving and faced with a patient who is difficult to communicate with in a clinical examination tend to go to pieces and start muttering about an 'unfair examination' instead of concentrating on analysing what the problem in communication is, establishing a differential diagnosis, and then looking to see how communication could be improved.

Some patients are difficult to understand because they have problems with articulation or mutter or whisper; some because they talk too loudly, fast, or both; some because the words they use cannot be understood, or the words can be understood but not the sense, or the sense can be guessed at but the concepts are so alien as not to be comprehensible.

If faced with a patient with whom you cannot communicate (see Section 4P (p. 370) for the mute patient) do not panic. If you assess the patient carefully, you will usually be able to communicate with him to some extent, or at least work out why you cannot. Be prepared to get help—a speech therapist's advice can be invaluable, and recording the patient (on audio or, better, videotape) for later analysis can also be extremely useful.

Assessment

Be prepared to confront the patient with your difficulty and always try to determine if he can understand you (either verbally or in other ways) even if you cannot understand him. If he realizes that he is not being understood, does it distress him or does he not seem to care? If he appears to be using a private language does it clearly have meaning for him, and does he expect you to understand it? Try to communicate by writing if speech fails.

You will need to determine how long the patient has had the difficulty and whether it came on slowly or suddenly. An informed witness is therefore very necessary. You will need to determine whether the patient is deaf (or blind) and whether, if he is deaf, he uses sign language. Whether deaf or not, always sit in front of the patient with whom you are having communication difficulty, establish easy eye contact, talk slowly and clearly, and make sure the patient can see your gestures, facial expression, and your lips, and check that he is aware of your presence. Listen to his *language* carefully. Occasionally, the problem is that he is using extreme dialect or patois or has a very thick accent combined with excitement.

If you suspect an organic speech disorder then look to see if it is receptive as well as expressive, whether it is fluent, non-fluent (for example, telegraphic), or paraphrasic, and whether there is nominal dysphasia, good comprehension, and repetitive ability, visual and tactile agnosia, dyspraxia, dyslexia, dysgraphia, prosopagnosia, and anosognosia, as well as performing a careful examination of the rest of the patient's cortical function.

1. Patients whose speech is unclear or inaudible

Bearing in mind the above general points, if the patient is whispering try to find out why ('the voices' may be telling him to, or he may be frightened that he may be overheard). Encourage him to speak louder and indicate that it is safe to do so. If he is very frightened a reassuring touch is helpful (and indeed, much can be communicated through the medium of touch, even when there is no comprehensive speech at all).

Muttering may reflect extreme thought disorder (for example word salad), excitement (psychotic or otherwise), or an organic speech disorder (dysarthria, dysphonia, or dysphasia). Alternatively it may be due to loss of personal auditory feedback as in delirium, or may be due to affectation, or occur in response to hallucinatory commands, or it may be meant to deliberately confuse not just the person talking to the patient but supposed unseen listeners. Confrontation and encouragement to speak more clearly often helps. Sometimes a few words can be heard clearly against the muttered background.

If you think that inaudibility or lack of clarity is due to dysarthria, then look for evidence of intoxication or of a local (or general) neurological or neuromuscular disorder. Look particularly for difficulty in swallowing, tongue movement, sensation and movement of the palate, phonation, extreme dry mouth, sialorrhoea, poorly fitting false teeth, or tardive dyskinesia.

2. Patients who are too loud or speak too quickly

Keep your cool and try to establish why the person is behaving in this way. Check for deafness and receptive or expresive dysphasia as well as running through the differential diagnosis of the excited patient (Section 4B, p. 130) and an examination of his speech (Section 3E, p. 79) looking particularly for pressure of speech, sudden shifts in topic, puns, clang associations, etc. Are shifts in topic understandable or not? Is there evidence of disordered syntax, neologisms, a 'private language', or other evidence of thought disorder? Is there an obvious (and often infectious) elevation in mood? Is the patient, though loud, *coherent* or is he just rambling with loss of determining tendency, or is he showing obsessional attention to detail? Will confrontation ('look, you are going so fast that I can't understand you') slow him down? Is he loud, noisy, *and* confused? Is he frightened and trying to drown out his 'voices'?

3. Patients who are articulating normally, but whose words cannot be understood

Is it organic (for example, jargon dysphasia) or is it a private psychotic language with word salad, neologisms, etc.? Make sure it is not just a patois—i.e., a private language that *can* be understood by the initiated (for example, rhyming slang or 'jive'). Is the patient aware that he cannot be understood? Does he seem to care if he does realize it? Can you communicate in other ways? Is his written speech as incomprehensible?

4. Patients who are articulating normally and whose words can be understood, but whose sense cannot

Is there a private meaning (thought disorder with neologisms, private syntax, etc.)? Is it an organic disorder, for example, telegraphic speech or a receptive dysphasia? Does the patient realize he cannot be understood? Does he show distress if he does or is he not surprised? Can he communicate in other ways (for example, writing)? Is he forgetting where he started from (dementing speech—such patients often show 'organic orderliness' as well)? Is he so preoccupied with his thought content (i.e., an overvalued idea) that he cannot keep it out of his discourse? (like King Charles's head in the memoirs).

Differential diagnosis

Organic mental illness

1. delirium
2. dementia.

Speech may be incomprehensible in delirium because of muttering or incoherent due to excitement, or the patient may be so overactive and his speech to fast that sense cannot be made of it. If the patient has had a cortical stroke, he may be showing an organic speech disorder in addition to excitement and delirium, which can make diagnosis difficult. As the delirium clears, however, the speech disorder will remain in this case. Focal encephalitis (for example, herpes simplex) may sometimes present in the same way.

Many patients with dementia may have difficulty in communicating, particularly those with Alzheimer's disease and multi-infarct dementia in which organic speech disturbance (for example, nominal dysphasia) may be part of the presenting symptoms in the setting of the primary intellectual loss. This is usually easy to recognize. What often happens, however, is that a primary speech disorder due to a focal cerebral lesion is misdiagnosed as a dementia or even as a thought disorder, which is why psychiatrists must be familiar with neurological causes of speech and communication difficulty.

Psychotic illness

Formal thought disorder is common (but not invariable) in schizophrenia, particularly talking past the point, loss of determining tendency, derailment, poverty of ideation, neologisms, and idiosyncratic speech leading in its extreme form to word salad. Thought withdrawal and insertion, although delusional experiences, may present as an apparent speech disorder.

Affective disorder

1. hypomania
2. depression.

Hypomania is often accompanied by rapid excited speech, words fizzing from the patient like sparks from a catherine wheel. There is pressure of speech, clang associations, flight of ideas, puns, etc. Very occasionally the patient's mind is so active that he, as it were, has no time to take a thought before a new one comes and he therefore becomes mute.

Muteness, of course, is also found in depression, and retardation can look like poverty of ideation. Some patients who are agitated can become incoherent and therefore appear thought disordered as can those who are so preoccupied with their delusional experiences that they talk of nothing else.

Intoxication

Acute intoxication with alcohol can lead to dysarthria and incomprehensibility as can intoxication with other substances. Psychomimetic intoxicants give rise to a brief psychosis, but rarely to a psychotic thought disorder. They produce changes in inner experience of reality that may lead to incomprehensibility as the victim tries to explain his experience to others but cannot find the words or expressions to do it.

Neurotic disorder

The actively anxious may become difficult to understand and hysteria may cause disordered speech such as 'speaking in tongues', although in particular circumstances this interesting phenomenon is accepted as normal. Patients with obsessional verbal rituals may occasionally be thought to be speech disordered. Gilles de la Tourette syndrome (disguised coprolalia and multiple tics) is a variant of this, although probably has an organic aetiology.

Personality disorders

There is no particular speech disorder to be found in the personality disordered, although incoherence through fright, speaking in tongues, strange speech in the intoxicated, and brief reactive psychosis may occur. Deliberate obscurity of speech can be found in those who wish to cloak their real purpose, even from themselves, but this is the world of politics and administration!

Management

Basically, the management of the speech disordered is of the condition that causes it, if possible. Psychotic speech often responds well to antipsychotic medication and mania will resolve with treatment. Organic speech disorder responds well to time, encouragement, and specific exercises. Speech disorder, of whatever cause, responds well to patient listening but badly to impatience.

F Patients who are confused or who have poor memory

- Have a high index of suspicion in any patient that you see that an organic element may be present, and look for memory/cognitive impairment.

- Confusion is not always obvious.

- Impaired memory, perplexity, failure to comprehend surroundings, restlessness, suspiciousness, mis-identification of people, or rising agitation suggest developing acute brain disturbance.

- If any impairment on organic screen (see Section 3C, p. 70) do *mini mental state* examination as it is semi-quantifiable.

- Formal memory tests are available, but you will need the help of a clinical psychologist.

- Always perform a careful neurological examination including tests of cortical function (speech, visual fields, parietal/frontal lobe testing, hearing) and a *thorough* medical examination.

- Take the patient's temperature.

Routine laboratory investigations

- Full blood count and indices, ESR or viscosity, B12, folic acid.

- Urea, electrolytes, calcium, phosphate, albumin/globulin, alkaline phosphatase, bilirubin, liver enzymes, blood sugar, and thyroid function tests.

- Urinalysis and culture.

- Serological tests for syphilis.

- Electroencephalogram.

- CT of brain and skull.

- Chest X-ray.

Other laboratory investigations when appropriate or indicated

Blood gases, sickling tests, serum magnesium and occasionally other metals, such as copper/ceruloplasmin, aluminium, manganese, lead, mercury, and arsenic, ammonia, cortisol, porphyrins, blood/urine for intoxicant and illicit drug screen, HIV testing, and lumbar puncture.

Differential diagnosis

1. Delirium

May be mild, or may start with mild confusion and then take two or three days to become severe. Most causes are not in the brain. Do not assume that there is a single cause.

Causes

1. alcohol-related delirium (delirium tremens, Wernicke's);
2. infection (few systemic signs in the old, and remember exotic diseases like malaria and typhoid);
3. anoxia/failure of cerebral blood flow (prolonged hypotension, loss of cerebral perfusion due to cardiac dysrhythmia, hypertensive encephalopathy, myocardial infarction, lung disease, CO_2 retention);
4. vascular (subarachnoid haemorrhage, subdural haematoma, cortical stroke, sickle cell disease, TIA);
5. acute brain disease (encephalitis/meningitis, cerebral abscess, focal encephalitis, AIDS, concussion, postictal, nonconvulsive status, collagen disease (SLE, PAN), cerebral tumour);
6. metabolic disease (liver failure, acute renal failure, hypoglycaemia, hyperglycaemia, dehydration, overhydration (water intoxication), hyponatraemia, hypernatraemia, hypocalcaemia, hypercalcaemia, hypomagnesemia, hypermagnesemia, hypophosphataemia, hyperphosphataemia, pancreatitis, porphyria, Wernicke's encephalopathy, pellagra);

7. endocrine disease (Cushing's syndrome, Addison's disease, myxoedema, severe thyrotoxicosis, hyperparathyroidism);

8. postoperative delirium (delirium tremens, blood loss, anoxia (myocardial infarction, pulmonary embolus, collapse/consolidation), infection, dehydration, electrolyte imbalance, reaction to medication, 'pseudodelirium').

2. Dementia

Try to recognize remediable/arrestable causes as soon as possible. Investigate all patients of whatever age thoroughly. Look long and hard for depression. Assess social behaviour and competence.

Causes

1. primary degenerative dementia (Alzheimer's)
2. multi-infarct dementia
3. subcortical dementias
4. Pick's disease
5. infective dementias (including AIDS)
6. normal pressure hydrocephalus
7. toxic encephalopathies
8. endocrine dementias
9. cerebral tumours
10. drugs/intoxicants
11. depression
12. traumatic encephalopathy.

Psychotic illness

Chronic schizophrenia can easily be mistaken for dementia and vice versa.

Affective disorders

Depressive pseudodementia (perhaps 20 per cent of dementias).

Intoxications

Alcoholic dementia, Korsakoff's syndrome.

Acute situational reactions

Pseudodelirium.

'Neurotic' illness

Simulated dementia (Ganser syndrome), functional acute memory loss.

Management

Find the cause and reverse it. In delirium, nurse the patient in well lit quiet surroundings. Put up a drip, give intravenous glucose (not in severe liver disease), and parenteral vitamins. Restrain and tranquillize if necessary (diazepam, heminevrin, or haloperidol intravenously). Good nursing essential. In dementia, habit and memory training important—the patient is often less disabled at home.

Setting the scene

Depending on where and with whom you work, patients with confusion or poor memory may be an everyday problem or you may very rarely see them. They are the bread and butter of psychogeriatrics and form an important part of the work of the liaison psychiatrist. They are also relatively common in general psychiatric practice and in the field of alcoholism. But, even if you work in a field in which they are comparatively rare (such as psychotherapy), it is important to be alert to recognizing the sometimes quite subtle signs of confusion and to be able to recognize that a patient's memory ability is outwith the normal limits for his age.

There is a skill in recognizing the early signs of confusion or delirium and it is important to acquire it.

Heading off delirium tremens before it has gone too far, or recognizing Wernicke's encephalopathy early, can prevent much distress on the ward and prevent the patient from suffering irreversible brain damage. In any patient that you see you should have a high index of suspicion that you may be dealing with organic brain disease, or with physical disease masquerading as psychiatric illness.

Confusion may sometimes be very obvious, with the patient clearly being totally disorientated, having no retentive memory, and being completely out of touch with his surroundings. It may, however, be subtle so that it takes you a long time to realize that the patient has a minor contraction in consciousness and a critical, if difficult to detect, unawareness of what is going on around him. Confusion may also present as a wild excitement (Section 4B, p. 130) or as an apparent psychotic state with vivid visual and sometimes auditory hallucinations (Section 4C, p. 143) so that the underlying brain disorder is not immediately apparent. Confusion may also be covered up by confabulation so that until you know the patient well (particularly the life events he has had in the preceding few days) you may be misled.

The use of empty stock phrases and social but meaningless speech may also lull your critical faculties to sleep. You may also have unrealistic expectations of the patient's performance not realizing that the patient has always been mentally handicapped or glibly ascribe the patient's memory problems to 'old age', thereby missing some remedial cause for the patient's failing memory. Serious psychiatric disorders such as depression can also present as apparent confusion or as memory impairment. When faced with a patient who has an apparent confusion or memory impairment, you therefore face wide diagnostic possibilities and the patient will need careful assessment.

General assessment

In assessing any patient with any condition, a high index of suspicion should be maintained for the presence of organic brain disease. Memory impairment, perplexity, failure to comprehend surroundings, restlessness, suspiciousness, misidentification of people whom the patient should know, and rising agitation are particular signs of possible developing acute brain disturbance.

Section 3C (p. 70) outlines the usual cognitive screen that is suggested should be used on any patient during the assessment of mental state. If, during this screen, you pick up an indication that there may be cognitive impairment, it is better to go on to a quantitative screening assessment (particularly because you will want to look at changes over time). For this the **mini mental state** is ideal and is presented below.

Mini mental state examination

1. Orientation

Ask the date, the day, the month, the year, and the time. Score one point for each correct answer. (5)

Ask the name of the ward, the hospital, the district, the town, the country. Again score one point for each correct answer. (5)

2. Registration and calculation

Name three objects and ask the patient to repeat these. Score three for all correct, two if only two correct, and one for one correct. (3)

Ask the patient to subtract 7 from 100 and to repeat the subtraction four more times (93, 86, 79, 72, 65). (5)

Recall—ask for the three objects to be named again. (3)

3. Language

Ask the patient to name two objects shown to him (for
example, pen, watch). (2)

Score one point if he can repeat 'no ifs, ands, or buts'.
(1)

Ask the patient to carry out a three stage command, for
example, 'take a piece of paper in your right hand, fold
it in half, and put it on the table.' (3)

Reading—write in large letters 'close your eyes' and
ask the patient to read and follow this. (1)

Writing—ask the patient to write a short sentence. It
should contain a subject and a verb and make sense.
(1)

Copying—draw two intersecting pentagons, each side
about one inch and ask the patient to copy it. (1)

The total possible score for this 30.

In tests of memory it is most important to ask questions to which you know the answer (for instance, do
not ask the number of the Queen's children if you
yourself do not know how many she has, and do not
ask the patient what he had for breakfast unless you
happen to know—we will be surprised if you do). The
advantage of using a quantitative assessment like the
mini mental state examination is that you can chart
the patient's progress and as you develop experience
you can have an agreed cut-off point in your mind for
abnormality (say a score of 25).

Formal memory tests are available, although these
require experience and skill if the results are to be
meaningful and they are therefore best performed by
clinical psychologists or psychology technicians. The
Wechsler adult intelligence scale is useful and there
are many other standardized memory tests available. If
you think that they are necessary, either to help in the

diagnosis of your patient's memory disorder or to provide a basis for comparison later, then you should
discuss with a clinical psychologist what the most
appropriate test is to use.

Patients with confusion or apparent memory disorder
need a careful neurological examination, including tests
of cortical function such as tests for agnosia, dyspraxia,
speech, the integrity of the visual fields, hearing, etc.
They also need a careful medical examination, particularly of the respiratory, cardiovascular, and abdominal
systems as often the clues to the aetiology of the patient's problem may be found there. Always take the
patient's temperature (a veterinary nurse, subject to brief
episodes of withdrawal and auditory hallucinations was
diagnosed as having a recurrent affective disorder and
only received the correct diagnosis (and treatment) of
her brucellosis when her temperature was taken during
one of the episodes—it was 40.5°C).

In addition to routine biochemical and haematological
screening, it is appropriate to carry out thyroid function tests, serum vitamin B12 and folic acid levels,
and, if appropriate, blood gases and blood ammonia. In
confused patients an EEG is often helpful (and occasionally so in people with memory impairment). Although it may be misleading, computed tomography of
the brain is usually indicated, as is a chest X-ray.

Differential diagnosis
Organic mental states

1. delirium and confusion (acute brain syndrome);
2. dementia and memory impairment (chronic brain
   syndrome).

Delirium

Delirium may present insidiously with only a mild
confusion or (particularly if its development has gone

unnoticed) may present explosively with agitation, gross psychomotor activity, and hallucinations. Since the key to managing delirium is recognizing the cause and removing it as rapidly as possible, the differential diagnosis of delirium is important. Most causes of delirium are not found in the brain itself. Disorder in other systems is a far more likely cause of it and it should also be recognized that delirium is much more likely to occur in people who are already compromised in some way. Delirium may well be multifactorial (for example, the alcoholic who also has pneumonia) and discovery of one cause for a patient's delirium should not prevent a search for others.

1. Alcohol-related delirium

Classically, alcohol delirium (delirium tremens) is associated with acute alcohol withdrawal or with a sudden reduction in alcohol intake in people who normally have a heavy alcohol intake. Usually, but not necessarily, this occurs in people who one might class as being alcoholic. Some people who work in hot dusty jobs such as foundry workers may, however, take their necessarily heavy fluid intake as beer, say up to 20 pints a day, and such people are not alcoholic in the currently accepted sense, but, when suddenly deprived of alcohol, may develop a withdrawal syndrome. It is also important to recognize that delirium tremens may sometimes occur in people who continue to drink heavily, either because deficiency of the B-complex vitamins has reached a critical point or because they have developed an intercurrent infection. Sometimes the true cause of delirium tremens is masked by the development of coincident disease in chronic heavy drinkers, such as pneumonia or pancreatitis.

The full blown syndrome of delirium tremens is ushered in by one or two days of rising agitation, rising pulse rate, and coarse tremor followed by suspiciousness, irritability, and misidentification of people and surroundings. These are warning signs and should be responded to rapidly. If necessary, one should go back over the drinking history again carefully and get evidence of the patient's level of drinking from elsewhere. In these patients, frank paranoid ideas can develop quite suddenly accompanied by usually vivid and often threatening visual hallucinations plus excitement and psychomotor overactivity. Occupational delirium may be seen, in which the patient recreates a fragment of his normal occupation. For example, an alcoholic railway guard admitted for observation after a fall began marching up and down the orthopaedic ward shouting 'right away!' and whistling piercingly as he tried to order his train from what he regarded as his local station. A former pilot jumped through the ward window into the cockpit of his waiting Spitfire in his attempt to get at the oncoming Germans, who for reasons best known to themselves were coloured green and two inches high.

In addition to agitation, tremor, tachycardia, confusion, visual hallucinations, and excitement, tonic clonic seizures commonly occur and marked dehydration may be present. Look particularly for ataxia, nystagmus, lateral rectus palsy with weakness or absence of conjugate gaze, and peripheral neuropathy. These are the features of Wernicke's encephalopathy, which needs emergency treatment with thiamine intravenously. Liver function should be assessed as accurately and as quickly as possible (as to some extent treatment will depend on the result). At a later stage, when the patient has recovered from the acute delirium, a full mental state, cognitive function, and neurological status examination, needs to be made to detect other neurological disorders that may be associated with alcoholism.

It is very important to remember when treating what appears to be an obvious delirium tremens due to alcohol withdrawal, that other factors, such as a chest infection, liver failure, and gastrointestinal bleeding, may be playing a part in the condition. An accurate drinking history is necessary, but may not always be obtainable. (The aetiology of recurrent excitement and hallucinosis in a 'respectable' single lady of middle years was only determined during a home visit, when 134 empty gin bottles were discovered in her kitchen cupboard. She had always strenuously denied taking alcohol and had primly reprimanded her doctor for being so suspicious.)

2. Infection

Young children with acute infection (such as measles or chickenpox) often hallucinate and become confused, but this very rarely presents a management problem, often passes unrecognized, and may even appear charming. (A four-year-old girl's conversation with the fairies at the end of the bed during her attack of measles may be taken for no more than delightful fantasy.) Such delirium may, however, occasionally presage a serious complication of the infection, such as measles encephalitis, and if the condition does not disappear rapidly as the temperature falls then further investigations should be done.

In elderly people, delirium is often due to hidden infection, usually of the lungs or of the kidneys, and in such people there may be very few systemic symptoms or signs of the underlying infection. The pulse rate may be normal and there may be no increase in temperature, and a serious infection may merely present as a delirium, which, of course, may be 'written off' as being due to 'old age' or to dementia and the remedial cause not looked for. (One only has to think of a subdural haematoma to realize how dangerous this dismissive attitude of mind can be.)

Most patients with infective delirium, however, will

have obvious signs of infection with local signs, fever, etc. In these days of rapid travel, it is important to think of possible exotic illnesses such as malaria or typhoid fever in delirious patients who have recently returned from abroad. Such diseases may well present as delirium, and only a careful search will reveal physical signs such as rose red spots to reveal the underlying aetiology of the delirium.

3. Anoxia

Acute anoxia (or acute on chronic anoxia) often gives rise to delirium. If it is accompanied by marked psychomotor overactivity, the patient will be compromised even further and will therefore need treating swiftly. Failure of cerebral blood flow due to prolonged hypotension or frequent prolonged changes in cardiac rhythm, or occurring in a patient in shock who remains upright, may cause delirium. Hypertensive encephalopathy is an often unrecognized cause of delirium and also needs emergency treatment.

Acute cardiac failure, such as may occur in myocardial infarction, may give rise to delirium, which may be the presenting feature, particularly if the infarction is otherwise silent. Anoxia, due to lung disease or carbon dioxide retention, may also give rise to delirium. ('Blue bloaters' and 'pink puffers' are both at risk.) In patients with chronic respiratory embarrassment, even a mild chest infection may be enough to trigger delirium.

4. Other vascular causes

Subarachnoid haemorrhage, although more usually presenting with headache and prostration, may occasionally present with delirium. Chronic subdural haematoma (particularly in the elderly) may give rise to a fluctuating confusion with the responsible head injury long since forgotten. Cerebral infarction may also give rise to delirium. If it occurs in a silent area of the brain, it may not present with a characteristic hemiplegia or speech difficulty, but may present with sudden excitement and confusion. These so called *cortical strokes* should be high on your list of possibilities and are often not recognized as a cause of a patient's condition. Sudden delirium in Negro patients exposed to a change in oxygen tension, such as in high altitude flying, should raise the possibility of sickle cell disease. Transient ischaemic attacks sometimes present with delirium with minimal physical signs.

5. Acute brain disease

Brain infections, either generalized as in meningitis or encephalitis, or localized as in cerebral abscess, are a possible cause of delirium and may (particularly with encephalitis) be ushered in by a prodromal psychiatric disorder, such as hallucinations, delusions, anxiety, or depression. Only later does confusion begin to develop, and later still do signs of severe cerebral derangement, such as myoclonic jerks, seizures, and coma occur. A focal encephalitis, such as herpes simplex encephalitis, can commonly present as a delirium. Successful treatment of cerebral syphilis with penicillin may be accompanied by an intense delirium (the so-called Herxheimer reaction). Concussion producing swelling of the brain and disorganization of cerebral function may result in delirium, which may be difficult to manage. Acute cerebral infections related to AIDS (for example, toxoplasmosis) may become an important cause of delirium. Computed tomography will usually reveal the cause.

Occasionally, postepileptic delirium can occur, often with wild excitement and aggression. Very occasionally, complex partial or subconvulsive general status, which may go on unrecognized for several days, will present with confusion and hallucinations. Usually it occurs in a patient with known epilepsy, but occasionally, particularly in middle-age, it may arise *de novo*. Collagen disorders with associated inflammation of the cerebral blood vessels (such as in polyarteritis nodosa or systemic lupus erythematosus) may also give rise to delirium and may be the presenting sign of the illness, occurring before the systemic disease has been diagnosed. Cerebral tumours rarely present as delirium, although occasionally acute pressure changes or haemorrhage into the tumour may precipitate an acute confusional state.

Dementia may be accompanied by episodes of acute confusion and delirium, either because of the nature of the dementing illness itself or because the dementing person has suffered some intercurrent upset. A sudden worsening of confusion in the dementing patient should make you look hard for evidence of intercurrent infection, myocardial infarction, hypertensive crisis, uraemia, cortical stroke, etc.

6. Metabolic disorders

Acute, or acute on chronic, liver failure can give rise to portal encephalopathy with confusion and delirium. The patient is often quite wild and treatment is difficult. The patient may be jaundiced and have other signs of liver failure, such as a flapping tremor, ascites, and (if you are lucky enough to detect it) foetor hepaticus. Chronic, slowly progressive uraemia does not usually cause much in the way of mental disturbance until the urea levels are very high, but *acute* renal failure will often give rise to delirium.

Hypoglycaemia, either due to overenthusiastic treatment of diabetes or to the rare insulinoma or functional hypoglycaemias, is an uncommon but important cause of delirium since, if recognized and treated early, response is dramatic, but if left too late irreversible brain damage may occur. If you are in the slightest doubt about whether a patient's delirium might be due to hypoglycaemia, it is usually safe to give an intravenous bolus of glucose, although it is not safe to do so in advanced liver failure. (It should be given with thiamine if you suspect vitamin deficiency from any cause.) Hyperglycaemia may also cause delirium, although it is only likely to happen in patients with diabetes. Recovery from the confusion caused by hyperglycaemia is slow, even if the hyperglycaemia is corrected.

Fluid and electrolyte changes, dehydration, over-hydration, hypo- and hypernatraemia, hypo- and hypercalaemia, hypo- and hypermagnesemia, and (possibly) hypo- and hyperphosphataemia, can cause delirium and may be responsible for the delirium seen in acute pancreatitis, although this may be due to infection or to toxic products entering the bloodstream. Porphyria is a rare cause of delirium in the United Kingdom, although it should be thought of in any patient who has bouts of delirium with intervening periods of normality accompanied by abdominal pain, vomiting, and neurological symptoms.

Delirium can occasionally occur in malnutrition, particularly thiamine and nicotinic acid deficiency (Wernicke's encephalopathy and pellagra).

7. Endocrine disease

Severe Cushing's syndrome may present with delirium as may Addisonian crises. Myxoedema may present as an acute delirium with hallucinations, confusion, and sometimes paranoid delusions (myxoedema madness), and extreme thyrotoxicosis (thyroid storm) may occasionally present as a delirium. Hyperparathyroidism may present as delirium (often accompanied by a previous history of muscle weakness, anorexia, vomiting, and generalized fatigue) if calcium levels are high enough.

8. Postoperative delirium

This may be florid with psychomotor overactivity, paranoid delusions, and hallucinations, or more commonly present as paranoid delusions and confusion. Postoperative delirium is a common complication of surgery. It is often multifactorial and needs to be dealt with quickly. In the acutely confused or delirious postoperative patient look for:

1. delirium tremens;

2. blood loss;

3. anoxia (from any cause including silent myocardial infarction, pulmonary embolus, or silent collapse or consolidation of a lung);

4. infection (including subphrenic abscess—'pus somewhere, pus nowhere, pus under the diaphragm');

5. dehydration, overhydration, or electrolyte imbalance;

6. untoward reactions to medication (for example, pentazocine or sedating patients in pain without giving analgesia).

Some patients who were frightened before an operation, are terrified in the intensive treatment unit, are in pain and exposed to constant light, develop a kind of *pseudodelirium* with confusion and behavioural disturbance interspersed with withdrawn periods—a psychological reaction to the experience.

Investigation of delirium

All patients with delirium need careful examination of their mental state and a careful general medical and neurological examination (this may not be possible until the patient has been restrained and sedated (see Section 4J, p. 301)). In addition, the following investigations should always be performed unless the cause of the delirium is obvious and you are sure it is the only cause:

1. patient's temperature and pulse rate at least four-hourly;
2. full blood count and platelets (including looking for sickling when appropriate);
3. urea, electrolytes, blood sugar, liver function tests, albumin and total proteins, calcium, phosphate, thyroid function tests, and, if appropriate, tests for porphyria, serum magnesium, and blood gases.
4. blood should be taken for drug and intoxicant screening and blood cultures if infection is suspected;
5. urine should be examined for evidence of infection, sugar, and protein;
6. chest X-ray may be indicated, and if the patient can cooperate an EEG may be extremely useful and computed tomography may also be useful in some cases. Lumbar puncture (if you can exclude raised intracranial pressure) is sometimes necessary—skilled help will be needed if the patient is uncooperative.

Dementia

Dementia is the most likely cause of chronic confusion or of memory loss. In the initial assessment of patients, it is particularly important to try to distinguish those causes of dementia that are remediable or which may need urgent treatment. Often the diagnosis is based on a balance of probabilities and may take some time to be arrived at. It is made not only by performing a full neurological and psychiatric examination but also by consideration of the patient's past history and other medical evidence. Although perhaps commoner under the age of 65, remediable causes of dementia exist at all ages and any patient, no matter what age he is, needs his newly presenting dementia thoroughly assessed. Argument still exists about whether the presenile form of Alzheimer's disease (i.e., occurring under the age of 65) is the same condition as Alzheimer's disease occurring in those aged over 65. Alzheimer's disease presenting under the age of 65 is much more likely to have florid neurological symptoms and focal signs.

Aetiology of dementia

1. primary degenerative dementia of the Alzheimer type;

2. multi-infarct dementia;

3. subcortical dementias (Parkinson's disease, Huntington's chorea, Wilson's disease, etc.);

4. Pick's disease;

5. infection (Creutzfeldt–Jakob disease, neurosyphilis*, AIDS dementia, and chronic infections* like toxoplasmosis, fungal infection, etc.);

6. normal pressure hydrocephalus* (ataxia, incontinence, and dementia), both idiopathic and secondary;

7. toxic encephalopathies* (chronic hepatic* and renal failure*, chronic cerebral oedema,* chronic electrolyte disturbance*, chronic anoxia*, Wernicke's syndrome*, Korsakoff's syndrome*, non-Korsakoff's alcoholic dementia, vitamin B12 deficiency*, folic acid deficiency* (possibly), aluminium toxicity* (dialysis dementia), chronic lead*, mercury*, manganese*, and arsenic* poisoning, some industrial solvents;

8. endocrine dementia, hypothyrodism*, Cushing's disease*;

9. cerebral tumours* (slow growing tumours in any area, particularly if accompanied by cerebral oedema; other neurological symptoms may be absent and there may be no headache or visual disturbance);

10. drugs*; occasionally long-term use of certain drugs in toxic doses such as phenytoin, the bromides, and anticholinergic drugs, may give rise to a chronic dementia-like syndrome; phenytoin also causes cerebellar damage, which may become irreversible;

11. depression; pseudodementia* related to depressive illness may account for up to 20 per cent of patients of presenting with dementia and must never be forgotten;

13. chronic traumatic encephalopathy following head injury or repeated head injuries (as in boxing).

* These are the potentially reversible or arrestable causes of dementia that need to be rigorously excluded.

In the course of a chronic dementia, remediable causes of a sudden worsening of the dementia may occur, such as intercurrent infection, myocardial infarction, etc.

Assessment of dementia

The assessment of a patient with apparent dementia must be thorough and include a detailed neurological and psychiatric assessment, including any previous psychiatric history looking especially for previous alcoholism, noting the way the dementia presented (slow, rapid, or explosive in onset), and its course since presentation (rapid deterioration, sudden onset with comparatively little change, slow, relentless deterioration, or progressive and stepwise degeneration). Focal and neurological signs and symptoms must be looked for including movement disorders, myoclonus, parkinsonian symptoms, incontinence, ataxia, delirium progressing to dementia, ophthalmoplegia, and nystagmus. Look for specific signs of regional cortical impairment, such as parietal lobe signs (language dysfunction,

agnosia, apraxia, memory for faces, etc.) and frontal lobe
signs (sensory inattention, grasp and sucking reflexes).

The usual laboratory investigations include full blood
count and indices, folic acid and B12 levels, (sickling
tests when appropriate), urea and elelctrolytes, calcium,
phosphate, (magnesium, aluminium, manganese, arsenic, ammonia, lead, and mercury levels occasionally),
liver function tests, thyroid function tests, and serological tests for syphilis. An electroencephalogram may
be helpful (including visual evoked responses to flash
and pattern if available). Computed tomography of the
brain and skull is indicated, and it may rule out certain
remedial causes of dementia, such as hydrocephalus,
but may be misleading. The place of magnetic resonance
imaging in assessing dementia is at present uncertain.

Baseline assessment of social behaviour, competence
in the tasks of daily living (dressing, keeping clean,
managing money, etc.), and behaviour towards others
should be made. Some baseline assessment of intellectual function (for example, Wechsler adult intelligence scale) should also be made in cooperation with
clinical psychologists. Both baseline assessments are
needed to provide evidence of change in the future.

Psychotic illness

1. schizophrenia
2. schizophrenia with affective component
3. paranoid psychosis.

Psychotic illness (particularly schizophrenia, and most
commonly when chronic or when associated with
paucity of ideation or thought disorder and a lack of
interest in what is going on around the patient) may
occasionally be mistaken for dementia. Many patients
with chronic schizophrenia have an altered time sense,
and because of this or because of delusional systems

they may give inappropriate or incorrect answers to tests of orientation, or may be uncooperative with cognitive testing. Thought disorder is often mistaken for dementia.

Affective disorders

Depression

Depression, which untreated may last for months if not years, may easily be mistaken for dementia. Pseudodementia is one of the commonest causes of an apparent dementing state. This condition can occur in all ages, but is particularly easily missed in the elderly. Be especially suspicious of those patients who seem to be taking an unduly gloomy view of their decline in intellectual powers, who appear to have a diurnal variation to their cognitive impairment, or in whom cognitive impairment fluctuates. Also, be suspicious of those patients who are grossly impaired on some tests but not on others, or who appear to have depressive symptomatology (like delusions of guilt, unworthiness, or self-blame) mixed up with their cognitive impairment. Although depression and dementia can exist side by side (and patients who retain some insight into their failing cognitive powers may become depressed), if you are suspicious that you are seeing a pseudodementia it is worthwhile vigorously treating the patient for depression. Remember that cerebral atrophy on computed tomography may be particularly misleading.

Intoxication

In addition to Wernicke's and Korsakoff's syndromes, some chronic alcoholic patients develop a chronic dementia. Unless treated quickly with thiamine, Wernicke's encephalopathy is irreversible. Korsakoff's syndrome, which may be accompanied by a peripheral neuropathy, is characterized by loss of short-term retentive memory and may be accompanied by confabulation, which is often misrepresented as a deliberate covering of memory gaps by use of the patient's imagination. Almost certainly confabulation is actually the recounting of true memories that happen to be 20 or 30 years out of date (for example, the patient who tells you that he is in hospital in Cairo, when you ask him the name of the place where he is at the moment, may well have been in hospital in Cairo some 30 years ago). The prognosis both of Korsakoff's syndrome and of ordinary alcoholic dementia and cerebral atrophy is often better than usually indicated, although recovery is often slow.

Heavy cannabis ingestion can produce a state of apathy that may be mistaken for dementia. It is uncertain whether cannabis actually causes dementia in its own right. Repeated heavy use of solvents may occasionally give rise to an encephalopathy, as can certain prescribed drugs.

Acute situational reactions

These may sometimes be so extreme or bizarre, or the patient may be so temporarily out of touch with his surroundings, that a spurious impression of delirium can be given. This may account for some cases of apparent delirium occurring in such places as intensive treatment units or postoperative delirium.

'Neurotic' illness

If a patient is extremely anxious and terrified, he may be so little in contact with his surroundings or be paying such little attention to the examiner as to give an erroneous impression of delirium. Dissociation states may also present as memory loss. The sudden onset of total amnesia, particularly in the young (including disorientation for person), is usually dissociative (or deliberate). In middle-aged patients, **transient global amnesia** must be carefully excluded. Hysterical pseudodementia with apparent memory loss and fantastic answers, like 'five' to a simple question such as 'how many legs has a donkey?'—the so-called Ganser syndrome—is usually seen as related to hysterical dissociation, although the Ganser syndrome may be deliberate and appear in prisoners. In our experience, the Ganser syndrome may also accompany organic mental states including cerebral tumours. Deliberate and conscious simulation of dementia may occur. Continued contact with the patient will usually reveal inconsistencies in the clincal picture that makes the diagnosis obvious, but carefully exclude depressive illness as depression may make the patient tell you he is faking even when he is not.

Personality disorder

Since those who are personality disordered often indulge in illicit substances and intoxicants or have repeated head injuries, they may show evidence of organic brain impairment from time to time, or may suffer from recurrent hysterical dissociation.

Management

The management of acute confusion or delirium involves trying to accurately diagnose what the cause of the delirium is so that it may be removed as quickly as possible, and applying restraint (either physical or chemical) judiciously and sparingly with due regard for the cause of the delirium. For example, in severe anoxia or in portal encephalopathy it is important to avoid using medication if at all possible but instead to treat with oxygen in the first example, and to evacuate the gut and sterilize it (using neomycin) in the second.

In most delirious patients, it is useful to put up a drip as many are dehydrated (but beware of accidentally overhydrating the patient precipitating heart failure). An intravenous bolus of glucose (not in those with liver failure) and parenteral vitamins, including thiamine, will usually do no harm and may do some good. If alcoholic delirium is suspected, give a loading dose of intravenous vitamins straight away as this may prevent much disturbance. It is useful to do this also in alcoholics in whom delirium tremens seems imminent. If infection is suspected get immediate medical advice about the best way of treating it.

Since attention span and memory is short in delirium, make sure that reassurances and comfort are repeated as necessary and if possible have one or two nurses detailed to look after the patient continually so that he is nursed by familiar faces. Nurse the patient in good, but not glaring, lighting, avoiding shadows, and keep the patient's surroundings as quiet as possible (we all know how difficult this is in the average medical or surgical ward).

Medication may have to be given to calm the patient. If an alcohol withdrawal syndrome is suspected, then it is probably better to use diazepam, chlordiazepoxide, or chlormethiazole (Heminevrin) as these drugs are anticonvulsant. All three are potentially habituating or addictive and so a large dose should be used to start with (say up to 100 mg of chlordiazepoxide a day orally), but the dose should be rapidly tailed off and the medication withdrawn within about ten days. Haloperidol or droperidol can be given intravenously if necessary. They are reasonably safe, even in the physically ill, and given intravenously are unlikely to produce acute parkinsonian reactions, except in the elderly or in those whose basal ganglia are already compromised (see Section 4J, p. 301 for advice on restraint and emergency medication). Reassess the patient frequently and reduce any psychotropic medication as rapidly as possible, consistent with the safety of the patient and other people. In patients with delirium or dementia due to hypothyroidism, thyroxine supplements must be given in very low doses to start with.

The immediate management of dementia is to try to recognize any remedial causes, to treat them as rapidly as possible, and to recognize and treat any underlying depression. Medication at the present time is unlikely to alter the course of dementia, but good consistent nursing care aimed at reteaching lost social and personal skills and which stimulates the patient's memory as much as possible, is essential. Remember that the patient who may appear very demented in hospital may be much more competent in his own familiar surroundings.

G Patients who are sad

- Sadness can be a reaction, exaggerated or not—this is a value judgement—or can be imposed from within, i.e., an illness.

- Sadness carries many physical symptoms with it, conversely, physical illness can cause sadness.

- Sadness can be masked or hidden; some people cope with it better than others.

- A sad person may make you feel sad, hopeless, or angry, or wish to escape from his grief.

- Sad people have poor judgement and you may need to prevent them from making wrong decisions.

- Sadness and anxiety can look very similar.

- Sadness has a mortality and morbidity rate.

- Full psychiatric and physical history is mandatory.

- Look for affect-laden delusions and hallucinations, and assess suicidal risk thoroughly—record your findings.

- Suicidal people may be a risk to others.

- Note any changes in appetite, weight, sleep pattern, libido, concentration, memory, and pleasure in life.

- Is there diurnal variation?
- What drugs is the patient taking?
- Is there a relation to the menstrual cycle?
- Physically examine the patient thoroughly.
- In a first depression haematological/biochemical and thyroid screening is needed, and in the middle-aged B12/folic acid, syphilitic serology, and chest X-ray should be performed.

Differential diagnosis

1. organic brain diseases (remember pseudodementia!)
2. physical illness:
   carcinoma/lymphoma
   infections
   endocrine disorders
   metabolic disorders
   nutritional disorders
3. medicinal drugs:
   steroids
   antihypertensives
   CNS drugs
   anticancer drugs
4. psychotic illness
5. affective illness
6. intoxication
7. situational reaction (grief and mourning)
8. personality disorder.

Management

- Identify the suicidal. Get to know the patient. Delay treatment for a few days if in hospital as spontaneous recovery is possible. Grief must be supported and talked through. Depression needs chemical treatment. All patients need explanation and rehabilitation on recovery.

Setting the scene

Sadness is a universally experienced emotion—we have all felt it. Some of us have, or will, experience it very keenly, usually in response to situations that we would expect to make us feel that way (though the grief is no less painful for all that). A few of us will experience sadness to a degree when it becomes overwhelming, or its intensity and pain passes without the understanding of those fortunate enough never to have experienced it. Sadness, of any degree of intensity, may appear to have arisen spontaneously, or may appear to be of an intensity out of proportion to the events apparently causing it. You must always remember that this is a value judgement, and until you have a large and universal experience of life, value judgements are like rapids in a river, often shallow and usually treacherous.

Grief and mourning can be suspended or controlled, only to spring up many months later, often when the person is least prepared for it, triggered off by a chance remark or a passing memory. Grief can be intense and overwhelming and therefore look like an illness. For one reason or another it may not remit because the mechanisms that allow the natural resolution of grief have failed to operate. Sadness then can be a reaction, exaggerated or not, or it can be imposed from within, an illness.

It can also look like a physical illness because it often carries somatic symptoms with it. Many people with pathological sadness feel ill rather than depressed, and many people who are physically ill, whether or not the illness is a mortal one, feel sad. Depression is often accompanied by somatic complaints, particularly pain, shortness of breath, gastrointestinal symptoms, and fatigue.

Many people feel ashamed of being sad and will put on a brave face and you will need to be able to see behind the mask that the patient is presenting to the world. How well people cope with sadness depends on their personality (both genetically determined and acquired), their previous life experiences (particularly of loss and at what age it occurred), and their upbringing. The same biological degree of depression may seem to barely ruffle the existence of one person, who accepts it with stoic calm, but may seem to have completely destroyed the sanity of another patient, who might seem to have been completely overwhelmed by the experience.

As mentioned previously, there is undoubted infectivity of affect. When interviewing or counselling a depressed patient you may go through a bewildering variety of emotional reactions to the patient, such as, irritation with his slowness and hopelessness or empathically related feelings of sadness and despair that the patient will never get better (because, like him, you have got his problems out of proportion). If you find naked grief unpleasant to be with, you may wish to detach yourself from the patient and fail to recognize the seriousness of the patient's feelings or of the threat that they pose to his life.

There is one other aspect of depression that is important. It is one of the very few psychiatric conditions in which it is both permissible and necessary that, at least for a while, you take over some aspects of the patient's decision-making as his jaundiced view of his life may make him make fundamental changes in it that he will regret when he has recovered. This loss of ability to see himself and his life realistically also means that his account of his relationships, his past life, and present circumstances will be jaundiced and 'seen through a glass, darkly,' and you will need to make allowances for this when assessing him.

Another difficulty of assessment in depression is that it is often contaminated or associated with anxiety, and it is sometimes difficult to tell which is the predominant affect. The two can look very similar and they share some common characteristics (early morning waking, expectant dread, etc.). You do need to try to decide which is the predominant affect, and treat that rather than trying to treat both.

Depression has a mortality rate both in terms of suicide and also of the loss of fighting spirit and the will to live, which means that the patient may not be able to overcome coincidental physical illness. Depression also has a strong morbidity rate, and morbidity extends to those who live with the patient.

Assessment of depression

Also read Sections 3D (p. 75), 4B (p. 130), 4D (p. 153), 4H (p. 215), and 4P (p. 370).

A full psychiatric history and assessment is obviously mandatory in a patient with depression, particularly looking at the patient's past history and experiences, which may explain the aetiology of his depression. His previous psychiatric history is also important in assessing the prognosis of his depression. It is important to pick up, for instance, episodes of affective change that have previously occurred in the patient without being formally treated or recognized.

A full examination of the patient's mental state is necessary, looking particularly for delusions and hallucinatory experiences (which may not be volunteered). Depressive psychotic experiences are affect-laden (delusions of self-blame, guilt, unworthiness, hypochondriacal delusions, etc.). These will both influence your immediate management and tell you something about the suicide risk that the patient poses (see Section 4H (p. 215) for full assessment of the suicidal patient). The severely agitated or retarded patient may be difficult to assess (Section 4B (p. 130) and 4P (p. 370)). In addition to assessing the patient for suicidal risk (remember to record your findings clearly), you will need to look at his potential risk for aggression. Anger is often a contaminating emotion in the depressed and depression may well release previously inhibited behaviour such as aggression. The sudden onset of unexpected anti-social behaviour in someone of previously good character is often caused by a depressive illness (see Section 4J (p. 288)). The depressed patient may be a risk to others if he is suicidal, particularly his family (see p. 232).

It is particularly important to look at the biological changes that may take place in depression and enquire about the patient's appetite, any changes in weight, changes in sleep cycle, particularly insomnia and early morning waking or hypersomnia, and diurnal variation in depressive symptoms. Diurnal variation can be misleading. If you only assess patients in the afternoon you may seriously underestimate how depressed they are. Changes also take place in libido, usually in a downwards direction, but occasionally a kind of frantic indulgence in sexual activity is used by some people as a defence against depression. Concentration and memory may be impaired and will need careful asssessment, particularly if you are dealing with a possible pseudodementia.

Another characteristic symptom of depression is **anhedonia** or loss of pleasure in the patient's usual pursuits ('How weary, stale, flat, and unprofitable, Seem to me all the uses of this world'). You will pick this up more from the patient's description of his life than from asking him directly whether he has it. If you are satisfied that you are dealing with depression you obviously need to look to see if you are dealing with a bipolar or unipolar depression. Careful enquiry about whether the patient has ever had any, even mild, episodes of hypomania is important.

Because of its association with physical illness and because many physical illnesses can present with a depression-like syndrome, a full medical and neurological examination is necessary, particularly if you are investigating a first episode of depression. Certain screening investigations are mandatory, including full blood count and indices, biochemical profile, and thyroid function tests. In the middle-aged and elderly, assessment of serum B12 and folic acid levels is important, as is a chest X-ray and a serological examination for syphilis, plus examination of the pupils and proprioception. If a full physical history and examination suggests the possibility of an underlying disease, then other investigations may well need to be done, although it must be recognized that many patients with depression have physical symptoms (particularly gastrointestinal, respiratory, cardiovascular, and pain). These symptoms, plus the weight loss that the patient may well have experienced, may give a spurious impression of physical illness, particularly cancer, when no such illness exists.

Depression may be associated with physical illness in several ways:

1. As a true component of the illness due to changes in neurotransmitter status (as in Cushing's syndrome).

2. Depression may resemble the symptoms of illness so closely as to be mistaken for it (as in myxoedema) and vice versa.

3. Depression may occur as a complication of the illness or as a reaction to it (as in ME).

4. A drug used to treat illness may cause depression (for example, steroids).

5. More than one factor may operate.

Despite the earnest endeavours of many research psychiatrists there are as yet no biological tests for the presence of depression itself. The decision about how many physical investigations to undertake in a depressed patient can be very difficult. There is also no infallible way of recognizing those patients who are particularly at risk of killing themselves (see Section 4H, p. 215) A full drug history is also necessary in assessing patients who are depressed.

Differential diagnosis

Organic mental states

1. delirium (acute brain syndrome)
2. dementia (chronic brain syndrome)
3. other physical illnesses
4. medicinal drugs.

Delirium

Depressive symptoms may occasionally contaminate delirium, and conversely a severe agitated depression, in which the patient cannot concentrate and appears disorientated, may be mistaken for delirium. Depression is also part of the aftermath of other delirious illnesses. Some medical illnesses which can cause delirium can also cause depression (see below). As indicated earlier, mania can look like delirium and hypomania that drops rapidly into severe depression may be diagnostically puzzling.

Dementia

Dementia and depression can be very difficult to distinguish and pseudodementia is an important part of the differential diagnosis of dementia (see Section 4F, p. 173). Many patients who are dementing pass through depressive episodes, particularly if they retain some insight into their failing powers. Because both conditions are common, both may exist side by side. The commonest mistake to make is to misidentify a depressive illness as a dementia (the patient's loss of interest in his surroundings, apparent memory impairment, and poor concentration being mistaken for dementia). Occasionally the mistake can be the other way round: an early dementia can look very like depression, the emotional lability of early dementia being mistaken for diurnal variation.

Many of the neurological conditions that cause dementia can also cause depression and again the two conditions may occur side by side, which can make assessment difficult. Although cerebral syphilis is rare nowadays, it still occurs and usually presents as a depression with dementing features and therefore still needs to be considered in the differential diagnosis of this syndrome. Most patients with cerebral syphilis will have pupillary signs: a few will have negative syphilitic serology and so if you are still suspicious cerebrospinal fluid serology will need to be done. Depression can occur in multiple sclerosis and may occur early. Depression is much more common than would be expected by chance in Parkinson's disease, and bradykinesia and lack of facial expression may be common to both conditions. Depression is common in cerebrovascular disease, is extremely common after strokes, and may contaminate multi-infarct dementia. Depression is very usual in Huntington's chorea and many patients with the condition have episodes of depression before the chorea appears. Central nervous system intoxication with heavy metals (for example, lead and manganese) may also give rise to depressive symptoms, with or without signs of organic impairment.

Brain tumours may cause depression without physical signs. Headache, poor concentration, and slowing of thought processes due to raised intracranial pressure may easily be thought to be depressive symptoms and a tumour overlooked. Frontal meningiomas and tumours of the corpus callosum are particularly likely to present with affective symptoms.

Medical illnesses

A wide variety of medical illnesses may be associated with, or cause, depressive symptoms and there may be little in the way of physical signs or physical symptoms, apart from depression, to aid you. Many patients with depression have unnecessary physical investigations performed because they have physical symptoms, but often necessary physical investigations are not done in those patients who actually do need them. Neoplasms often present with depression. This is particularly true of carcinoma of the head of the pancreas (physical symptoms of this neoplasm often present very late), and carcinoma of the lung. Some carcinomas of the lung produce secondary endocrine changes or are hormone secreting. Metastatic spread of many cancers can cause symptoms resembling depression. Lymphomas also commonly seem to cause a depressive syndrome. These depressive syndromes occur in distinction to the fatigue, anorexia, and weight loss that many cancers cause and, of course, the understandable depressive reaction to knowing that one has cancer.

Infections are also associated with depression. Infectious mononucleosis, hepatitis, and tuberculosis are the commonest, but viral encephalitis may often be ushered in by a prodromal depressive phase. Some illnesses are followed by depression when they resolve. The classical example is influenza. Although there have been some studies that have thrown doubt on the relationship between depression and influenza, a severe depression following closely upon influenza is clinically well recognized and is associated with a good prognosis. Some authorities now ascribe myalgic encephalomyelitis (ME) to the effect of a chronic viral infection, but many psychiatrists would see it as a state of demoralization, anxiety, and depression following the virus infection, which tends to become self-perpetuating. The general debility and weight loss of AIDS can also be mistaken for depression.

Endocrine disorders may also present with depression. Cushing's syndrome is particularly likely to be accompanied by a severe psychotic depression and depression can also be the presenting feature of Addison's disease and hyperaldosteronism (Conn's syndrome). Depression is part of the differential diagnosis of hypothyroidism. The apathy, slowing down, poor memory, and sluggishness of somebody with myxoedema can look very like a depression, although patients with myxoedema do not usually feel depressed. Paradoxically, thyrotoxicosis often presents with depression rather than agitation or excitement. Hyperparathyroidism is often accompanied by depressive illness, and depression may be the presenting symptom of it. Hypopituitarism (again with apathy, sluggishness, and general slowing down) may closely resemble depression, and some patients with acromegaly have an associated severe depression. Some metabolic disorders, particularly uraemia and rarely hypokalaemia and hyponatraemia, may be mistaken for depression. Epilepsy is often accompanied by depression, either as a prodroma to the ictus, as an aura, as the ictus itself, or postictally. Depression is also very likely to occur as epilepsy resolves.

Collagen disorders, particularly systemic lupus erythematosus and polyarteritis nodosa, may be associated with depression, and in the elderly temporal arteritis may be ushered in by a depressive syndrome.

Nutritional and deficiency diseases may also present with, or be associated with, depression. Vitamin B12 deficiency (combined degeneration of the cord) is often associated with a depressive syndrome that may be the presenting feature, and it is possible that folic acid deficiency may also be. Pellagra and thiamine deficiency may be associated with depression: some patients with depression may have scurvy.

Depression is also associated with the menstrual cycle. Recurrent severe premenstrual depression does occur. As a depressive illness resolves in a woman (particularly puerperal depression), premenstrual re-exacerbation of the depression may occur long after the main depression has resolved. In middle-aged women it can sometimes be difficult to distinguish between a depressive illness and the symptoms of the climacteric (depression is certainly a menopausal symptom). Puerperal depression is well recognized but has to be distinguished from the almost universal experience of a sudden brief letting down of spirits following childbirth, which produces exhaustion and tearfulness, usually on the third day post-partum. Puerperal depression may be contaminated by psychotic symptoms or by mania and tends to come on about ten days post-partum.

Medicinal drugs

Some medicinal drugs can cause depression. The mechanism seems to be twofold. The drug may have an effect on the neurotransmitter systems that seem to be involved in the regulation of mood states and therefore cause direct lowering of mood (for example, steroids). Other drugs do not have a direct effect on transmitter systems, but do cause lethargy and other symptoms that resemble and can be mistaken for depression. Withdrawal of some psychoactive drugs may also give rise to a usually short-lived depressive reaction. It is sometimes not clear which particular mechanism is operating. Drugs that are most commonly associated with a true or a pseudodepressive reaction include:

1. corticosteroids;
2. oral contraceptives;
3. antihypertensive drugs, particularly reserpine, methyldopa, beta-blocking drugs (occasionally), clonidine, and guanethedine;
4. psychomimetic drugs;
5. levodopa;
6. morphia, pentazocine, and other opiate-like drugs;
7. anticonvulsants, particularly phenobarbitone, phenytoin, primidone, and possibly vigabatrin; all anticonvulsants can cause depression if blood levels enter the toxic range; remember that successful control of epilepsy may lead to severe, if transient, depression;
8. withdrawal of amphetamine, cocaine, and anorectics;
9. anticancer drugs (like vincristine); it is difficult to know if this is a true drug effect or just an unpleasant side-effect of the drug, or due to the disease the drug is treating;
10. some psychotropic drugs, particularly neuroleptics (for example, chlorpromazine, haloperidol).

Psychotic illness

1. schizophrenia
2. paranoid states
3. reactive psychosis.

Many patients with schizophrenia have episodes of depression or sadness. Sometimes this is due to the patient's appreciation of what has happened to him, or is due to the medication that the patient has been given, but there is a biological link between depression and schizophrenia and it can be difficult to decide if one is dealing with a primary schizophrenia in which there is a marked affective component or vice versa. Unfortunately, many depressed patients acquire a spurious label of schizophrenia because they are deluded or hallucinated (or both) and the affect-laden quality of the experience has not been appreciated. Mania is often mistaken for schizophrenia (see Section 4B, p. 130). In such patients a sudden swing to depression is not surprising. Generally, if you have a patient with apparent schizophrenic symptoms who has an obvious and clear-cut depression as well, you are probably dealing with a primary affective disorder and should treat it as such.

Depression is often accompanied by paranoid delusions, and before making a diagnosis of a primary paranoid disorder you should be very certain that you are not really dealing with a depressive illness. An acute reactive psychosis often has strong affective symptomatology as well, and it is important to decide whether you are dealing with a depressive reaction rather than a psychotic one.

Affective illness

1. mania

2. depression.

Primary affective illness is obviously the most likely diagnosis in anybody whom you see with a depressive state, but it is important to try to distinguish between bipolar and unipolar affective disorder (see Section 6B, p. 455) as this will to some extent influence your management of the patient and the prognosis that you give to him. Mania and depression can occasionally exist side by side. Such mixed affective states, in which the patient has symptoms of both mania and depression, are not uncommon.

Intoxication

Many people drink when they are depressed. There is a subgroup of alcoholics who seem to have a primary affective disorder with secondary alcoholism. They help to brighten up the otherwise gloomy prognosis of alcoholism and are worth looking for. The management is that of the primary affective disorder. More commonly, alcoholics have episodes of depression that are usually reactive to the changes in their social circumstances and to other disasters that alcoholism brings with it. Depression may be a symptom of alcohol withdrawal. The early stages of an alcoholic dementia may need to be distinguished from depression.

Heavy cannabis use can occasionally induce a true depressive illness, and it is difficult to distinguish it from the apathy, withdrawal, and loss of interest in normal pursuits that heavy cannabis smoking can produce. Conversely, however, heavy use of cannabis may be for the self-treatment of depression, as may the abuse of drugs of addiction such as heroin. Opiate withdrawal may give rise to depression. Prolonged abuse of solvents can also lead to withdrawal depression and possibly occasionally to a true depressive illness.

Patients withdrawing from psychoactive drugs such as cocaine or amphetamines may pass through profound periods of depression, and this also applies to patients withdrawing from anorectic drugs. The depression may reach suicidal intensity and is probably related to changes in neurotransmitter function.

Acute situational reaction

Loss, whether or not anticipated, leads to grief. Although we tend to see grief only related to bereavement, grief reactions occur following the loss of other valued objects (such as pets, personal possessions, etc.) and following loss of function or disfigurement due to physical illness, whether permanent or not (for example, following mutilating operations such as mastectomy, or the loss of a limb, or the loss of a function or faculty previously valued, such as sight or hearing, or being able to walk as far as one likes).

Grief is ushered in by denial. There is a period of struggle as the loss is slowly accepted. The predominant affects of grief are anger and sadness. The anger may express itself as anger at the person or object that has has been lost, or anger at whatever agents are thought by the sufferer to be responsible for the loss. Bereavement anger is often directed against doctors, and at times has led to violence.

The depression of grief may be intense and certainly as intense as that found in endogenous depression, is often accompanied by somatic symptoms (which the sufferer may well misinterpret as symptoms of illness), and is usually accompanied by weight loss, sleep disturbance, and feelings of guilt and remorse. In other words, grieving can resemble depression extremely closely. Grief, however, has a natural history and your approach to it should be very different since it is not an illness. It is important to help the grieving person talk through it, to discharge the emotion that he feels, to cry, and to eventually let go of the lost object.

Intense grief is usually felt for up to six months, although unfortunately many lay people assume that it will resolve much sooner. A full return to normal mood may not occur for a further six months after that. 'Stuck grief' occurs when it is clear that the natural resolution process has not occurred, so that long after the usual resolution time the person remains grief stricken and cannot 'let go' of the lost object. A kind of shrine is made of the dead person's effects, and he is still talked of as though he were still alive. If after a year it is clear that natural resolution of grief has not occurred, then formal grief therapy may be needed for this 'ossified grief', particularly as it may well affect others, such as dependent children. In a society like ours, which allows little external manifestation of grief and which no longer has grieving rituals, intolerance of grief is common. Since young people may have little direct experience of grief, it is important that young psychiatrists learn about it as soon as possible so that it does not become overmedicalized. During periods of grief the body's natural defences are probably less effective, and grief carries not only a morbidity rate but also a mortality rate.

Neurotic disorder

Although the concept of 'reactive' and 'psychotic' depression is no longer entertained by most psychiatrists, there is no doubt that many depressions, of what ever intensity, are associated with a significant degree of environmental stress or maladjustment to the stresses of life. The classical depressive response that can be seen as reactive to life circumstances is a depression whose intensity fluctuates (but does not show diurnal variation), is often contaminated by anxiety and other neurotic symptoms, tends to be associated with overeating, weight gain, and excessive sleeping, and is not accompanied by psychotic manifestations of depression such as delusions or hallucinations. Although you will recognize individuals who seem to have the characteristics of this kind of depression, many people whose depression is probably a reaction to environmental or personal circumstances have depressive symptoms that are indistinguishable from those of depression occurring as an illness. Often, it is only when the patient has recovered from the depression that you really understand whether or not environmental factors were related to it. Even if it is clear that the patient's depressive symptoms do relate to external or internal stress, you may still need to treat the depression medically before the patient can cope with the cause of his depression. You must always remember that many people who are depressed will give you what sound like very rational reasons for being depressed, but which both you and they realize were totally false once they have recovered. It is probably better to regard all depression as containing both reactive and endogenous elements, at least until you know the patient very well.

Personality disorders

Many people who are personality disordered, and therefore often in conflict with their relatives or society, will suffer short-lived or sometimes more prolonged depressive episodes, which at times can be severe. Since those who are personality disordered often have less control over their behaviour, sudden changes in mood are very likely to lead to impulsive attempts at suicide, or even attacks on other people.

Management

The immediate management of sadness is to try to determine the differential diagnosis, to remove any obvious causes of the sadness, and to decide whether one is dealing with a depressive illness. You have to protect the patient from harming himself or harming others and from making irreversible life decisions whilst depressed, and you have to look at what supports he or she has in the community. The severely depressed will often need to be admitted to hospital for a short while unless a full home treatment service is available. The relatives of the depressed person will also need to be supported. It should be remembered that although you can recognize certain factors in the patient's background and clinical presentation that make suicide more likely, you can only imperfectly predict who is going to attempt suicide and who is not, and you will need to re-examine and re-evaluate the patient from time to time.

You will also need to decide if the depression is severe enought to warrant electroconvulsive therapy (ECT) or whether drug treatment alone will be sufficient. If you admit a severely depressed patient to a ward it is helpful to delay medical treatment for a few days whilst you get to know the patient. You may find that an admission to hospital will actually help the depression to spontaneously resolve (see Section 4H below for full advice about managing the suicidal patient).

H Patients who attempt or threaten suicide or self-harm

- You are responsible for the patient you assess until he has been transferred or discharged.
- Every suicidal attempt, no matter how apparently trivial, warrants full assessment.
- Delay *full* assessment after an attempt until the patient has physically recovered and is not confused.
- Beware the brief cathartic effect of a recent suicide attempt on mood in the depressed.
- Do not be punitive, but do not reinforce attention-seeking behaviour.
- Most people who kill themselves have told someone of their intention.
- Repeated attempters, whatever their motive, often eventually succeed.
- Multiple methods in the same attempt or violent methods suggest a strong wish to die.
- Most overdoses are with prescribed medication—watch your prescribing!

- The differentiation between those who were genuinely trying to die and those who were not is often difficult—do not let anyone tell you it is easy!

Assessment of self-harm

- What was the method?
- What was the motive (cessation intended, subintended cessation, intended interruption, intended continuation)?
- Did the patient know of the likely effect of what he took?
- Was the attempt concealed or openly revealed?
- Was it planned or impulsive?
- Was there a note—what does it say?
- What was the patient's state of mind at the time of the attempt, and leading up to it?
- Does the patient regret the failure of the attempt?
- Is he glad to be alive?
- What does he feel about how near he came to death (if he did)?
- Is there an expressed intent to try again, or the reverse?
- What is the patient's mental state now?
- Perform full psychiatric history and examination.
- Is there a previous history of attempts?
- Is there a family history of suicide?
- Is there a history of previous psychiatric illness?
- Has the patient a present psychiatric illness?
- Has the patient a significant physical illness?
- Any delusions of guilt, unworthiness, or self-blame, or of hypochondriacal or paranoid delusions?

- Are there command hallucinations?
- Any evidence for personality disorder or alcoholism?
- Has the attempt changed the patient's situation or family dynamics?
- What is the immediate risk of him trying again?
- Any risk to others?
- Remember that both the patient and his relatives may not be telling you the whole truth.

Threatened self-harm

- Do not make promises you cannot keep.
- Do not reinforce manipulative behaviour.
- Assess mental state and psychiatric history carefully—a few such patients may be mentally ill.
- Try to talk down.
- Rehearse more acceptable methods of coping with the problems.
- If the threat is clearly manipulative and the patient has no psychiatric illness and other attempts have failed, you may need to call his bluff (consult with others before you do), or he may need to be restrained by the police.
- If violence is threatened to others, treat seriously (particularly if children are involved).
- Is the patient psychiatrically ill? Can he be talked down or offered alternative ways of coping with his problems?
- If this is not possible, or the person is not psychiatrically ill, overpower and subdue as soon as it can be done without risking the safety of those threatened.

- If children are threatened, involve social services as well as police.
- You have a common-law duty to save life: you can impose life-saving treatment on those who are refusing it after an attempt at self-harm.

Assessment of suicidal risk

- Always do this in every patient you see and record that you have done so in the notes.
- Most psychiatrically ill patients have thought of suicide—do not necessarily believe those who say they have not.
- If the patient has suicidal feelings, how strong are they?
- Do they fluctuate (and if so why)?
- Can they be resisted?
- Has the patient thought of a method or made definite plans?
- How much risk does the patient think he is to himself?
- Any command hallucinations?
- Any delusions (particularly guilt, self-blame, unworthiness, paranoid, or hypochondriacal)?
- Is he agitated?
- Any evidence of personality disorder or alcoholism?
- Any previous attempts?
- Any family history of suicide?
- Any physical illness (real or imagined)?
- What are his social supports?
- Is he alone, widowed, divorced, or separated?
- Any recent loss or bereavement?

- Remember to assess homicidal as well as suicidal risk.
- Beware *sudden* 'recovery' from depression and those who, although depressed, deny suicidal thoughts.
- The retarded depressive is at risk as he recovers.

Conditions associated with increased risk of suicide or self-harm (including accidental harm)

1. delirium
2. dementia
3. physical illness (and the terminally ill)
4. schizophrenia
5. paranoid psychosis
6. reactive psychosis
7. mania/hypomania (particularly during mood switch)
8. depression
9. alcoholism and drug addiction
10. the personality disordered
11. acute situational reactions (and bereavement)
12. some neurotic disorders.

Management

- Identify the risk as well as you can.
- If the risk is severe, admit the patient to hospital (or to formal home treatment)—compulsorily if needed.
- Make sure the severely at-risk patient is never left unsupervised (even when apparently asleep or in the toilet) until the risk of suicide has clearly gone. This supervision should be done in the general hospital until transfer to psychiatric care.

- If the risk of suicide is less, the patient can be managed at home *providing* that there is adequate support and supervision.
- Treat the underlying illness vigorously.
- If there has been recent self-harm and the patient is not admitted, then make sure relevant community services, social services, and general practitioner know.
- See the patient within a few days in the out-patient clinic yourself to check that relevant supervision is taking place at home.
- Do not withdraw support too soon—many patients will be at risk of further attempts for several months.

Setting the scene

Successful suicide is extremely distressing. There is a natural sadness that one feels for the person beset with such misery that he felt compelled to kill himself. There is the anguish of relatives, felt with the particular keenness and shame that suicide brings with it. Those professionals who knew the patient feel a bitter sense of loss and have a sharp sense of failure that they could not prevent the suicide from taking place or recognize what the patient's intent was. Suicide always brings recrimination in its wake. The guilt and anger of relatives will understandably be directed against the medical and nursing staff. There is the unpleasantness of an inquest, and often witch-hunting by administrators and senior staff who have long since forgotten, or who have never known, how difficult it is to prevent somebody determined on killing himself from doing so.

It would be possible, using the most rigid and repressive regimen, to prevent more suicides than customarily now occur in our hospitals and among patients in our care in the community. Such an environment would, however, be so deleterious to the care and cure of other patients that it would be counter-productive. We have to accept a balance between repression and liberty in managing people with mental disorder, some of whom may try to kill themselves, and we have to recognize that we have to take some risks. We cannot restrain everyone who has had vague thoughts of suicide. Out of the mass of patients presenting to us we have to try to recognize those patients who are at most and particular risk of suicide, to restrain them as humanely as we can, and to treat them so that the illness abates and the risk resolves as quickly as possible. In every patient we therefore have to try to assess suicide risk. This is very difficult and it is not an exact science. Even the most experienced of us will make mistakes and nowhere is Hippocrates' adage 'judgement difficult, experience treacherous' more true than in the assessment of suicidal risk.

There are several important general points to be made about assessing suicidal risk and assessing those who have recently attempted suicide. The first is that the decision to end one's life, or an actual attempt to do so, is often cathartic. Shortly before the attempt, or directly after it, the patient may appear cheerful and relaxed. You may be misled into thinking that his depression has lifted or into believing his protestations that he does not know why he took the overdose, that it was silly, and he will not do it again. Some patients will deliberately try to mislead you. Be suspicious of sudden recovery from depression or of the patient with a clear-cut history of depressive illness who, post-overdose, smilingly tells you 'it's all right now'. Keep him under careful review.

A problem also occurs if the patient has overdosed and is in a state of confusion. Although some authorities suggest that this is the best time to interview someone who has overdosed as one is most likely to hear the truth, in our experience this is not the case. You may have to delay assessment until the patient has recovered his wits.

Another problem about assessing people who have attempted suicide, or who appear suicidal, is our own natural feelings about the act. Threats of suicide may make you feel anxious (because you fear blame if the patient succeeds) or you may feel angry with the patient giving way to what you consider (making a value judgement) to be minor problems. It may take great control, when dragged out of bed at 3 a.m., to continue to be pleasant to and properly assess a teenager who has apparently taken a handful of pills after a tiff with her boyfriend. Such a patient, however, does need full assessment as there may be more to the story than meets the eye. Although you should not reinforce attention-seeking behaviour, you should not be punitive and should ensure that you really are dealing with such behaviour. You will also need to cope with the anxiety of other professionals who will be keen to remove the potentially suicidal patient from casualty or from the medical ward and who may pressurize you into making premature decisions before you have made a full assessment or have been able to arrange proper aftercare. Resist such pressure firmly but politely; you are responsible for the psychiatric care of the patient until formal transfer has been made into someone else's care.

Another problem in assessment is that relatives, who feel ashamed that they have allowed a family situation to develop to such a point that one of the family members has needed to draw attention to the problem by overdosing, will themselves often dissemble and may not tell you the whole story. This is particularly true of the parents of adolescents who overdose. It is vitally important to talk to the adolescent on his own, and if possible, interview a family member who is not directly involved (such as an aunt or a family friend). 'I don't know what has made her do that, doctor,' says mother, 'she has everything she wants.' (Everything, you think to yourself, except the freedom to be herself.) The patient's own shame or remorse may prevent him from telling you things you should hear. Fear of reprisal (as in the sexually abused) may also prevent disclosure of information.

There is a generally held distinction between those who attempt suicide and actually kill themselves and those who, although they were apparently attempting suicide, were not really trying to die but were merely expressing a 'cry for help' or trying to manipulate people around them. Our own impression is that the distinction between these two groups is becoming increasingly blurred and, relying as it does on value judgements, is a treacherous one to make. Every suicide attempt, no matter how apparently trivial, needs careful assessment. At least half of the people who attempt suicide and fail will try again. Those who repeatedly attempt suicide (usually people with personality disorders or who are living in appalling social circumstances) will often eventually succeed. Nearly every successful suicide victim has disclosed his intention to someone within a short time of killing himself.

It is particularly important to remember that patients do not know as much pharmacology as you do, and what might seem to be a trivial overdose of a mildly poisonous sedative to you, might genuinely have seemed to be a lethal dose to the patient. Patients who are found quickly after an overdose may not have planned it that way, or may have made a very serious attempt but panicked after the attempt (perhaps the subjective symptoms of poisioning were unpleasant) and thus sought help. They may well try again.

Most attempts at suicide in our society are made by overdoses of medication. Sadly, most of this is prescribed medication, usually antidepressants or tranquillizers, given to patients by unwary doctors. A sizeable proportion of overdoses are of over-the-counter analgesics (many lay-people still do not know of the potentially lethal nature of paracetamol). Occasionally, other substances are taken, such as industrial substances, rat poison, etc. Many overdoses are taken in combination with alcohol. It is often difficult to determine whether the alcohol has been taken to give the patient 'Dutch courage' or whether it disinhibited a pre-existing suicidal intent.

A small proportion of people who attempt suicide do so by other means. Violent methods, such as hanging, suffocating, drowning, shooting, falling under road vehicles or trains, usually indicate a serious intent to die, although this is not invariable. Following the detoxification of coal gas and the introduction of North Sea gas, suicide attempts using this method have diminished considerably. Gassing using the exhaust of an internal combustion engine in a confined space is still comparatively common and again usually serious.

Wrist slashing, often multiple, is another common method of self-harm. It can be difficult to distinguish between the person who genuinely believed that cutting his wrists would lead to death and the person who was merely making an appeal attempt (or uses it as a means of releasing tension). The depth and the severity of the wounds may give you some indication (particularly if arteries and tendons were severed, or if the patient used the Roman method of opening an artery and then lying in a warm bath to keep the artery open). Those who survive throat cutting are usually serious in their attempt, as are those who threw themselves from buildings or into canals, rivers, or ponds, or who waded into the sea. You should take such methods as a prior indication of the seriousness of the attempt no matter what the patient says on recovery. Patients who use multiple methods are also usually determined to die. For example, a farmer patient of ours took 100 aspirin tablets, and on finding himself alive some hours later he shot himself in the abdomen with his shotgun. Still alive, he then crawled to the top of his silage pit and threw himself in. He survived all this and following treatment of his depressive illness was able to return home.

Assessment of the attempted suicide

It is customary to divide those who have attempted suicide into four groups. The first group (**cessation intended**) is when it is very clear that the attempt was a serious and determined attempt to end the patient's life, which only failed by accident and which may well be repeated. In the second group (**subintended cessation**) the attempt was clearly serious and well made, but there seems to have been indifference as to whether the person survived or not, and the outcome was left to fate. Such attempts are not uncommon, particularly in adolescents undergoing an existentialist crisis. The motivation is to try death—if death does not come then they carry on. Such attempts are not usually immediately repeated. The next group (**intended interruption**) is when death itself was not intended, although may, of course, accidentally occur. The person was intending a short remission or respite from his problems by a brief withdrawal from reality. This usually occurs in those with overwhelming social and emotional problems, but may also occur in the mentally ill. In the last group (**intended continuation**) there is clear evidence that the attempt was not made **as a** threat to life but as a signal of stress, as a piece of manipulation or as an appeal, and not even as a temporary withdrawal from reality.

It is often possible to determine (from the method used, the degree of concealment, the circumstances of

226 | Practical Psychiatry

the attempt, and the patient's mental state at the time) which group your patient falls into, but there are pitfalls. In particular, after the attempt the patient may dissemble and make it seem to be far less serious than it was. In addition, you will therefore also need to look critically at the patient's social, personal, psychiatric, and medical history and, of course, make a full examination of the patient's present mental state and his mental state prior to the attempt. This should be done in all patients who have made an attempt on their lives no matter what you feel the motivation was.

It is important to also try to determine the attitude the patient has to not dying and to being alive. By and large most people will show some relief at not having died, and only the very depressed or the very determined will express disappointment (but remember the cathartic effect of a suicide attempt and the false cheerfulness it may produce). In the first few days after a suicide attempt, many patients will report that its objective has succeeded in that there is a sudden change in family dynamics, or difficult social and emotional circumstances are brought to the attention of others and some relief seems indicated. This is often only short-lived. Many families find it difficult to change their ways permanently, and those who have attempted self-harm often find it difficult to change their behaviours or their own attitudes and may be tempted to resort to it again if things go wrong. You can easily be misled into thinking that the person whose episode of self-harm seems to have produced a change in other people's behaviour, or in his circumstances, is less likely to attempt further self-harm than those whose appeal attempt has failed. There is good evidence that this is not so, and both groups are just as likely to overdose again.

You should make a careful note of the circumstances surrounding the attempt. Some attempts are obviously preplanned and prepared and done in secret, with obvious attempts at concealment (for example, booking into a hotel miles away from home to take the overdose, or taking it concealed in dense woodland or a garden shed). Some attempts, on the other hand, are clearly unplanned and often impulsive with no attempt at concealment (indeed sometimes the attempt is flaunted in the faces of relatives or ex-lovers). Although an impulsive attempt suggests that the attempt is less serious, this is not always so. Sometimes a chance opportunity presents itself to the deeply depressed patient and is taken without forethought.

The patient's state of mind at the time the attempt was made may also be deduced from the contents of any suicide note. It is important to get hold of such notes, although they will often be concealed by families, or their importance overlooked by ambulance men, policemen, or nurses in casualty. Suicide notes are of three basic types: (1) distressing, often incoherent, cries of despair and pain, indicating that the sufferer can no longer go on; (2) more detailed, often rational and clearly thought out, almost altruistic explanations of intent, and often with careful disposals of property; and (3) messages, which are intended for relatives or significant others, which illustrate an aggressive or manipulative element to the suicide attempt ('now you will be sorry', 'now you will take me seriously'). Whether or not someone leaves a suicide note is not in itself indicative of the seriousness of intent, but does give you some idea of what he was feeling at the time.

The method used, the circumstances in which it was used, and the content of any note may therefore give you some idea of the seriousness of the intent of the suicide attempt itself. There are, of course, pitfalls as mentioned earlier, that should make you cautious about putting too much weight on the decision that the attempt was not a serious one, and you will still need to assess the patient carefully.

Part of the task of your assessment is to try to recognize those people who are at immediate risk of attempting self-harm again. Those with a severe mental illness will obviously remain at risk until the illness has been treated and relieved, and they represent about a tenth of people who attempt suicide. There is also a group of repeated self-harmers, often suffering from alcoholism or personality disorder, for whom self-harm has almost become a way of life (and, eventually, sadly often a way of death). They seem to have a short fuse in terms of reacting to unpleasant circumstances, and reach for the razor or the bottle of pills without pausing to think of the consequences. Such patients often present to their local casualty department several times a year and may eventually (often by accident) kill themselves. They usually reject support and counselling in between attempts, and seem to learn little from what intervention can be offered (nevertheless you should offer it). There are some people who, having harmed themselves and having learnt of the unpleasant consequences of the act, do not do it again, particularly if they are offered short-term help and support with ongoing problems. There is also a group of people who, for a variable period of time (perhaps a few months to a year), are at risk of further self-harm following the first attempt, usually whilst some more long-term life crisis is taking place. During this time, two or three further attempts may be made, but the life crisis then resolves and they are no longer at risk. Such patients need medium-term support, which is often helpful.

If any patient has attempted to end his life by means of taking psychotropic medication, both you, and anyone you refer the patient to, should be very careful about prescribing more psychotropic medication. This should only be used in those who are clearly mentally ill and in need of drug treatment, and they should be closely supervised.

Patients who threaten self-harm

Occasionally, you will be presented with the clinical problem of a person who has presented in casualty (or in his doctor's surgery or in a social services office) threatening to harm himself. Rarely this may be a person who recognizes that he has deep-seated suicidal urges and is genuinely requesting help (for example, a person with command hallucinations, or who is trying to resist depressive suicidal urges). More commonly, however, you are faced with a person who is using the threat of self-harm to raise anxiety in others to try to manipulate them or to change his circumstances. Assess such patients carefully to exclude the presence of mental illness. Try to talk the patient out of his expressed intent and help him look at other ways of solving his particular difficulty. Occasionally, a short-term crisis intervention admission is useful, or intensive work may need to be done with the patient in his own home. Above all, do not make promises that you cannot keep.

In some circumstances, however, if you are satisfied that the patient is not mentally ill and is in full possession of his faculties, his bluff should be called (though do not do this until you have discussed it with your consultant and the patient has also been assessed by social services). Although attempted suicide is not a crime, and nor is threatening it, such behaviour may, under certain circumstances, be considered to be a breach of the peace. In rare circumstances it might be justifiable to call upon the police to help restrain and contain the individual. Remember that the press quite enjoy situations in which the police earnestly talk somebody out of threatening to jump from a high building or some other dramatic suicide attempt, and the fuss and attention that this causes may reinforce the patient behaviour. Occasionally, 'paradoxing' the patient may be of value. For example, 'OK, fine. You are an adult and if you want to kill yourself, go ahead—I won't stop you,' but do not do this until you are experienced or unless you have consulted your consultant as it can backfire!

The above general advice also applies to a person who threatens violence to others as a means of getting his own way. Talk the person down if you can, but do not give way. It is important to be extremely firm otherwise you will merely reinforce the behaviour. If the person is not mentally ill, have him charged with threatening behaviour and removed by the police. On no account allow yourself or your colleagues to be used as punchbags. If a parent is threatening to harm his or her children, inform the duty social work team and police at once so that, if necessary, the children can be removed to a place of safety (whether or not the parent is mentally ill—do not gamble with children's lives).

You may sometimes be asked to *certify* a patient who has taken an overdose and is now refusing necessary treatment (including stomach washout). Detaining such a patient is not needed. Doctors have a common-law duty to save life. Providing that you can justify the treatment (i.e., it is not punitive and is particularly lifesaving) the patient's wishes should be ignored and the treatment carried out by force if necessary, without having to decide if the patient is mentally ill enough to be detained.

Assessment of suicidal risk

You should ask some questions about suicidal risk of every patient that you see, no matter what his presenting complaint and no matter what seems to be wrong with him. Do not fear that by doing so you will put the idea of suicide into his head. It is already there. Most people welcome honest discussion about self-destructive feelings. Make sure that you record clearly and accurately the patient's response to your questions in the notes that you make.

Most people will have at least contemplated the idea of suicide, particularly if they have a severe psychiatric illness. It is better, when you are beginning, to assume that everybody poses some risk. The real skill comes in recognizing those patients in whom the risk is greater than average and cannot be ignored.

Try to establish the strength of any suicidal feelings that the patient has, whether they wax and wane or are fairly consistent. Does the patient feel that he can resist them (remembering that if his psychiatric condition worsens then his resistance may be easily overcome)? Does the patient have command hallucinations, or delusions of guilt, unworthiness, and self-blame, or paranoid or hypochondriacal delusions? This increases the risk of suicide considerably. The personality disordered are also more likely to indulge in impulsive attempts at suicide, as are those who are alcoholic or subject to swift and sudden changes in mood. Ask the patient about how he rates his own risk of suicide—this may surprise him, but may help him to see what your concerns are. Check to see if he has made plans or thought of methods.

The patient's social supports are also important. Patients who are living with supportive families are less likely to harm themselves than those living alone, or who are separated or divorced or who have had a recent loss. A past family history of completed suicide is a powerful pointer to possible suicide attempts in the patient, as are previous attempts at suicide by the patient himself. If the patient is physically ill, particularly if he has a disabling or painful physical condition, there is a markedly increased risk of suicide. This is particularly true for those who are terminally ill (or believe themselves to be).

A very full assessment is needed to try to determine the risk of suicide for a particular individual. This comprises a full developmental and family history, a personal history, the previous psychiatric and physical history, the present physical and mental state, and an enquiry into the patient's present social circumstances. By and large, successful suicide occurs in older isolated men. The majority of people who successfully kill themselves are probably suffering from a definable mental illness when they do so. A small proportion of people who successfully kill themselves are physically ill at the time, some of them mortally so.

People who are suicidal may also be homicidal and their families and dependants may be particularly at risk. The truly suicidal may well dissemble and conceal their intent from you. Often you will need to be guided more by your own instincts, by the depth of depression that the patient has, and by the other factors in the patient's previous history, mental state, and present social circumstances, than by what the patient says. Be particularly careful of the 'smiling' depressive, or the patient who, although severely depressed, denies ever having had the slightest thought of suicide.

Despite many attempts, there is as yet no foolproof biological way of detecting those who are suicidal. Many attempts have been made to try to measure the risk of suicide using biological markers or tests, but these have not yet proved to be clinically practicable. The biological features of depression, such as weight loss, early morning waking, etc., merely give a clue to the severity of the depression. It is the delusional content of the depression and a history of past attempts or completed suicide in the family, that is helpful. Patients with agitated depression are perhaps more at risk than average because the agitation is an indication of the intolerable nature of the experience. Patients who are very retarded are often more at risk as the retardation recovers after treatment commences. Always be particularly careful of the patient who, after a long spell of depression, suddenly improves.

Differential diagnosis

Organic mental states

1. delirium (acute brain syndrome)
2. dementia (chronic brain syndrome)
3. other physical illnesses
4. medicinal drugs.

1. Delirium

Patients in the grip of delirium may kill themselves. Sometimes this is accidental or occurs in response to the patient's attempts to escape from terrifying hallucinations, but occasionally it may be deliberate as depressive feelings may contaminate delirium. It may also result from self-neglect. All patients with delirium should be considered potentially at risk of self-harm and should be continually watched.

2. Dementia

Dementing patients not infrequently kill themselves. Sometimes this is by accident (confusion leading to some rash act or misjudgement), but usually it is due to the patient's awareness of his failing intellectual powers or due to the depression that may contaminate dementia. Patients with some forms of dementia seem particularly prone to self-destruction (particularly patients with Huntington's chorea or cerebral syphilis). Impulsive suicide attempts (sometimes successful) occur in the middle of catastrophic reactions.

3. Physical illnesses

Physical illnesses that are accompanied by depression pose a risk of potential suicide. Patients with severe, chronic, debilitating or painful illnesses are also much more likely to kill themselves. Although this is understandable, the correct response to the patient is to help him overcome the disability or to treat his pain, rather than to agree to the suicide. This is also true for the patient who recognizes that he is terminally ill and appears to be making a rational attempt at ending his life. Carefully check that he is not clinically depressed. If he is depressed, then treat it as you would treat any other depression. If he is not depressed, then he should be encouraged to think through the consequences of a suicide attempt, both for himself (and the potential effect on life insurance) and others (i.e., the emotional effect his suicide will have on his family). Often, if the patient can be helped to see that his fear of death can be faced and the unpleasant aspects of dying relieved and that he will die with dignity, then his perceived need for suicide is usually lessened. You are treating the fear of the process of dying rather than of death itself. If, after counselling, the non-depressed dying patient still wishes to speed his exit from this world, it is up to your conscience as to whether you stand in his way or not.

4. Medicinal drugs

Medicinal drugs present powerful opportunities for self-destruction. (You must always think carefully about how much of a drug you should prescribe to a potentially suicidal patient, and make sure that others have control of it and that it is really being taken and not stored for future use.) Many medicinal drugs also cause depression and therefore may cause suicidal feelings (see Section 4G, p. 197). Sometimes successful treatment of a disease with a drug may temporarily release depression due to complex psychological or neurophysiological mechanisms. A very good example of this is the successful control of epilepsy, which may release short-lived but powerful depressive feelings.

Psychotic illness

1. schizophrenia
2. paranoid states
3. reactive psychosis.

Patients with schizophrenia, paranoid states, or reactive psychoses are very much at risk of suicide. There are several reasons for this and in assessing patients with these conditions you need to look at all of them. Firstly, depressive episodes are very common in all three psychoses (or depression may be the primary cause of the apparent psychosis). Psychotic patients in the middle of a depressive down-swing are probably more at risk of killing themselves than the average patient who is merely depressed.

Secondly, some patients with psychotic experiences have command hallucinations that instruct the patient to perform self-destructive acts. These may not only be directly suicidal ones but also ones, which if acted upon, would lead to death or serious injury. For example, a patient of ours heard a voice that told him that 'inner cleanliness comes first'. He interpreted this to mean that he was to swallow lavatory bleach, which he accordingly did.

Thirdly, many patients with chronic schizophrenia have enough insight to realize how much their lives have changed and are uncomfortably aware of their unhappy existence and the effect their negative symptoms of schizophrenia have on others. In despair they may therefore take their lives.

Affective illness

1. mania
2. depression.

In this country, primary affective illness is undoubt-edly the commonest cause of attempted and completed suicide, and probably the majority of people in this country who kill themselves are depressed when they do so. Suicide and attempted suicide occasionally occur in patients who are manic. Accidental death can result from the patient's exalted view of his powers or his own strength. Depressive symptoms are sometimes mixed in with manic symptoms, or suicide occurs at the transition point between mania and depression or when the patient becomes aware of what he has done in his manic state (such as spending all his money).

In depressed patients, apart from the patient's own expressed intention, a previous history of suicide at-tempts, a family history of completed suicide, coexisting alcoholism, command hallucinations of self-destruction, and delusions of guilt, unworthiness, self-blame, and hypochrondriasis are pointers to an increased suicide risk. The risk of suicide is also increased in those patients who live alone, have suffered a recent loss, are male, middle-aged, unsupported by relatives, or who have significant physical illness. Patients who strongly deny suicidal intent, suddenly become more cheerful, are agitated, or are recovering from retarded depres-sion, are also particularly at risk. Patients who have good family support or who are living with people who can supervise them and their medication, or who, despite suicidal feelings, have a reason for continuing to live (such as children, religion, a sense of shame about suicide) are less likely to kill themselves although if the depression worsens the risk will suddenly worsen so that even low risk patients need to be kept under close supervision until the illness has resolved.

In women with puerperal depression, it is important to remember that not only are they very likely to be suicidal but they may also be a risk to their young children, with the deluded belief that they are taking the child into a better world or protecting it from the horrors of this one. Be particularly wary of the woman who, shortly after childbirth, consistently presents her child to a doctor, convinced that there is something wrong with it when in fact there is not. Such a mother, in the midst of her depression, may have the delusional belief that there is something seriously wrong with the child and that it is best to put it out of its misery. Even the sanest of mothers will from time to time harbour aggressive and resentful thoughts against a much loved child. These aggressive impulses are much harder to resist if the mother is in the midst of a severe depression or has poor control over her aggressive instincts.

Intoxication

People with alcoholic problems are prone to suicide. Alcohol may in itself release suicidal behaviour in the predisposed because of its disinhibiting effect on behaviour. People who are alcoholic are often prone to prolonged or short-lived episodes of depression during which suicide may occur. Many people who are alcoholic have poor impulse control and respond to transient changes in their feelings or social circumstances with attempts at self-harm. Many alcoholics come to realize the mess and wreck that they have made of their lives and of their family's lives and attempt to kill themselves in fits of remorse. Acute intoxication contaminates many overdose attempts, and many people who successfully kill themselves are intoxicated when they do so. Often this is just an indication of 'Dutch courage' rather than true alcoholism.

Suicide attempts are also common in opiate abusers, again partly because of the chaotic lifestyle and social disturbance of such people, partly because the personality disordered tend to be drug abusers, and also because of the sudden intense changes in mood that such drugs can induce. Cannabis use is not usually associated with attempted suicide. Solvent abusers who are using the drug to solve personal problems may, of course, use it for self-destruction. Suicide may occur as part of the withdrawal from psychoactive drugs such as cocaine or amphetamines, and many patients intoxicated with psychomimetic drugs, particularly PCP or LSD, may be accidentally killed because of their unfounded belief in their own powers (such as being able to fly from high buildings) whilst intoxicated. Intoxication itself may release sudden intense depressive feelings.

Acute situational reaction

Attempted or completed suicide may occur during intense grief or following loss. The recently bereaved, particularly if they have little support during their grief and bereavement, are particularly vulnerable to committing suicide. Those who have lost dignity, a reason for living, important personal possessions, or who have lost function or are disfigured due to physical illness, whether permanent or not, are more at risk. The mortally ill are also particularly prone to suicide, and it is important to explore these feelings when counselling the physically ill.

Neurotic disorder

People who are anxious, reactively depressed, or in the grip of what appear to be uncontrollable obsessional symptoms, are more prone to suicide than would be expected by chance. Attempted suicide, often of an appeal nature, is common in these conditions. Full assessment of suicidal intent is necessary. Patients with conversion disorder (hysteria) may be at risk of suicide if they 'lose face' by suddenly losing their conversion symptoms. You should never attempt to relieve conversion symptoms (say by hypnosis) unless, at the same time, you are prepared to help the patient deal with the situation that has caused the conversion symptoms in the first place.

Personality disorder

As already indicated, the personality disordered, who often have a low tolerance of frustration and stress and who tend to be impulsive, are very prone to make attempts at suicide, some of which succeed (sometimes by accident and sometimes by design). Repeated attempters tend to come from the ranks of the personality disordered and, as already indicated, many of these patients will eventually succeed in killing themselves. Since they tend to reject help, treatment is difficult and takes a great deal of patience and effort. Many of these patients remain at a high risk of suicide for a very long period of time.

Management

Those who have attempted suicide and failed must be assumed to have been making a determined effort to kill themselves until they have been fully assessed by someone competent to do so. In some hospitals, overdose assessment is done by specially trained psychiatric nurses or social workers, and it is important that they have immediate psychiatric back-up and support. In perhaps a tenth of patients who attempt suicide, the risk of a further suicide attempt in the immediate future is high, and most are suffering from a recognizable psychiatric illness. Such patients will need to be admitted to hospital or supervised at home by a home treatment team. The patient may well need to be detained under the Mental Health Act.

Those patients who are considered to be a serious suicidal risk must be supervised 24 hours a day by someone competent, and not allowed to be on their own under any circumstances (this includes supervision when apparently asleep, in the toilet, or in the bath). The supervisor must not allow himself to be distracted from the constant watch on the patient, and immediate help must be at hand at all times. It is also important to make sure that the patient is similarly supervised within the general hospital until his physical state is such that it is safe to transfer him to a psychiatric facility. Be particularly careful not to discharge patients who have taken paracetamol overdoses too soon from a general hospital, and likewise patients who have taken overdoses of tricyclic medication, as they may remain at risk of sudden arrhythmias for some days after the overdose.

Patients who are judged, following self-harm, not to be a severe suicidal risk can go home. Provision should be made for short-term supervision of the patient (in terms of providing support and counselling to help him deal with the immediate crisis that has caused the overdose or to provide out-patient care of any psychiatric illness). For some patients, faced with what appear to be overwhelming problems, short-term admission for crisis intervention may be necessary. If you yourself will not be responsible for the patient's aftercare following discharge from hospital, make sure that the general practitioner has been informed and put the patient in touch with the appropriate community psychiatric services. It is useful, if at all possible, to get a member of such services to visit the patient in hospital before he is discharged, although this will depend on local custom and practice.

It may be appropriate to refer the patient to the local social services department for hostel accommodation if there are good reasons for the patient not going home (as in the sexually abused). Special services exist in large cities for those people whose attempts at self-harm were the result of a clash between two cultures. If you are responsible for a patient's aftercare (or until other arrangements have been made) arrange an early out-patient appointment, within a few days of discharge from the hospital, until you are sure follow-up of that patient in the community has occurred. All patients should be encouraged to contact their appropriate community service or general practitioner if the same circumstances arise again, rather than resorting to another episode of self-harm.

The management of people who are found to be potentially suicidal during mental state assessment depends on the severity of the suicidal urges and on the degree of support that the patient will receive in the community—support also means supervision. The moderately suicidal can be managed in the community providing that their condition does not worsen, that they are living with relatives who are prepared to take responsibility for the patient's medication and are prepared to act in a supervisory role, that there is good communication between community support services and the general practitioner, and that the patient is seen regularly. If a patient is living on his own, has a non-supportive family, or is severely suicidal, then he should be admitted to hospital (compulsorily if necessary) or have the full support of a home treatment service. The psychiatric illness should be vigorously treated and full precautions against suicide (being under observation night and day and never being left alone) should be undertaken. Precautions should only be relaxed when it is clearly safe to do so (apparent sudden improvement in the patient should not be one of the indications for relaxing precautions). It should be remembered that a constant suicide watch on the ward is draining of resources and is exhausting. Nursing

staff will need support from the medical staff. Lesser
degrees of supervision may be appropriate and a joint
nursing and medical decision about the degree of risk
for each patient must be formally made and *recorded*.

In the psychiatrically ill who pose a less immediate
suicidal risk, it is nevertheless important that they are
supervised frequently and that their mental state is
monitored carefully, in case there is a sudden unexpected worsening of their illness, until full recovery is
reached. Do not withdraw support too soon as many
patients will remain at risk for a few months until the
crisis in their lives has finally resolved.

If the worst happens

Let us hope that you do not have to read this section,
but most of us will experience the unpleasantness of a
patient we know personally, killing himself. Such an
experience is shattering to morale for all ward or community staff who will be shaken by feelings of grief
and self-blame (often reinforced by criticism (justified
or not) from relatives, the press, and senior staff and
administrators who will be trying to protect their own
shortcomings). The fact that there is to be an inquest
often prevents staff from offering support or condol-
ence to the relatives of the patient, and scapegoating
and recrimination may seriously affect staff morale.
There is also the effect of the suicide on fellow patients,
who are often highly disturbed by it and need support
at the very time when the ward or community staff feel
impotent because their judgement has been called into
question. It is most important to remember that on a
ward (or within a therapeutic group) one successful
suicide may beget others and suicide precautions will
need to be intensified for a while.

You will need to talk your own feelings out and look
critically at your own actions (however painful, you
have to learn from your own mistakes and misjudge-

ments). You will also need to help counsel staff, encourage morale, and make sure that the events are discussed with the patients on the ward who will also need support. If it is impossible to support the relatives of the deceased (or if you are prevented from doing so, make sure that someone in the community or the GP is doing so), however critical they are of you and your colleagues. Above all, allow time for grief.

Make sure that you write an accurate, complete account of the events that led up to the suicide while they are fresh in your memory, leaving nothing out, and sign and date it. If you feel that staff shortages, sloppy procedures, or maladministration led to the disaster then say so, but be able to justify it. Do not let you own feelings of self-blame allow you to be a scapegoat, but admit mistakes if you made them. You will learn from the experience, but it is a very unpleasant way of discovering how difficult the assessment and care of the suicidal can be, and how often those really detemined to die will do so, no matter what you do.

Patients with attack disorders (fits, faints, and funny turns)

- Do not accept other doctors' diagnoses—assess the patient yourself.
- Distinguishing between epilepsy and non-epilepsy is often difficult and takes time—it may be impossible.
- Observe seizures carefully—do not suppress them.
- Listen to seizures as well as looking at them.
- Do not diagnose attacks as epileptic unless you are certain that they are.
- Using videotape, see as many different seizure types as possible as it aids history taking.

Assessment of a seizure

- What kind of seizure was it?
- Make allowance for witnesses' fear, and get them to describe what they actually saw (not what they think they ought to have seen).
- What was the patient doing before the attack?
- Any warning or premonition? Any change in breathing, colour, consciousness, staring, automatism, etc?
- What was the exact sequence of the attack from start to finish?
- Try to witness an attack yourself (or employ a competent witness or use videotape).
- Take blood 20–30 minutes after the seizure for prolactin levels.
- Be aware of the wide variety of seizure types (Table 4.1, p. 251): frontal lobe seizures can look very bizarre.
- *Most* epileptic seizures are brief: *most* non-epileptic seizures are prolonged.
- Most non-epileptic seizures are emotional, but organic non-epileptic seizures occur (Table 4.2, p. 259).

Questions to ask oneself

- Is it epilepsy?
- What type of epilepsy is it?
- Is there evidence of an exogenous cause?
- Is there evidence of an endogenous cause?
- Is there evidence of active brain disease?
- Is there evidence of inactive brain disease or damage?
- Is there evidence of psychiatric illness or an emotional response to the seizures?

- Is there evidence of a reflex element?
- Is there evidence of family/social disturbance?
- Is there evidence of elaboration or secondary gain?
- Are there contraindications to certain treatments (age, childbearing potential, etc.)?
- Can the patient do anything about his attacks?

Investigations

- Full medical, neurological, psychiatric history, and examination.
- Full blood count, biochemical profile, and serology. Prolactin level after a seizure sometimes, or blood sugar during the attack rarely.
- EEG essential, but does not diagnose epilepsy. Several may be needed plus augmentation (sleep, etc.) or special electrode placements. Check response to hyperventilation and flashing light. Eight- or 16-channel ambulatory EEG monitoring if attacks frequent enough, and get good description of attack.
- CT in focal epilepsy or if evidence of coarse brain disease. MRI if cerebral lesion seriously suspected in a patient with a negative CT. Chest X-ray sometimes, skull X-ray rarely.
- Psychological testing may be needed as may be social and family assessment.
- Reinvestigate (including asking 'is it epilepsy?') if attacks do not come under control.

Differential diagnosis (see Table 4.2, p. 259)

1. delirium
2. dementia
3. other physical illness
4. medicinal drugs

    5. partial status

    6. subconvulsive status

    7. schizophrenia

    8. paranoid psychosis

    9. reactive psychosis

  10. mania

  11. depression

  12. intoxication

  13. acute situational reaction

  14. neurotic disorders

  15. personality disorders.

Management of epileptic attacks

- Only treat established epilepsy, and once it is clearly established treat it vigorously. Do not make the treatment worse than the disease.

- Have the least complicated drug regimen and try to stick to monotherapy.

- Use carbamazepine for partial epilepsy and valproate for generalized seizures as first choice.

- Withdraw all anticonvulsants slowly.

- Intoxication with anticonvulsants is common and may increase seizure frequency.

- One doctor only should be in charge of prescribing.

- Do not use benzodiazepines in epilepsy except as anticonvulsants (and then rarely).

Management of non-epileptic attacks

- Recognize the type of non-epileptic attack you are dealing with (see Table 4.2, p. 259).

- Do not confront the patient—let the patient save face.

- Operant conditioning and explanation are needed, as may be abreaction.
- Recognize primary gain and prevent secondary gain.
- Help the family as well as the patient.
- Anxiety management, cognitive therapy, and psychotherapy are all helpful.

Setting the scene

Sudden episodic changes in behaviour that are often of a dramatic nature and which are usually brief but occasionally prolonged, are a common problem in medical practice. Both lay-people and professionals find them difficult to cope with, and indeed physicians often attempt to remove such sudden changes in behaviour from their domain by labelling them as 'psychiatric'. Psychiatrists may, in order to remove them from their sphere of influence, label them as epileptic.

Sudden disruptive changes in behaviour, often of a convulsive nature, are accepted by many lay-people, particularly in certain cultures, as a socially sanctioned way of expressing emotion ('Surprised? I nearly had a fit'). Such a sudden change in behaviour, or a convulsion, may result from organic pathology (usually, but not invariably, epileptic) or may be a distorted expression of emotion, and either kind may present to the psychiatrist. Epilepsy itself may be accompanied by emotional distress or by frank mental illness. It is our impression that this is an aspect of psychiatry that is often not properly addressed and in which mistakes can easily be made, particularly because convulsive behaviour causes anxiety even in trained professionals. Their response is often not to critically look at the behaviour in front of them, but to intervene and to try to suppress it (often nowadays with medication). Vital opportunities for observation are therefore lost.

Not all convulsive behaviour is epileptic, and not all strange bizarre behaviour is necessarily psychogenic (up to a fifth of people who are labelled as having chronic intractable epilepsy in fact have some other condition). Do not take a previous diagnosis for granted. When you are faced with that pejorative label of a 'known epileptic', look at the facts critically. If somebody carries a diagnosis of a non-epileptic attack disorder, make up your own mind about the diagnosis, no matter how eminent the authority who has declared that the patient's attacks are not epileptic. Look at the evidence put forward to support that diagnosis.

Distinguishing between epilepsy and non-epilepsy is not easy and will often take time, but it is particularly important that you do not diagnose epilepsy until you are certain it exists. The problem is that you will find great pressure on you to 'do something', particularly if you are faced with a patient who has convulsive or frightening behaviour. The primitive strength of the compulsion to suppress seizures, which exists in all of us, but particularly in some nursing staff and in most lay-people, is intriguing (there are theses to be written on the ethology of convulsive behaviour). When faced with someone who is having an attack in front of you, restrain yourself, step back, prevent others from interfering, and look critically at what is happening. If posssible, try to get a video recording of the behaviour, especially if it is often repeated and if you are unsure what it is (lightweight portable video recorders or camcorders are readily available, and you will sometimes find that relatives themselves can provide video recordings). Video recording is particularly useful at night if patients are having attacks apparently in sleep. If someone is having a puzzling 'convulsion' in front of you, shut your eyes for a short moment and *listen* to what is happening—non-epileptic seizures often have characteristic sound effects.

As quickly as you can, look at videotapes of the common types of epileptic and non-epileptic seizures. As with movement disorder it is very difficult to take a history of a convulsive event and understand what the witness is trying to tell you if you have never seen something like it before.

What kind of seizure is it?

This is the first question to ask. To try to make this diagnosis you will need to take a history from witnesses first of all. Bear in mind, however, that witnesses are unlikely to be medically trained and will often have been frightened by what they have seen, and their fear will distort the account of what happened. Witnesses who have seen many attacks may also have developed a stereotyped (usually repressive) response to them, and may no longer be looking at them critically. They will tell you that the patient was having a convulsion because that is what they have been led to believe. In such circumstances it may be useful to show the witness a videotape recording of a convulsion and ask him if what he saw looked like what he is seeing on the videotape. Be patient, be painstaking, and take the witness through the attack from beginning to end.

The person who has had the attack may be able to give you some information, particularly of any regular warning signs or other events that occur before the seizure, and of how he feels afterwards. It is unlikely that he will remember anything of the actual convulsion. If he is describing a partial seizure, he may have had an altered time sense so that the seizure actually seems much longer or much shorter than it really is. He may remember parts of the seizure but not all of it (say, remembering hearing a snatch of music, but not the automatism that occurs, during the attack). Try to witness an attack yourself (particularly if certain stimuli precipitate an attack, such as overbreathing). At least try to get someone professionally trained to see it, but make sure that they do not interfere with it. Admitting the patient to hospital for a short while for observation may be useful, but often both genuine epilepsy and non-epileptic attacks will cease for a while if the patient is admitted to the safe and secure environment of hospital. Observation in hospital only works if you can persuade your colleagues not to restrain the patient and not to inject him with diazepam every time he convulses. Video monitoring at home is often an acceptable substitute for hospital admission.

There are certain ancillary aids that will help you in making a diagnosis. Ambulatory EEG monitoring (with 8 or 16 channels) is possible. It can be continued, if the patient is having sufficiently frequent seizures, until at least one (preferably more) seizures are recorded. In special centres telemetered ambulatory EEG will be available with concomitant video recording.

If a patient has a convulsion whose nature you are unsure of, then taking blood to estimate serum prolactin 20 minutes to half an hour after the attack can be helpful. If it is an epileptic convulsion, there will be a very characteristic rise in prolactin concentration at this time. It is important to record a baseline prolactin level at another time to compare with the apparently elevated one.

Only diagnose epilepsy if the diagnosis is beyond reasonable doubt. You should seek advice if you are unsure and delay making a diagnosis as the passage of time will usually reveal what you are dealing with. In order to diagnose epilepsy you need to be aware of the wide variety of seizure phenomena (see Table 4.1).

Two patterns of epileptic discharge are generally recognized: those arising initially in the cortex (**partial seizures**), and those that apparently arise in the brain stem and which spread to the cortex (**primary generalized seizures**). Partial activity may spread to the brain

Table 4.1 International classification of epileptic seizures (From *Epilepsia*, (1981). **22**, 489–501).

1. Simple partial seizures (consciousness not impaired)

(a) With motor signs

    (i)   focal motor without march
    (ii) focal motor with march (Jacksonian)
    (iii) versive
    (iv) postural
    (v) phonatory (vocalization or arrest of speech).

(b) With somatosensory or special sensory symptoms (elementary hallucinations, for example, tingling, light flashes, buzzing)

    (i)   somatosensory
    (ii) visual
    (iii) auditory
    (iv) olfactory
    (v) gustatory
    (vi) vertiginous

(c) With autonomic symptoms or signs (including epigastric sensation, pallor, sweating, flushing, piloerection, and pupillary dilatation)

(d) With psychic symptoms (disturbances of higher cerebral function)

These are much more commonly part of complex partial seizures

    (i)   dysphasic
    (ii) dysmnesic (e.g., *déjà vu, jamais vu*)
    (iii) cognitive (e.g., dreamy states, distortion of time sense)
    (iv) affective (e.g., fear, depression, rage)
    (v) illusions (e.g., macropsia)
    (vi) structural hallucinations (e.g., music, visual scenes)

Table 4.1 (*cont.*)

2. Complex partial seizures

With impairment of consciousness: may begin with simple symptomatology

(a) Simple partial onset followed by impairment of consciousness

- (i) with simple partial features (A1–A4) followed by impaired consciousness
- (ii) with automatisms

(b) With impairment of consciousness at onset

- (i) with impairment of consciousness only
- (ii) with automatisms

3. Partial seizures evolving to secondarily generalized seizures (GS)

Generalized seizures may be manifested as tonic clonic, clonic, or tonic

(a) Simple partial seizures evolving to GS

(b) Complex partial seizures evolving to GS

(c) Simple partial seizures evolving to partial seizures evolving to GS

4. Generalized seizures (convulsive or non-convulsive)

(a) Absences

- (i) Typical absence (with 3 cps spike wave on EEG)

  impairment of consciousness only
  with mild clonic component

Table 4.1 (*cont.*)

---

       with atonic component

       with tonic component

       with automatisms

       with autonomic components

  (ii) Atypical absence (generalized absence but without classical 3 cps spike wave)

     changes in tone more pronounced than (a) (i)

     onset/cessation not abrupt

(b) Myoclonic seizures (single or multiple jerk)

(c) Clonic seizures

(d) Tonic seizures

(e) Tonic clonic seizures

(f) Atonic seizures (astatic: may occur with any generalized seizure)

5. Unclassified seizures

---

stem and induce a generalized seizure (**secondary generalized epilepsy**). This distinction between partial and generalized seizures is clinically useful but somewhat artificial, and some doubt exists as to whether it is entirely accurate.

Partial seizures when **simple** are characterized by a phenomenon occurring that reflects the function of the part of the cortex in which the seizure starts, but in which the patient retains full awareness and consciousness. **Complex** seizures occur when, in addition to the local phenomenon, there is abrogation or impairment of consciousness of varying intensity. Simple partial seizures may become complex, and both may be followed by a secondarily generalized convulsion (and are then usually called an aura). Both are usually brief and stereotyped, but may occasionally be prolonged (partial status).

Most partial seizures originate in the temporal or frontal lobe, although may also occur in the parietal or occipital lobes. Since epileptic activity spreads quickly through pathways in the brain, the clinical phenomenon of a partial seizure may not always accurately reflect its site of origin. Some partial experiences are so alien as to be impossible to describe.

Table 4.1 lists some of the phenomena that can occur in a partial attack. A patient having a partial complex seizure may only have a distorted or fragmentary memory of the experience, and a subsequent secondary generalized tonic clonic seizure may wipe out all memory of the attack.

Focal motor seizures may be parietal or frontal in origin, and may include loss of ability to move the part, tonic spasm, or clonic jerking. Postictal paralysis is common. Versive seizures are usually frontally based, as are seizures in which the patient falls and lies still. Phonation during a seizure usually implies a frontal origin, although formed speech may imply a temporal lobe origin. Unilateral motor movement or versive seizures usually imply an epileptic origin on the other side of the brain, *but not invariably so*, and localization may be misleading. Frontal discharge on one side may give rise to a bilateral motor automatism with flailing arms and bicycling movements of the legs, and it is often mistaken for hysteria or deliberate disability.

Somatosensory symptoms are usually parietal in origin. Occipital discharge gives rise to elemental visual phenomena, such as flashes of light or blobs of colour in the visual field, although occasionally ictal blindness can occur (and can be difficult to distinguish from migraine). Elemental auditory hallucinations can occur and are usually temporal in origin as are gustatory or olfactory phenomena (usually originating in the uncus). Ictal tastes and smells are usually unpleasant, but can be pleasant or indescribable. Ictal vertigo (which occurs with no warning, stops suddenly, is usually brief, and is a true vertigo) is said to imply a bilateral temporal lobe discharge.

Autonomic changes are common accompaniments to partial seizures. The very common epigastric rising sensation can easily be mistaken for anxiety and vice versa, and pallor and sweating mistaken for syncope. Autonomic symptoms are likely to be temporal in origin as are most of the ictal disturbances of higher cerebral function that usually occur as part of a complex partial seizure (but which may occasionally occur without an alteration in conscious level). Table 4.1 lists the commoner types.

Complex partial seizures may start with immediate abrogation of consciousness or with a simple partial seizure (of any kind) after which awareness is lost so that the patient may remember some of his experience but have no recollection of the rest of it. Complex partial seizures may be accompanied by automatism, i.e., a stereotyped piece of behaviour, usually primitive, such as lip smacking, swallowing, fidgeting, or aimless searching, although occasionally more organized behaviour occurs like undressing. Many people, after a complex partial seizure, are temporarily confused.

The commonest type of generalized seizure is the tonic clonic seizure in which there is loss of consciousness and sudden intense spasm of all the muscles of the body (tonic phase), which may last several seconds. If standing, the person falls stiffly and may emit a characteristic cry as air is forced out of the lungs through a closed glottis. There may be loss of control of bladder and bowels, although *frequent* faecal incontinence raises the suspicion of a non-epileptic attack. Characteristic rhythmic jerking of the head and limbs then follows (the clonic phase), which sometimes is more prominent on one side than the other. It usually ceases within a couple of minutes, sometimes suddenly, but often with a characteristic dying away. It is important to see several videotaped examples and to have the clinical picture fully in your mind's eye.

During the seizure the patient is not effectively breathing and may go blue, and there is characteristically an increased production of saliva, which appears at the lips and may be bloodstained due to the characteristic bitten tongue. These bites occur along the side of the tongue and are deep, and sometimes the insides of the cheeks are bitten. This may also happen in complex partial seizures (little nips of the tip of the tongue or inside the lips are not usually epileptic in origin).

The attack often ends with a characteristic gasping intake of air (during the attack there are gasping expulsions of air that may be mistaken for breathing). There may be coughing and choking as the accumulated secretions are cleared away. The patient will be dazed and confused for at least a short while after the attack and may wish to sleep. He may occasionally vomit. Although vomiting may be a regular accompaniment of a complex partial seizure (more commonly retching than vomiting), an apparent convulsion in which retching or vomiting features regularly is often a non-epileptic attack.

Pure tonic or pure clonic seizures may occur, and are usually briefer than a clonic tonic seizure and usually occur in the severe deteriorative epilepsy syndromes of childhood. Atonic attacks consist of a sudden loss of consciousness accompanied by a sudden loss of muscle tone so that the victim (usually a child) falls and may be hurt. There may be a massive myoclonic jerk that throws the child off balance so that he falls (**retropulsive attack**). Myoclonic jerks, sometimes focal, sometimes of the upper body or of the whole body, can be single or multiple and are usually accompanied by a loss of awareness, but not always. They often occur in the early morning. Other movement disorders may be mistaken for them and vice versa (see Section 4O, p. 359).

Generalized absences may be simple, complex, or atypical. A simple absence (**petit mal**) consists of a sudden loss of contact with the child's surroundings, which may be accompanied by minor myoclonic jerking of the eyelids, and which is brief (but may be very frequent), and of which the child is almost invariably unaware. Simple absences are usually easily provoked by hyperventilation and are characteristically accompanied by generalized 3 cps spike wave activity in the EEG. Atypical absences are similar, but tend to persist beyond childhood and, unlike simple absences, are relatively resistant to treatment and the patient is often aware of them and may be briefly confused after them. They are, however, not accompanied by the characteristic 3 cps wave EEG activity, but by polyspike and wave forms. Some authorities believe that these absences are of cortical or subcortical origin. Complex absences are more common than simple absences, are often symptomatic of brain damage, and are accompanied by other generalized epileptic activity, such as myoclonic jerks, retropulsive attacks, or atonic attacks. Children with frequent such attacks are often in need of head protection and may become progressively retarded.

Convulsive status epilepticus (recurrent tonic clonic seizures without recovery of consciousness between attacks) is rare, but is a medical emergency when it does occur. When arising *de novo*, it is usually the result of some cerebral catastrophe. In patients with established epilepsy it usually suggests poor compliance with treatment, although some patients with frontal epilepsy or with generalized epilepsy with widespread metabolic or structural abnormality are particularly prone to it. Patients in convulsive status need immediate admission for intensive treatment and EEG monitoring (*pseudostatus* is not uncommon). Non-convulsive generalized status and partial status will be described later.

A tonic clonic seizure may, of course, result from severe syncope that produces such a profound change in brain function that an epileptic seizure occurs (this is particularly likely to happen if the patient in syncope does not actually fall but for some reason remains standing or sitting). Tonic clonic seizures due to sudden cerebral ischaemia, cardiac dysrhythmia, or hypoglycaemia may also occur—symptomatic epilepsy. Occasionally, paroxysmal dyskinesias (see p. 363) may be mistaken for epilepsy.

The differential diagnosis of non-epileptic attacks (Table 4.2)

Convulsive behaviour, often mistaken for epilepsy, can occur because of emotional causes, or may occasionally be deliberate. Deliberate simulation of a convulsion is uncommon except in people in prison or in those who wish to gain shelter for the night or wish to obtain phenobarbitone. Occasionally simulation is part of a dissociative mechanism so that the patient is not consciously aware of his imitation of an epileptic seizure. People who are deliberately simulating epilepsy have often practised and make quite a good job of it. Those who unconsciously simulate epilepsy usually simulate the layman's idea of what epilepsy is and therefore

Table 4.2 Classification of non-epileptic seizure disorders

1. Convulsive

(a) Physical

(i) convulsive syncope

(ii) cardiac dysrhythmias (e.g., Stokes–Adams attacks)

(iii) sudden cerebral ischaemia

(iv) hypoglycaemia

(v) paroxysmal dyskinesias

(b) Psychogenic

(i) deliberate simulation (malingering)

(ii) unconscious simulation

(iii) convulsive 'tantrum'

(iv) convulsive 'abreaction'

(v) pseudostatus epilepticus

2. Syncopal (collapse but no convulsion)

(a) Physical

(i) syncope (including postural, cough, micturition, and stretching)

(ii) drop attacks of the elderly (aetiology unknown)

(iii) cardiac dysrhythmias

(iv) aortic stenosis

(v) atrial myxoma

(vi) 'grey out'

(vii) mitral valve prolapse?

(viii) basilar migraine

(ix) cataplexy

(x) narcolepsy

(xi) transient ischaemic episodes

(xii) colloid cyst of third ventricle

Table 4.2 (*cont.*)

    (xiii) decerebrate attacks
    (xiv) akinetic mutism/coma vigile

(b) Psychogenic
    (i)   emotional syncope
    (ii) hyperventilation (panic attack)
    (iii) breath holding (in children)
    (iv) 'swooning'

3. Partial and prolonged

(a) Physical
    (i)   partial status
    (ii) non-convulsive (generalized) status
    (iii) cataplexy
    (iv) transient ischaemic episode
    (v) cortical stroke
    (vi) transient global amnesia

(b) Psychogenic
    (i)   catalepsy
    (ii) anxiety phenomena (e.g., depersonalization, derealization)
    (iii) fugue
    (iv) unusual tics
    (v) Gilles de la Tourette syndrome
    (vi) rare movement syndromes (e.g., jumping Frenchman of Maine)
    (vii) episodic dyscontrol syndrome

4. Sleep attacks

(a) Hypnopompic/hypnogogic hallucinations

(b) Sleep paralysis

Table 4.2 (*cont.*)

(c) Night terrors

(d) Nocturnal anxiety

(e) Sleep walking (and variants, including violence)

(f) REM sleep disorder

(g) Hypnogenic paroxysmal dystonia

(h) Multiple sleep myoclonus

---

tend to give a rather noisy and violent performance, the whole thing being rather overdone. At first it is surprising that epilepsy is ever simulated since it seems to convey so much social disadvantage, but on occasions an epileptic seizure (or its imitation) may prove deliciously disruptive or help the victim to escape from some threatening social situation. Simulation is common in people who also have epilepsy, which is why it is most important not to reinforce seizure behaviour in people with epilepsy (for example, by giving a child who has a seizure in the classroom the rest of the day off from school).

There are two forms of convulsive behaviour that often get mistaken for epilepsy. One, usually occurring in the underprivileged or the brain-damaged, is nothing more or less than a childish **tantrum** appearing in an adult. The victim, often with a piercing scream, throws himself to the floor and thrashes and kicks, often banging his head on the floor in rage and becoming much worse if restrained. Such behaviour is similar to that seen in young children in whom it is labelled bad behaviour and, providing that it is not reinforced, usually ceases. In adults it is often labelled as epilepsy and is therefore rewarded and continues.

In women who have been sexually abused or traumatized, a **convulsive abreaction** often occurs. This piece of behaviour (familiar to Freud, Charcot, and other nineteenth-century psychiatrists) consists of back arching and stiffening followed by a convulsive struggle with breath holding, gasping, and pelvic thrusting. In our experience it often occurs at night, and vomiting may also occur. It actually looks like a symbolic expression of sexual intercourse (and sounds like it if one listens to it rather than looking at it). It usually gets mislabelled as epilepsy, and its sad symbolism is not understood. It is usually responsible for the increasingly recognized condition of pseudostatus epilepticus, in which this behaviour occurs continually despite (or possibly because of) large doses of intravenous diazepam or other benzodiazepines. It needs to be carefully distinguished from frontal lobe partial seizures in which back arching and vigorous *scissoring* of the legs can occur.

Some patients *collapse*, but do not convulse and may appear to be unconscious for varying lengths of time after collapsing. Epileptic drop attacks are usually brief, the patient suddenly falls and has no recollection of falling. Unless he hits his head and renders himself unconscious for a short while, he will usually awake quickly. Most epileptic drop attacks are generalized seizures and therefore in addition to the drop and the absence there may be myoclonic jerking. Some patients in fact fall because they are thrown backwards or sideways by a massive myoclonic jerk. The absence and drop may be accompanied by a tonic seizure or a clonic seizure. Complex partial epileptic drop attacks can occur and are usually frontal in origin. In generalized drop attacks the person is usually stiff and rigid during the fall. In partial drop attacks the fall may be floppy rather than stiff, and the patient may remain unconscious for varying lengths of time. He will then usually awake confused. One of the difficulties in diagnosing brief epileptic drop attacks is that falling, particularly falling involving striking the head, produces so much artefact in ambulatory EEG records that the record cannot be interpreted.

There are many physical causes for sudden loss (or apparent loss) of consciousness with collapse but no convulsion. **Syncope**, including syncope that occurs on suddenly standing up from a recumbent posture, or during coughing, trumpet playing, micturition, and stretching, must be the commonest. Syncope is usually preceded by a feeling of light-headedness. People who faint are often slightly stiff and there may be some twitching, occasionally damage to the tip of the tongue occurs, particularly if the head is struck forcibly, and there may, on occasion, be micturition. Unconsciousness may continue for some time if injudicious attempts at first aid are made, which include raising the patient's head. There is, of course, intense pallor and a slow pulse rate.

Middle-aged and elderly people, particularly women, may also have drop attacks that usually occur whilst the person is walking (it is often described as like being struck from behind). The patient is conscious as she falls and often injures herself. The cause is unknown.

Cardiac dysrhythmias, including the classical Stokes–Adams attack, may cause sudden loss of consciousness with falling and a variable length of unconsciousness after that, without a convulsion. The onset is abrupt, and the patient has a greyish pallor and a very slow pulse. When the pulse rate returns to normal, there is often a sudden flushing of the face. Occasionally, a change in cardiac rhythm is less sudden and a 'cerebral grey out' may occur in which the patient loses consciousness more slowly and may stagger and have time to sit or lie down before passing out. Both aortic stenosis and an atrial myxoma may also produce sudden loss of consciousness with syncope, particularly on exertion. It may thus occur if the patient is very anxious. It is presently uncertain whether the rather fashionable diagnosis of mitral valve prolapse is associated with syncope (or anxiety).

Migraine occurring in the vertebral or basilar circulation may also give rise to syncope and collapse into unconsciousness. Sometimes this is preceded by occipital hemicrania, but sometimes it is the presenting symptom of the migraine so that it is after the patient recovers consciousness that he experiences headache and vomiting. This is often mistaken for epilepsy.

Narcolepsy is sometimes mistaken for epilepsy or for some other cause of syncope. The irresistible desire to sleep is usually well described by the patient before he does fall asleep, but occasionally efforts to stay awake may give rise to hallucinations, eye rolling, and slurred speech before he falls asleep, and the diagnosis may be difficult to make. Likewise, **cataplexy**, which is part of the narcoleptic triad, particularly if it occurs during strong emotion or during laughter, may be mistaken for emotional syncope. The history from the patient will, however, reveal that he was actually quite conscious as he collapsed, unlike in syncope.

Transient ischaemic episodes may result in falling unconscious and being unconscious for a varying length of time. Often, of course, when the patient recovers there will be some transient neurological symptom that will make the diagnosis fairly obvious. A colloid cyst of the third ventricle, which produces sudden collapse and unconsciousness, particularly on certain movements of the head, is very rare and may take a long time to diagnose. It is, of course, one of the causes of akinetic mutism and coma vigile (see Section 4P, p. 370 on the mute patient) that enters into the differential

diagnosis of syncope although, of course, such attacks
are usually very prolonged. Damage around the third
ventricle or in the midbrain may also give rise to decer-
ebrate attacks, which can look very like tonic seizures.

Sudden collapse with apparent unconsciousness is
often also due to **emotional causes**. The commonest is
emotional syncope. There is no doubt that some people
have a genuine syncope that is triggered off by some
emotional precipitant. This may be a visit to the dentist,
the threat of bloodletting, or some other feared situation, and is often very easily mistaken for epilepsy,
particularly if injury occurs or there is some twitching.
Sudden collapse may occur in a **hyperventilation** attack
in which there is a rising feeling of anxiety with accompanying unconscious overbreathing, followed by
tingling of the extremities, stiffening of the fingers, and
unconsciousness. The patient will often then lie unconscious for two or three minutes without breathing.
The tingling and the stiffening often causes these attacks to be mistaken for epilepsy. In our experience
this is one of the commonest emotional attacks to be
mistaken for epilepsy. Breath holding in children, which
occasionally occurs in adolescence, is sometimes followed by cyanosis and eventually leads to convulsive
movements. It is also common and easily mistaken for
epilepsy.

The other syncopal phenomenon that is common in
our experience is what we term the '**swoon**'. The patient, usually at moments of stress (or occasionally
following the intrusion into consciousness of unpleasant memories or thoughts), closes his eyes, sinks to the
floor, and lies inert for varying lengths of time, quite
floppy, usually resisting attempts at eye opening, and
often having curious eyelid flickering (because he is
taking surreptitious peeps at his surroundings). Anybody who has seen children 'play dead' will recognize
this phenomenon.

Occasionally, attacks resemble those of partial epilepsy, or may be prolonged. Partial epileptic attacks, whether complex or simple, are usually brief. Phenomena that occur during a partial attack may be similar to phenomena that may be a normal experience or that may occur as part of psychiatric illness, such as hearing a voice, depersonalization, *déjà vu*, etc. If it is epilepsy, there is usually clouding of consciousness, which makes the diagnosis fairly obvious, particularly as there is an abrupt onset and abrupt cessation. Even if there is no clouding, as in a simple partial seizure, something else recognizably epileptic will usually be occurring at the same time. The experience is often slightly alien from the normal experience and is usually very intense. If, for example, someone has recurrent attacks of a feeling of *déjà vu*, and if all he gets is a feeling of *déjà vu*, and if the experience, although real is not very intense, and there is no clouding of consciousness, no pallor, flushing, lip smacking, chewing, or automatism, and the person has a perfect recollection of the feeling afterwards, it is unlikely to be epilepsy.

Occasionally, a partial phenomenon, usually accompanied by some clouding of consciousness and with a subsequent imperfect memory for the event, may continue for long periods of time and sometimes even days. **Complex partial status** (and occasionally **simple partial status**) is rare, but can occur (it used to be called a twilight state) as can **non-convulsive generalized status**.

Transient ischaemic episodes or **cortical strokes** may be mistaken for psychiatric phenomena and may, of course, produce symptoms that continue for some time. **Transient global amnesia**, the aetiology of which is unknown, is a sudden profound transient loss of memory from which full recovery occurs. Such memory loss in a comparatively young person can be mistaken for a hysterical amnesia.

There are, of course, many psychogenic causes for partial or prolonged phenomena. **Catalepsy** is currently thought to be psychogenic, although it may well have an organic component (see assessment of the mute and stuporose patient, Section 4P, p. 370). Common anxiety phenomena, such as **depersonalization** or **derealization**, may be prolonged and may be mistaken for epilepsy, particularly if they occur as part of a panic attack and there is a strong autonomic component to them.

Most fugues, in which the patient wanders away in a confused state, are psychogenic and usually relate to dissociative phenomena or to severe depression, but may occur in organic states, particularly epilepsy.

Tics are thought to be of psychogenic origin, although blepharospasm and hemifacial spasm have an organic basis as do the dystonias, which may be focal. Some tics are rather unusual, may continue for some time, and may be mistaken for focal epilepsy. **Gilles de la Tourette syndrome**—repeated tics plus vocal ejaculations (usually swearing or coprolalia, or a repetitive noise)—is also thought to be psychogenic, although there is growing evidence that it may relate to specific biochemical changes in the brain. It may, on occasions, be thought to be deliberate, or may be mistaken for epilepsy as may the other rare movement syndromes (such as the jumping Frenchman of Maine, etc.). Some patients have unprovoked (or minimally provoked) sudden episodes of rage and aggression, and such patients often have abnormal EEGs. Such **episodic dyscontrol syndromes** are often miscalled epilepsy, but are not, as true ictal rage is different (see Section 4J, p. 298).

Attacks occurring in sleep may also sometimes appear to be psychogenic or related to epilepsy, and are sometimes difficult to recognize for what they are unless sleep EEG recording can be done (see Section on sleep disorders, 4M, p. 332).

What to do during the attack

During a convulsion, apart from protecting the patient from injury to the head and putting the patient in the recovery position afterwards, little needs to be done. It is useful to observe whether the patient is actually breathing during the convulsion and to check his pulse rate and colour. Apply very gentle restraint to see if this increases the severity of the seizure (if it does you are unlikely to be dealing with an epileptic seizure). The progression of the attack should be noted: whether there is a tonic phase followed by a clonic phase and whether there is confusion afterwards. Take blood for a prolactin level 20–30 minutes after the attack has finished if you have any doubts as to what it is. Crying or sobbing during or after the attack, shouting, biting (either onlookers or the patient himself), back arching (once the tonic phase has subsided), pelvic thrusting, gasping, and striking out are suggestive but not conclusive of a non-epileptic attack. The patient whose convulsion seems to carry him from one side of the room to the other or who resists eye opening is probably not having an epileptic seizure.

In patients apparently having a syncopal attack, check the pulse, and if it is slow note how quickly it recovers (in partial seizures there is sometimes a transient cardiac dysrhythmia but usually the pulse rate is quite fast). Look critically at the breathing before, during, and after the attack. Characteristically, patients with hyperventilation attacks will describe that they were struggling or gasping for breath during the attack. Do not attempt to lift the patient until the attack is clearly over in case it is a true syncope. Check the level of consciousness, gently open the eyes, check pupillary responses (resistance to eye opening usually indicates that the patient is conscious), and enquire of the patient, after the attack is over, what recollection he has of it.

Do remember during both convulsions and syncope to go on talking to the patient as though he can hear you. Check to see if you can modify the attack by what you say. It is always worthwhile saying firmly, but politely 'OK, that's enough. Now stop it.' Psychogenic attacks will sometimes stop if you do this, and rarely, you can stop epilepsy in this way.

Investigation

If you decide that the patient's attacks are of an epileptic nature then they will need investigation even if you are not going to treat them. Investigation is aimed at answering the following questions:

1. **What type of epilepsy is it**? Is it simple partial, complex partial, partial with secondary generalization, or is it primary generalized? (See Table 4.1 (p. 251) for the present international classification of epileptic disorders). By and large, partial seizures, whether or not they are secondary generalized, need more extensive investigation than primary generalized seizures as they are more likely to have a pathological cause.

2. **Is there evidence of an exogenous cause**? For example, tricyclic antidepressants and some neuroleptics, or following the swift withdrawal of drugs such as barbiturates, benzodiazepines, or alcohol.

3. **Is there evidence of an endogenous cause**? For example, cardiovascular disease, Stokes–Adams attacks, transient ischaemic episodes, or recurrent hypoglycaemia.

4. **Is there evidence of active progressive coarse brain disease**? For example, raised intracranial pressure or active change in brain structure due to tumours, infarcts, abscesses, or inflammatory diseases such as herpes simplex encephalitis.

5. **Is there evidence of inactive brain disease or damage?** If the integrity of the cortex is altered by congenital or acquired brain damage, particularly if this occurs in certain areas like the temporal cortex, epilepsy is likely to follow. Epilepsy in patients with severe brain damage is much more difficult to control and so brain damage is a prognostic factor both for control of the epilepsy and rehabilitation as the brain damaged also need particularly skilled rehabilitation.

6. **Is there evidence of psychiatric illness or an emotional response to the seizures?** It is often difficult to control epilepsy unless coexistent psychiatric illness is also treated. Many patients are understandably anxious about having seizures and this needs management as anxiety increases seizure frequency. Patients who are significantly depressed are not likely to respond well to attempts at rehabilitation unless the depression is treated.

7. **Is there evidence of a reflex element?** Some seizures only seem to occur following specific stimuli, for example, flickering or flashing lights. Other epileptogenic stimuli include music, immersion in hot or cold water, reading, writing, etc. The stimulus often has an emotional association (for example, musicogenic epilepsy). The importance of recognizing reflex epilepsy is that environmental manipulation or behavioural methods are often more useful than anticonvulsants in treatment.

8. **Is there evidence of family/social disturbance?** A family's attitude to seizures may unwittingly perpetuate them by increasing anxiety levels in the patient and may also encourage the appearance of non-epileptic behaviour. Likewise, social disturbance may, by increasing anxiety, increase seizure frequency. Relatives (and society) may also stig-

matize the person who has epilepsy, or worse, over-protect him (overprotection causes more lasting damage than the epilepsy itself).

9. **Is there evidence of elaboration or secondary gain**?
Some people with brief seizures elaborate on them and display a great deal of histrionic behaviour afterwards. It is very important to recognize the elaboration for what it is and not to try to treat it as though it were epilepsy. Epilepsy itself can acquire secondary gain (epilepsy in schoolchildren is often 'rewarded' by the child being removed from the classroom instead of being ignored). Secondary gain can also increase the frequency of non-epileptic seizure disorder, or cause it to appear for the first time.

10. **Are there contraindications to certain treatments (pregnancy, age, etc.)**?

11. **Can the patient do anything about his attacks**?
About a third of people with genuine epilepsy can acquire at least some control over their seizures, and in patients with intractable epilepsy much effort can be usefully employed in teaching self-control techniques. Some people can induce their seizures, and self-induction may be a particular problem, which has to be resolved with behaviour therapy, in children and adolescents.

The initial investigation of a patient with epilepsy starts with performing a full medical, neurological, and psychiatric history and examination. Certain screening tests are then usually undertaken including a full blood count, B12 and folic acid levels, biochemical profile, and serology when indicated (it is important to establish a baseline before treatment begins).

A chest X-ray may be indicated in the middle-aged and elderly, and in all heavy smokers, patients with obvious weight loss, and with evidence of possible cardiovascular disease. Skull X-rays rarely reveal any useful information.

It is usual to carry out an EEG examination. In uncomplicated epilepsy the yield from such an investigation (particularly if it is only done once) is often low. It is most important to realize that a normal EEG does not preclude the diagnosis of epilepsy—the diagnosis of epilepsy is a *clinical* decision based on an account of the attack. Only about a third of people with epilepsy have interictal abnormalities in their EEG. You may well need to augment EEG examination by sleep deprivation or by a sleep record (natural if possible).

In a routine EEG, the response to overbreathing is recorded as this will often bring out seizure activity. It is also usual to record a patient's response to various frequencies of flashing light and sometimes to pattern, particularly if he has primary generalized epilepsy. An EEG may show interictal epileptic activity, which although not diagnostic of epilepsy, may help to localize where the epilepsy is coming from (once you have made the clinical diagnosis) or may show other abnormalities (if, for instance, the patient has encephalitis or a space-occupying lesion). The interpretation of an EEG is a skilled task. The person making the interpretation needs as much information as you can give him, including a full description of the attack (not just '?fits'), and a record of the medication that the patient is taking. *Do not stop medication before the EEG*, although do try to avoid giving benzodiazepine drugs to people who need an EEG examination.

Ambulatory EEG records need careful interpretation as they are very prone to artefact, particularly that caused by falling or movement. Chewing, for instance, produces artefact in the record that looks very like epileptic activity. The person who is going to interpret the EEG for you needs a very accurate description of what the patient was doing during the attack, and you need a witness who, during the attack, can press the event marker on the recorder so that it is marked on to the EEG record. Conventional ambulatory monitoring (although very useful) can be unhelpful in simple partial attacks, and may also be normal during epileptic attacks that originate in the frontal lobes (such attacks can look very bizarre indeed) so a normal EEG during some types of seizure is not complete evidence that the attack is a non-epileptic one.

Some epilepsy centres have combined telemetered EEG recording with simultaneous video recording, and occasionally, special electrode placements (such as through the foramen ovale or laid on the dura mater under the skull) are needed to record epileptic activity that is hidden from conventional scalp recording.

Computed tomography (CT) of the brain and skull is indicated if the epilepsy is focal (either clinically or on the basis of EEG examination), or if there is a suspicion of active or coarse brain disease. Magnetic resonance imaging (MRI) is indicated if one is strongly suspicious of the presence of a cortical abnormality despite a normal CT investigation, or to clarify the results of CT investigation. Only very occasionally is other neuroradiology, like angiography, now indicated (usually when a small vascular lesion is suspected). Other physical investigations like 24-hour ECG monitoring is sometimes very useful, and this can be combined with a 24-hour EEG recording. Occasionally, blood sugar sampling during an attack with plasma insulin estimation is necessary.

Psychological testing of cognitive function and memory to provide a baseline before treatment is sometimes indicated and is particularly useful in planning rehabilitation. Social and family assessment by a skilled community worker is vital in many cases of epilepsy in terms of understanding the impact of the seizures on the family, educating the family, and helping to minimize the stigma of epilepsy, and preventing over-protection. People with epilepsy should learn that they have to take risks if they are going to live a normal life and not overprotect themselves or allow other people to overprotect them.

If you are dealing with a patient who has already been investigated, further investigation is often not necessary if you are satisfied that it is epilepsy you are dealing with. It is appropriate to reinvestigate if the patient's attacks fail to come under control despite appropriate and adequate anticonvulsant treatment, or if attacks reappear after a period of good control, or if the style of attack changes. Attacks that do not come under control with treatment need careful re-evaluation in terms of whether they are epilepsy or not, whether the most appropriate medication is being used, and whether there is some underlying process in the brain that is causing the attacks. This is also true if attacks reappear after a period of good control or if attack style changes. It is most important to remember that rein-vestigation includes asking the question 'Is it epilepsy?' When epilepsy starts, attack style may take some time to establish itself, and changes in anticonvulsants may lead to changes in attack style.

Differential diagnosis
Organic mental states

1. delirium (acute brain syndrome)
2. dementia (chronic brain syndrome)
3. other physical illnesses
4. medicinal drugs
5. partial status and subconvulsive generalized status.

Delirium

Epileptic delirium is usually indistinguishable from ordinary delirium, but occasionally may have a marked depressive element to it. A special type of postictal delirium is **epileptic furore** in which the patient is violently aggressive for a short while (and is best left alone to recover without restraint). In some patients delirium regularly follows seizures, in others it only occurs if several seizures occur close together. Whether delirium, which is usually brief, relates to continuing ictal discharge or whether it is due to exhaustion of cerebral neurons, is not known (it is not a condition in which it is easy to make EEG studies).

Other causes of delirium (Section 4F, p. 180) may themselves be accompanied by epileptic seizures, particularly those associated with alcohol or drug withdrawal or, of course delirium tremens. It may be difficult to distinguish whether one is dealing with a primary epileptic disorder with associated delirium, or vice versa, but usually in such cases time will tell.

Dementia

Some dementing syndromes have epileptic seizures as part of their symptomatology (for example, multi-infarct dementia or cerebral syphilis). There is controversy about whether epilepsy *per se* leads to dementia if seizures are frequent and cannot be controlled. There is a growing belief that under certain circumstances such a condition can occur, and may not just relate to structural change in the brain but possibly also to chronic neurotransmitter dysfunction. Many people with epilepsy are written off as demented when in fact they are depressed or are chronically demoralized, have specific learning difficulties, or are intoxicated with anticonvulsants. Many people with severe and intractable epilepsy are brain damaged, and people who are brain damaged have fewer cortical reserves with which to withstand further brain insult or the ravages of ageing and therefore will appear to dement earlier than the general population. Anyone with epilepsy who appears demented needs careful physical, neurological, and emotional assessment.

Other physical illnesses

Other physical illnesses that may give rise to psychiatric symptoms, such as liver failure, renal failure, hypercalcaemia, hypoglycaemia, etc. may also give rise to epileptic seizures. It is sometimes difficult to recognize that the seizure is secondary to the underlying disease, and not the cause of it.

Medicinal drugs

Epileptic seizures may be the result of your prescribing. Most antidepressants may cause epilepsy to occur for the first time in those with a low convulsive threshold, as will some neuroleptics. If seizures occur shortly after the prescription of an antidepressant or a neuroleptic, suspect the drug. Withdrawal of barbiturates and benzodiazepines, particularly if done rapidly, can also give rise to epileptic seizures.

Partial status

Partial status, in which there is a continuing epileptic discharge from part of the brain (usually one of the temporal lobes), is uncommon but can be diagnostically confusing. Such status may go on for several days or even weeks before resolving (sometimes ending with a tonic clonic seizure, sometimes spontaneously). There is usually some clouding of consciousness and confusion, although this may be minimal and may merely express itself as a difficulty in concentration. There are usually other symptoms present that can sometimes resemble psychiatric illness quite closely. There may be anxiety symptoms or depersonalization, derealization, the patient may feel (and look) quite depressed, or be hallucinated or excited, or may show continual automatisms or other behavioural changes. Partial status usually occurs in a patient who has a history of epilepsy, but not invariably. It should be suspected in any patient who has recurrent episodes of confusion with behavioural change, or episodes of emotional disturbance that seem to come on suddenly and end suddenly without any obvious environmental precipitant.

Subconvulsive generalized status

In this condition there is generalized subconvulsive epileptic discharge in the EEG, which gives rise to a characteristic obtunded state with fluctuating levels of awareness, confusion, and poor memory. The patient is usually mute, but will give some signs of awareness and can respond to some commands, although often only intermittently. This state may terminate in a tonic clonic seizure or may suddenly stop, it comes on suddenly, and may last for some time. It is commoner than realized. Although usually associated with a history of previous absences or tonic clonic seizures, it may arise *de novo*, and can even occur spontaneously for the first time in middle age.

Psychotic illness

1. schizophrenia
2. paranoid states
3. reactive psychosis.

People with epilepsy develop a paranoid schizophrenia-like state more commonly than would be expected by chance and, although still controversial, there is a relationship between the two conditions. Characteristically schizophrenia follows the onset of the epilepsy, but this is not invariable and some patients with schizophrenia may later develop epilepsy as people with schizophenia tend to have a lower convulsive threshold. Sometimes both the epilepsy and the schizophrenia are symptomatic of some other underlying condition, or epileptic seizures may occur in people with schizophrenia because of neuroleptic or anti-depressant medication. Patients with epilepsy who develop paranoid schizophrenia are said to have a better-preserved affect, and the condition has a good prognosis with both the epilepsy and the schizophrenia remitting, often within a short time of each other. Some patients with epilepsy who are said to be demented actually have a severe thought disorder.

Non-schizophrenic psychotic episodes, often with a paranoid flavour, are also common in epilepsy and are probably multifactorial in origin relating to med-ication, to epileptic changes in the EEG, and to life circumstances. They are often brief and resolve spon-taneously. Personality change of a sensitive paranoid type is said to be common in epilepsy and is of multifactorial aetiology relating to brain damage, re-jecting life experiences, chronic changes in transmitter chemistry, and possibly medication. Patients that do have a paranoid personality related to epilepsy often gradually worsen, and after some years a chronic paranoid psychosis with hallucinations and delusions emerges, but without the first rank symptoms of schizophrenia.

Psychotic states occurring in people with epilepsy should be treated with the appropriate antipsychotic medication, preferably non-sedative. Pimozide, halo-peridol, and sulpiride seem to be the most appropriate, although all three may increase seizure frequency. Sometimes one has to strike a balance between an increase in seizures and a decrease in psychotic phenomena.

Affective illness

1. mania
2. depression.

Mania

Hypomania may occur in patients with complex partial seizures if they have several seizures close together. The characteristic elevation of mood is accompanied by comforting hallucinations and delusions and wild excitement, often with a religious colouring. It usually settles rapidly if the seizures are brought under control. Occasionally, epileptic seizures can occur in the middle of a manic illness, particularly if the patient is oversedated, exhausted, or develops an intercurrent infection.

Depression

There is a very strong relationship between depression and epilepsy. Induced epilepsy is used to treat depression and conversely, as epilepsy resolves a transient, but severe, depression may occur. Depressive feelings may also occur regularly as prodromal symptoms to a seizure, as part of the aura, or as part of the ictal experience itself. Postconvulsive depression (presumably due to changes in transmitter levels in the brain) is also well recognized. Depression is certainly the commonest major psychiatric illness that people with epilepsy develop, and is almost certainly over-represented in people with epilepsy. Successful suicide is much commoner in people with epilepsy than in the general population, although there are obviously other reasons apart from depression for this, such as social stigma, access to powerful poisons, brain damage leading to impulsivity, etc.

Intoxication

Epileptic seizures are common in alcoholism (particularly in delirium tremens) and may occur as part of the syndrome of alcohol withdrawal. Some people who binge drink develop 'rum fits' during the binging. A few people with epilepsy are particularly susceptible to the effects of alcohol and may have seizures after even a small amount of alcohol, although most people with epilepsy can drink safely in moderation. Alcoholism, which leads to brain damage, may, of course, also lead to chronic epilepsy.

Overuse of all anticonvulsant drugs may lead to chronic intoxication with drowsiness, confusion, ataxia, and often, paradoxically, an increase in seizure frequency. Often this intoxication is blamed on the epilepsy rather than on the anticonvulsant, or is blamed on a developing dementia. You must always be particularly alert to the possibility that you are accidentally poisoning your epileptic patient. Intoxication can occur with more modern drugs, such as sodium valproate or carbamazepine, just as much as with the older ones. The use of more than one anticonvulsant drug at a time is particularly likely to lead to chronic intoxication. Ethosuximide may lead to a toxic psychosis as may vigabatrin, although sudden cessation of seizures may have a role in this.

Patients who abuse drugs of dependence may develop epileptic seizures as part of the withdrawal from these drugs. If the patient 'mainlines', epilepsy may occur as a result of metastatic infection in the lungs, the heart, or the brain. Acute overindulgence in drugs such as cocaine may also give rise to seizures in the susceptible.

Acute situational reactions

People with newly acquired epilepsy may pass through profound episodes of grief and anxiety and need support and counselling. The usual stages of the grief reaction, particularly denial, may be mistaken for hysteria or for other psychiatric illness. Failure to counsel and support the patient during this difficult phase may give rise to lifelong psychological handicaps, and may even help to perpetuate the epilepsy itself. It will also perpetuate overprotection of the patient.

Neurotic disorder

Anxiety is commoner in patients with epilepsy than would be expected by chance. Occasionally, anxiety is part of the prodrome before an epileptic attack. Anxiety is quite common as part of the aura of epilepsy, and may actually be part of the ictal experience itself. Postconvulsive anxiety is also well recognized. In addition to this, people with epilepsy are naturally anxious because they are fearful of their seizures and the effect that they have on themselves and on others. Phobic anxiety (which in itself will increase seizure frequency) is therefore very common in people with epilepsy and needs careful management. Epilepsy often starts for the first time in the predisposed during periods of stress. Careful anxiety management is therefore an important part of epilepsy management. Reactive depression is also common and needs counselling and support.

Conversion symptoms are commoner in people with epilepsy than would be expected by chance. This is especially true of pseudoseizures, which quite commonly occur in people who also have epilepsy. Other 'hysterical' symptoms may also be seen. This is often because people with epilepsy are socially disadvantaged, have inadvertently had their epilepsy 'rewarded', have not outgrown the manipulative mechanisms of childhood, or are chronically brain damaged and therefore do not have full control over their personalities. Drug intoxication may also produce pseudo-hysterical behaviour, and it may also occur in twilight states.

Obsessional illness is also slightly commoner in people with epilepsy than would be expected by chance, and has a complex and multifactorial aetiology. Sexual problems, particularly hyposexuality, are also said to be commoner in people with epilepsy. In our experience this is often due to the patient's fear of having a seizure during the act of lovemaking itself, although, particularly in men, endocrine factors (due to the effects of anticonvulsant drugs on testosterone production) may be partly responsible, as may other social factors (particularly in patients growing up disabled and disadvantaged who are not allowed to express their sexuality or are denied the opportunity to do so).

Personality disorders

There is no direct association between personality (disordered or otherwise) and epilepsy. As in any chronic medical condition, some patients who have grown up with it and never adjusted to it may show childish, attention-seeking, histrionic, or impulsive behaviour, and some patients who are brain damaged may show similar behaviour. It is often said that people with epilepsy are aggressive, but if one discounts occasional aggressive behaviour occurring either during the ictus or immediately after it and those who are brain damaged and who therefore have less control, there is actually no evidence that people with epilepsy are more aggressive (in fact the reverse may well be true).

There is no direct association between epilepsy and crime. Most people with epilepsy in prison are there for thieving as is everybody else. Very occasionally a crime may be committed during an ictus, in a twilight state, or in the confused period after the ictus. This is particularly unfortunate because the law may not recognize a sane automatism and patients suffering from such automatisms risk incarceration in special hospitals.

Management of epileptic attacks

Following investigation and the decision that one is dealing with epilepsy, one has to consider treatment. It is important to only treat established epilepsy, in other words, when it is clear that the epileptic seizures will show a conspicuous tendency to recur. Some people have one or two seizures that then stop of their own accord. They do not need treatment. It is therefore usual to treat only the second or subsequent seizures and not to treat the first, although there may be occasional exceptions to this. Someone having only very occasional nocturnal tonic clonic seizures, or someone with simple partial seizures, may not need treatment. Since all treatments carry a potential penalty with them, it is important that the treatment is not worse than the disease itself. Try to abolish the attacks without intoxicating the patient. This may not be possible and some people with epilepsy may have to accept that they will not get complete attack control without unacceptable side-effects. It is important to have the least complicated drug regimen in someone whose condition is going to be lifelong; giving him a drug that he has to take four times a day when he could equally well take it once or twice a day is senseless and cruel. Although you should be cautious about starting treatment, once you have done so be vigorous with it. Attacks that become established and do not respond to early treatment tend to stay.

Choose the most appropriate drug and gradually increase the dosage. Use a twice-daily regimen (you can use once-daily dosing with sodium valproate, clonazepam, and phenobarbitone) until either therapeutic blood levels are obtained or the limits of tolerance are reached. If you do this, the majority of patients will stop having seizures. It is sometimes necessary to give carbamazepine three times a day, although it is possible now to use a long-acting preparation twice a day.

The drug of first choice for partial epilepsy, at the moment, is carbamazepine, and the drug of first choice for generalized epilepsy is sodium valproate. Carbamazepine will usually be effective in patients that have partial seizures with secondary generalization. The second choice for partial seizures, with or without secondary generalization, is phenytoin, and for generalized seizures, particularly absences, it is ethosuximide. The third choice for partial seizures is primidone, and for generalized seizures it is clonazepam. Clobazam given intermittently is useful for treating cluster attacks or for predictably or regularly occurring seizures (as in premenstrual epilepsy). Its effect tends to wear off if it is given continually. Vigabatrin is a new drug for partial seizures which can be effective when other drugs are ineffective. Lamotrigine is another new drug, which seems effective in both partial and generalized seizures and may be an important drug for the future.

Carbamazepine may cause drowsiness and ataxia unless it is introduced slowly. Serious side-effects include intractable vomiting, water intoxication, and rashes. Sodium valproate may cause vomiting and anorexia. If this happens, stop the drug at once otherwise irreversible hepatic failure may occur. It may also cause an irritating weight gain and occasionally hair loss. Phenytoin dosage must be controlled by regular serum concentration monitoring. Primidone should be introduced slowly, like carbamazepine. It should not be used with phenobarbitone. Clonazepam can be difficult to use as it often causes ataxia and drowsiness, but can be effective when other drugs fail. Avoid phenobarbitone unless nothing else works, especially in children.

Avoid polypharmacy. If a drug does not work, introduce a second one. If it does not work when serum concentrations are within the therapeutic range, take it away again. If it does work, slowly withdraw the first drug. If polypharmacy is unavoidable, the best combination is probably sodium valproate and carbamazepine.

If you are managing a patient already stabilized and controlled on an unorthodox but non-intoxicating drug regimen, leave well alone. Patients with unilateral partial seizures resistant to medication may respond excellently to surgery, but careful preoperative assessment is needed.

Women taking oral contraceptives and anticonvulsants should take a preparation containing at least 50 micrograms of oestrogen (unless they are taking valproate, clonazepam, lamotrigine, or vigabatrin). If cycle control is not obtained in a woman who is taking the pill and an enzyme-inducing anticonvulsant (i.e., there is breakthrough bleeding) increase the oestrogen dose in the pill until cycle control is obtained.

Assume that all anticonvulsants may cause fetal malformation. Valproate and phenytoin are best avoided in women who may become pregnant unless their use is vital for controlling the epilepsy (since uncontrolled epilepsy in pregnancy is in itself damaging to the fetus). Women with epilepsy need preconception counselling.

Withdrawing even apparently useless anticonvulsants should be done very slowly (for example, 15 mg of phenobarbitone a month, 100 mg of carbamazepine a month, 50 mg of phenytoin a month, 200 mg of sodium valproate a month). Withdraw one drug at a time. Withdrawal fits are common with phenobarbitone, primidone, clonazepam, and carbamazepine, but can occur with any anticonvulsant. They do not necessarily mean that the epilepsy has returned. In patients whose epilepsy is controlled, withdrawal of drugs may be contemplated after the patient has been seizure free for at least two years. Recent evidence, however, suggests that withdrawal often leads to a return of seizures and it may be better to leave the patient on medication providing that he is not intoxicated.

Overuse of medication leads to intoxication. The patient often becomes so used to this that he ceases to notice it. Too much anticonvulsant may itself cause an increase in seizure frequency. It is best to regard epilepsy, in terms of its management, as a psychosomatic condition. Helping the patient to come to terms with the condition, counselling, anxiety management, education, helping the patient to regain his identity, and preventing overprotection are as important as drug therapy in the patient's management.

One doctor should be in charge of drug treatment and reviewing the patient. Other doctors who may be involved with the patient should not themselves alter the drug regimen. Prescription of other psychotropic drugs should be kept to a minimum, because of drug interaction problems. Some psychotropic drugs are epileptogenic. Use benzodiazepines sparingly in epilepsy, and then only as an anticonvulsant. Never use them as tranquillizers.

Management of non-epileptic seizures

Many patients with non-epileptic seizures will have originally carried a diagnosis of epilepsy. Direct confrontation with the fact that the seizures are not epileptic is often unhelpful. It is usually better to lead the patient to recognize himself that some, or all, of his attacks are not epileptic (many already know or suspect and may be relieved to be gently told). The attacks should be given a non-pejorative name like 'emotional attacks' and a positive attitude taken to them in terms of helping the patient to learn how to control them.

It is useful to look for precipitating factors and for primary or secondary gain from the seizure. You will often understand the attack's symbolic meaning as you get to know the patient. Abreaction is often useful, as is getting the patient to talk through his or her own attack whilst looking at it on videotape. Enquiry about sexual trauma, particularly incest, is often revealing, although do not expect information to necessarily be revealed to you at once. Look critically at whether intentional or unintentional reinforcement of the attack behaviour is taking place, either by the family or even by staff in the hospital.

It is best for yourself, staff, the family, and other patients on the ward to studiously ignore the attacks so that they are not rewarded. This often results in the frequency of non-epileptic attacks rising to a crescendo and then suddenly falling. Positive reinforcement should be given during attack-free periods. This operant conditioning is often successful, particularly if you are beginning to learn the reason for the attacks at the same time. Medication for epilepsy should be slowly withdrawn to avoid withdrawal seizures. If the pseudo-seizures are combined with epilepsy, then medication should be rationalized to monotherapy. If the patient can contain his pseudoseizures to socially acceptable times and they have an useful abreactive or tension-releasing effect for the patient, it may be better to allow the patient to have them. It is important to help the patient with pseudoseizures to save face with society, with his family, and even with himself in terms of losing his seizures. If you do not do this the attacks will continue.

Anxiety and panic attacks previously mistaken for epilepsy need intensive behavioural treatment, and occasionally antidepressants are helpful. The episodic dyscontrol syndrome is best helped by counselling, environmental manipulation, behaviour therapy, and, very occasionally, by major tranquillizers or by carbamazepine. Patients who 'swoon' are best helped by behavioural management (operant conditioning) coupled with explorative psychotherapy, particularly as some will be responding to the entry into consciousness of unpleasant thoughts or memories and hence abreaction can be helpful. 'Tantrums' respond to behavioural management, again particularly operant conditioning. Abreactive non-epileptic seizures are related to previous abuse and patients should be encouraged to talk out the underlying feelings rather than acting them out. Abuse counselling is often successful, although exacting for the therapist and time consuming. Unconscious simulation of epilepsy should be treated in the same way. It is important to discover the patient's need for the attacks, and abreaction (including hypnotic abreaction) is often very helpful. Patients who are consciously simulating epilepsy should be firmly discouraged from doing so.

Much of the behavioural treatment of non-epileptic seizures (anxiety management, operant conditioning, or abreaction) applies equally well to genuine seizures, and is better than too much medication.

J The violent or aggressive patient

- Most violence is predictable.
- Do not have a cavalier attitude to the risk of violence: assess it carefully.
- Aggression has cognitive, affective, and behavioural components. All should be taken seriously.
- Aggressive patients may cause a similar response in you.
- Take a careful history of the aggressive thought, feeling, or behaviour.
- What is its motivation and at whom is it directed?
- Premeditated or impulsive?
- Can the patient resist the impulse?
- Was it accompanied by strong affect?
- Can the patient remember the event?
- Was the event in conflict with the patient's value system?
- Any loss of self-esteem or of relationships?

- Carefully check for mood disturbance, paranoid ideas, suicidal feelings, delirium, and perceptual disorders (especially command hallucinations).
- Any evidence of organic brain disease or intoxication?
- Any previous history of violence or forensic history?
- Check factors that suggest increased risk of violence.
- Look for warning signs that violence is near.

Differential diagnosis

1. organic brain disease
2. psychotic illness
3. affective illness
4. intoxication
5. acute situational reaction
6. personality disorder (explosive disorder, antisocial personality disorder).

Management

- Do not be a hero: carefully assess possibility of 'talk down.'
- Confront and acknowledge patient's fear.
- Keep calm—do not shout—be firm.
- Do not make promises that you cannot keep.
- Use distraction when appropriate.
- Establish a dialogue and make sure you can still be observed when alone with the patient.
- Do not use restraint as a threat.
- If restraint is needed use six people and have a plan with you in charge. Talk to the patient.

- Restrain on a bed or floor and maintain hold until chemical restraint has worked.
- Use droperidol/haloperidol or diazepam intravenously.
- Once patient is calm, plan future management (including drugs).
- Talk over experience with patient and staff.
- You have a duty to warn people who may be at risk from your patient.
- Make sure that at some point the patient is searched thoroughly for a concealed weapon.

Setting the scene

The mentally ill inspire a fear of unpredictable violence in most of us. It is important, as a young professional, that you face this fear and recognize three important aspects of aggression that you will encounter in your work:

1. Violence is uncommon, but can occur.
2. Most violence is predictable. You will need to become skilful in recognizing the cognitive emotional and behavioural cues of impending violence, identifying the violence-prone patient, and the degree of *risk* a particular patient poses to yourself, other staff, the public at large, and relatives.
3. You will need to learn how to contain, defuse, and control violent situations so that neither you, other members of staff, the patient himself, or his family come to harm.

The degree of aggression that a society will tolerate varies from culture to culture and from time to time within that culture. Aggression is not always related to mental illness nor is it inevitably the province of the psychiatrist. When called to an aggressive incident as an emergency, it is pertinent to ask yourself if you should be involved, although you will often not know the answer to this question until you have assessed the patient's mental state.

Aggression has cognitive, affective, and behavioural components. In other words, you may be dealing with aggressive thoughts, delusions, hallucinations, fantasies, feelings, impulses, and actual acts of aggression. The three components may flow into each other but do not necessarily do so. They may be resisted by the patient or he may feel that they are outwith his control. He may feel compelled or directed to act on them or to experience them. He may find gratification in them. You should take aggressive threats, thoughts, feelings, and impulses, whether psychotic or not, as seriously as you take aggressive behaviour.

All of our brains contain neurochemical substrates and neurophysiological mechanisms for aggression: aggression is a natural part of all of us. As we grow up we learn controls over this natural animal aggression. These controls will not be learnt as thoroughly by some of us, often because aggression is sanctioned for an individual, or is rewarded, or curbs are not learnt due to emotional deprivation, or are obliterated by brain damage or changes in brain function due to intoxication or psychotic illness. Remember that the natural response to aggression (apart from fear) is also aggression. Aggressive patients may well make you angry and aggressive yourself. This is quite natural, but only rarely should you show it. Do not, however, feel ashamed or frightened of feeling angry. Acknowledge your feelings and remind yourself that the patient may be having a similar effect on others, and that others may be having a similar effect on him.

Assessing aggression

Every assessment of every patient you see should lead you to be certain at the end of it whether or not the patient has any thoughts of an aggressive nature, has feelings of anger or rage, or has or has not committed aggressive acts. Routine mental state examination and history taking should reveal this. Usually aggression is not a problem.

But if there is either a positive response to your routine screening or if you are assessing a patient following an aggressive act or the threat of one, then you need to carefully (and tactfully) assess the following factors. Getting as much background information as time permits is important, and an outside informant is necessary as the patient's previous history and social circumstances during growing up (about which he may not tell you) might contain many clues to the prediction of further acts of violence.

Take a careful history of the present act of aggression (or threat of it), its circumstances, apparent motives, and at whom it was directed. Was a particular person the target or was it random? Was it planned or premeditated? How sudden was the loss of control and how strongly was the patient able to resist the impulse? Was the act accompanied by strong affect (rage, anger, fear, depression, or elation)? Can the patient remember the circumstances of the act or is there true amnesia for it? Was the act in conflict with the patient's usual value system and beliefs, or was it in keeping with his milieu and previously held beliefs? Look particularly for recent loss of self-esteem, loss of purpose, or loss of a significant relationship. Try to get independent confirmation of reported acts of violence, as many young bravadoes may exaggerate or lie to impress you (particularly if you are female). 'Yeah, Doc, I've done violence,' needs confirmation, as do the lurid tales of the 'Falklands war hero'—men who have actually been in battle rarely talk of it.

Check carefully and thoroughly for mood disturbance, paranoid ideations (whether delusional or not), suicidal feelings, affect-laden delusions, and perceptual disorders, particularly command hallucinations, organic brain impairment, and delirium, intoxication, or evidence of drug abuse.

A careful history of previous episodes of violence or threatened violence is also needed, and whether such episodes fit into a pattern (for example, association with previous psychotic or hallucinatory episodes). A careful developmental and social history is also required, with particular emphasis on the forensic history. Often violence is superimposed on a pattern of repeated law breaking.

Factors associated with an increased risk of violence

These factors are only a statistical guide to risk. Sweet old ladies of impeccable breeding, class, and previous character can also be aggressive when mentally ill!

1. previous acts of aggression;
2. history of violent abuse in childhood; antisocial acts in childhood;
3. paranoid or antisocial temperament;
4. male sex and young;
5. history of antisocial acts, particularly driving offences;
6. low socioeconomic group; poor employment record; frequent change in domicile or employment;
7. present or previous history of alcoholism or drug abuse;
8. delirium or dementia;

9. hypomania;

10. loss of self-esteem or of a valued relationship;

11. a sense of grievance that cannot be assuaged.

Warning signs that indicate violence is near

1. aggressive paranoid ideation—whether delusional or not;

2. irritability; rising irritation or tension;

3. pressure of speech;

4. restless pacing;

5. shouting; loud voice; glaring eyes;

6. verbal threats, however delivered (*always take them seriously*);

7. no response to 'talking down';

8. intrusion into others' personal space;

9. your own 'gut feeling' that the patient is about to explode—trust it!

If violence seems imminent, withdraw and consider your next step carefully. The first thing to do, unless violence has already broken out, is to consider a differential diagnosis as this will affect your management. Your differential diagnosis will be based on the information you have collected already, and on your mental state examination of the patient.

Differential diagnosis of aggression

Organic brain disease

1. delirium (acute brain syndrome)

2. dementia (chronic brain syndrome).

Patients who are confused or who are misreading or misinterpreting their surroundings due to organic brain impairment, may often respond with aggression, particularly if aggression was already part of their personality structure or if they are subject to delusions or to disturbing and frightening visual hallucinations (like the old lady throwing bricks at Russian helicopters landing on her lawn). Patients with dementia are often subject to brief episodes of delirium and may also have delusional symptoms of a paranoid or morbid jealousy type, or may have *catastrophic reactions* of rage and frustration. Some forms of dementia particularly affect the frontal lobes leading to loss of control over impulses.

Aggression may therefore occur in all types of delirium and dementia (for a differential diagnosis see Sections 4F (p. 173) and 6D (p. 471).

It is important to remember that acute *medical* conditions can give rise to an acute brain syndrome and also need to be considered in patients who become aggressive after surgery. Aggressive outbursts occurring in patients on medical or surgical wards or in casualty may be due to:

1. *acute* (or acute on chronic) anoxia due to respiratory disease, CO_2 retention, myocardial infarction, etc.,

2. infection (lobar pneumonia, typhoid, etc.);

3. acute brain insult (for example, cortical stroke, brain abscess, encephalitis);

4. delirium tremens (due to failure to recognize the underlying alcoholism and applying preventive remedies early);

5. hypoglycaemia;

6. *acute* renal failure;

7. *acute* liver failure (portal encephalopathy);

8. unwise sedation of people in pain;

9. postictal states, non-convulsive status epilepticus, ictal rage (all rare).

This is why medical assessment is important in people with aggressive episodes or behaviour. Signs of brain impairment may be minimal or difficult to recognize against the background of excitement, but need to be assessed before you sedate the patient. Aggression is a symptom, not a disease.

Psychotic illness

1. schizophrenia
2. catatonic schizophrenia in the excitement phase
3. paranoid psychosis (often with preceding personality disorder).

People in the grip of a psychosis may be aggressive because of the pressure of their feelings (as in catatonic excitement), because of the nature of their delusional beliefs (as in all psychoses, not just the paranoid ones), or because of command hallucinations—'kill all queers' —that cannot be resisted. Violence in schizophrenia, unless a reaction to the torment of the experience, tends to be directed against particular groups or individuals, although it may look random if you do not know the delusional or hallucinatory experience that is driving the patient. Both forms can be extremely dangerous and are grounds for formal restraint of the patient. Although most people with psychotic illness are not dangerous, some are. It is part of your job to decide which is which. If you are in doubt get advice. Do not overreact so that you brand all psychotic people as dangerous, but do not underreact to those that are as you may be risking someone else's life if you do. You also have a duty to warn individuals that you consider may be at risk from the patient's delusional content or hallucinations. Do not have a cavalier attitude to danger when it really exists.

Affective illness

People who are hypomanic have a low frustration tolerance and are aggressive if crossed, or may have their natural aggression disinhibited, or may have aggressive delusions. The depressed may be aggressive to their loved ones when they are suicidal and, as with hypomania, depression may bring out previously concealed aggression. Paranoid delusions are common to both conditions and may result in aggression. Command hallucinations are rare in affective illness, but may occur.

Intoxication

Intoxication with many substances may result in aggression. This is particularly likely to happen in those whose characters already predispose them to it, and may much more readily occur in those who are brain damaged, in whom a little of the substance produces a dramatic reaction (**mania àpotu**). Illicit drugs are often contaminated so that unexpected reactions may occur.

Drugs associated with aggressive behaviour

1. alcohol
2. cannabis
3. amphetamines and other 'speed'-like drugs
4. cocaine and its derivatives like 'crack'
5. PCP (rare in UK)
6. paradoxical reactions to prescribed drugs like amitriptyline, benzodiazepines, antiparkinsonian drugs, etc.
7. solvents.

The importance of recognizing intoxications is so that they are not confused with mental illness and to remember that with supportive treatment most will settle quickly. Alcohol intoxication is, of course, the commonest and easiest to recognize (though often associated with other conditions such as head injury or with mental illness). Acute aggression with cannabis is rare, but can occur. Amphetamine-like drugs, cocaine, and its derivatives cause wild excitement in which judgement is suspended. They may be taken with a peer group for this purpose and seriously aggressive acts may result. PCP (phenocyclidine or angel dust), rare so far in the UK, is particularly likely to lead to unpredictable violence against the self or others. Markedly increased salivation is a useful sign of intoxication with this substance. Some prescribed tranquillizing or antidepressant drugs may produce paradoxical excitement and aggression in the elderly or brain damaged. Acute solvent abuse may lead to aggressive behaviour and may be taken with a peer group leading to gang violence.

Acute situational reactions

People, particularly those already predisposed or those from particular cultures, may react to overwhelming personal events, such as loss or grief, with violence or aggression. This is usually shortlived and burns out quickly, but may occasionally be longer lasting and directed toward particular individuals (as in jealousy states following perceived or actual loss of a valued relationship). Culture-specific aggressive states, such as 'amok', are very rare in this country.

Explosive disorder

Outbursts of rage and anger occur with little or no warning and may appear unprovoked. The patient may claim amnesia for the event, which will settle spontaneously unless provocation continues. They can be difficult to distinguish from the *rare* ictal rage, but this is *brief*, unprovoked, non-directed, and may follow, or terminate in, a tonic clonic seizure.

Antisocial personality disorder

Here mild provocation is followed by loss of control. Violence may become a way of life with little remorse (and sometimes vicarious enjoyment) and is comparatively unpredictable. Because of the potential damage to society such people may need to be detained for long periods of time.

Management

The principles of management are based on careful history taking, mental state examination, and assessment of risk, both to the patient and to others. It is important not to be a hero and not to try to deal with uncontrollable violence on your own. Most aggressive patients can be controlled without resorting to physical or chemical restraint, but a minority will need firm control using reasonable force.

Having arrived at a working diagnosis, your next step is to decide whether there is a reasonable chance that the excited and aggressive patient can be 'talked down'. If you think that he can be talked down, approach him in an open, friendly manner without hostility and avoiding a crowd of apprehensive onlookers. Nursing staff may well want to prevent you from doing so. If they are experienced, listen to their advice, but then make up your own mind. If they are merely frightened, ignore them and trust your reasoned judgement, but do ask yourself the question 'Is there a good chance I can talk this man down?' Acknowledge and quietly confront his fear, point out the effect that his anger is having on others, and offer, without giving promises that you cannot keep, to try to help resolve the situation. Keep a calm voice. Never shout back as this only makes the patient worse. Give any commands (for example, 'stop that') quietly, but firmly. Be prepared to show that you are considering the situation from the patient's point of view even though you cannot actually agree with it.

Distraction is a very useful manoeuvre with many patients, i.e., talking about something else other than what is troubling the patient. For example, psychiatrist (standing in a shop owned by a large, very aggressive manic butcher whose cleaver is poised menacingly) 'John, isn't that a new picture you've got?' Butcher (turning toward wall) 'Yes, I got that at Stafford Market. Do you want to see it?' Psychiatrist 'Yes please. Shall I hold that for you whilst you get it down?' (takes cleaver, butcher lifts down picture, and they are still discussing it animatedly as the psychiatrist leads him into the waiting ambulance . . .). Distraction works best in hypomania and in the organically impaired—do not try it on psychopaths!

Establishing a dialogue and making it clear that you are prepared to talk through the experience is very important, as may be finding somewhere quiet to talk, but in earshot of and in sight of others in case the situation gets out of hand. Helping the patient to see that he may be ill or in need of treatment is important and is done in the way you would with any psychotic or brain impaired patient. Indicate that you are prepared to help the patient talk out his aggression, but not act it out, and as quickly as possible try to relieve him of any weapons he may have. At some point always make sure that the patient is thoroughly searched for weapons —tragedies have occurred because this has not been done.

Make it clear that you will talk through his fears or tensions and will help relieve them, but that you cannot condone violence and that you will, with the help of others, restrain the patient if it is necessary, so that he is clear what the boundaries of behaviour are. Do not use restraint as a threat and do not suggest it until you have the immediate means of carrying it out.

Such an appeal will calm most patients and you can then institute treatment and further management, particularly if you have also calmed those around the patient. A minority of patients will need restraint, either because they will not listen or are too disturbed or psychotic to respond to reason. If this is the case, act decisively and swiftly.

Never attempt to restrain a patient on your own, and if you are threatened on your own, run away—that is practical common sense and not cowardice! The deranged are both stronger and less inhibited about hurting than you are. Always get help. It takes six fit people to restrain someone so that neither the person restrained nor those restraining get hurt or lose dignity. The six people involved need to plan what they are going to do before they start (to prevent an undignified scrum), and one person (you) needs to be in charge. Restrain in a calm, non-judgemental way. A large number of people is needed to avoid one of the restrainers being hurt because if this happens he will lose his temper and wish to hurt the patient. If you cannot muster such a team from within the hospital, or you are in the community, you will need to call the help of the police, but make sure they act under your command and restrain their enthusiasm for 'having a go'. They must realize that the patient is ill and not responsible for his actions. Tell them not to restrain the patient by asphyxiating him!

The team needs to approach the patient firmly, quietly, and purposefully. The one in charge should be talking to the patient explaining that they will need to restrain him for his own good and that they will not hurt him. This often calms the patient, who then submits. If not, he should be seized and put on the floor or on a bed, using pressure behind the knees to get him down. Each limb should be firmly held by one of the team and the fifth member should firmly hold the head (avoiding being bitten). You should not take part in the restraint, but talk to the patient as you prepare an arm for intravenous injection (see below). After the injection, continue to restrain the patient (but only using enough force to restrain) until it is clear that the treatment has worked and that he is calm and will not struggle. Gently move him to a bed, search him thoroughly for concealed weapons, and have the team remain with him until you decide on his future management.

Medication

Intramuscular injections of tranquillizers should not be used unless there is no way of giving an intravenous injection. Intramuscular injections take a long time to work, are irritating, and may be absorbed erratically so that the patient goes unconscious some hours after the injection. Liquid oral medication, if the patient will take it, is quicker, and an example of this is chlorpromazine elixir, which tastes quite pleasant (and looks a little like sherry) and which acts quickly. Intravenous medication, however, is usually indicated.

Your aim is to calm the patient as rapidly as possible, without producing unpleasant *sedative* side-effects that the patient will fight against. Intravenous diazepam is readily available, although it can damage veins and extravasation in a struggling patient is painful. Diazemuls should be used. In a very disturbed patient as much as 20–30 mg may need to be given, and there is therefore a risk of respiratory depression unless it is given slowly. Some patients are also further disinhibited by this drug. It has the advantage of being an anticonvulsant. It can be given rectally quickly and safely (as 'Stesolid') if you cannot find a vein.

Haloperidol injection for intramuscular use can also be used intravenously. Make sure that the depot form is not used by mistake. It provides rapid, safe tranquillization providing that it is given slowly. There is little risk of a dystonic reaction from a single intravenous dose. You may need to give a large amount (30 mg) in patients who are very disturbed or large. Droperidol is widely available in general hospitals as it is used in anaesthetics, if haloperidol is not available. Heminevrin is occasionally used intravenously in delirium tremens, but is best used well diluted in saline and is more suitable for maintainence therapy via an intravenous drip. Do not use intramuscular chlorpromazine, particularly in the unwell or in the elderly, as catastrophic falls in blood pressure may occur.

Future management

Once the patient is calm decide on a working diagnosis and plan of management. This will include planning further doses of medication to keep the patient calm. There is nothing more embarrassing than having to repeat the restraint procedure because the patient has become disturbed again, because no one has remembered to write up further doses of the necessary medication. You will need to decide if you have to formally detain him under the Mental Health Act. The patient need not be detained under the Mental Health Act for you to restrain him as you have a common-law duty to prevent harm both to him and to the general public, but you will need to spell out your reason for doing this in the notes.

You, or a deputy, will also need to talk to the patient, explaining what happened and talking him through any anger he feels about being restrained. You will also need to talk to the nursing staff (who may have feelings of failure or distress) and likewise to relatives. You will also need to talk through the incident with the nurses to see if they and you can learn from it in terms of prevention of similar incidents. You may also need to come to terms with the incident yourself and with any sense of failure that you may have.

Above all, do not be pushed into medicalizing non-psychiatrically determined aggression. Some people are dangerous and aggressive without being mentally ill, or are not suffering from a mental illness that can be treated. Their disposal should not be into the psychiatric service.

If your aggressive patient poses a particular threat to an individual (like a parent, spouse, or friend) because he has delusions or hallucinations about that individual that are of such a nature that he might act upon them, then you must clearly warm the threatened individual, and you have a duty to do so. You will need expert help to assess whether that risk continues once the patient is apparently better, and the patient must be kept under careful review.

Some patients with unresolved psychoses or aggressive personalities may be potentially dangerous for long periods of time. Make sure that such patients (many of whom may be referred for assessment to the forensic services) are known, and that members of staff are aware that they should not be seen on their own either at home or in the out-patients. If they attend out-patients, make sure that they leave the premises afterwards and are not seen at a time when most staff are leaving; make sure that there is an alarm system and that it works.

Do not go into unknown patients' homes on your own, particularly if you have been called to them because of acute disturbance. If you are working in the community, always make sure that your colleagues know where you are going and how long you are likely to be, and that checks are made if you do not return and have not indicated why.

If you are seeing a patient in seclusion in hospital or in custody in a cell, make sure that you either have an escape route or that you have an escort and are not locked alone in the room or cell with the patient (see Section 1B, p. 12).

K Patients with eating problems, weight control problems, and vomiting

Weight loss, appetite loss, and vomiting are potentially anxiety provoking, can have both physical and emotional causes, and need careful assessment.

- Full physical history and examination and vital signs.
- Assess endocrine function.
- Examine the skin carefully (and body hair).
- Are secondary sexual characteristics present and preserved?
- Check menstrual history.
- Check dental enamel, signs of chronic sinusitis, and parotid glands.
- Haematology and biochemistry screen, chest X-ray.
- Appropriate endocrine investigations including radiography.
- Full psychiatric history and examination.
- Any drug, laxative, or diuretic abuse?
- Assess attitude to weight and body shape.
- How is body size and shape perceived?
- Is there an intense wish to be thin or a fatness phobia?
- Assess eating behaviour. Is there calorie counting, bingeing, vomiting, or unpleasant feelings following eating?
- Are there food fads?

Differential diagnosis

1. organic brain disease
2. acute or chronic infection (including AIDS)
3. cardiac/respiratory disease
4. malignant disease

5. gastrointestinal disease (including malabsorption)
6. endocrine disease (thyrotoxicosis, pituitary failure, Addison's disease)
7. tumours of the hypothalamus/third ventricle
8. CNS stimulants
9. schizophrenia
10. mania
11. depression
12. anxiety
13. anorexia nervosa
14. bulimia nervosa.

Management

- Careful assessment. Admit the very severely under-weight or vomiting patient. Get the patient to keep a diary, and establish rapport. Use behavioural or cognitive therapy to help the patient make slow adjustments in the right direction.

Setting the scene

We live in a society that pays particular attention to a perceived ideal weight, and this social target is often far from the biological one that most people can reach. We also live in a society that sees good eating as a sign of good mental and physical health, in which the eating patterns of children often become imbued with emotional import, and in which the giving, sharing, and eating of food often seems to have strong emotional connotations of love and affection. Children rapidly learn that battling over meals and eating may gain them a great deal of emotional leverage against parents. Most of us have a rough idea of our body shape and weight and are aware if we are losing or gaining weight, but some people seem to lose the ability to make this value judgement of themselves and have a total misperception of their size and weight. Eating is often done for comfort in our society, and the unhappy will often overeat and gain weight, although some may stop eating and lose weight.

Changes in appetite, either decrease or increase, or sudden changes in the type of food eaten, are common presenting symptoms of psychiatric disturbance. Weight loss and, less commonly, weight gain may also be signs of psychological disturbance, but also occur in physical illness. Vomiting is another symptom that can be caused by emotional distress or illness (particularly anxiety), but may also have serious physical causes and therefore needs careful assessment.

You may therefore be presented with a patient with significant weight loss, which may be associated with loss of appetite or a normal appetite. You may be presented with loss of appetite, which is usually, but not invariably, accompanied by loss of weight. You may be presented with a patient who has significant weight gain, with or without any change in appetite. You may be presented with a patient who has a significant increase in appetite (or a patient that has a change in eating behaviour), which may or may not be accompanied by weight gain. You may be presented with a patient who has unusual food desires (**pica**). You may be presented with a patient who, with or without weight loss, complains of frequent vomiting. The patient may be indifferent to any of the above symptoms, may try to conceal them, or may be distressed by them.

Investigation of weight loss

The first important thing to remember when assessing such patients is that they often feel that they have no problem. They view their behaviour, weight, and attitude to eating as quite normal. It is often friends, relatives, or the family doctor who has persuaded them to attend your clinic, so the immediate problem is to establish a rapport with the patient and to develop a treatment plan that is acceptable to both yourself and the patient. It is vitally important to talk to relatives and get corroborating evidence of the patient's eating behaviour.

Physical

Include a careful history of the rate of weight loss. A careful history and examination is mandatory. In addition to a general medical and neurological screen, a careful endocrine assessment should be made. Record weight unclothed (as some patients with anorexia cheat by putting heavy objects in their clothing—one of our patients sewed lead shot in her underwear). Record future weights under similar standard conditions (same time of day, same machine, unclothed, empty bladder, etc.).

Examine the colour and warmth of the skin (excess pallor suggests hypopituitarism, cyanosed extremities suggests peripheral vascular stasis, orange colouration of the palms suggests carotinaemia, brown pigmentation of the skin suggests Addison's disease, warm skin plus high pulse rate suggests thyrotoxicosis). Look at hair distribution. Is there fine downy hair on the cheeks and back? See if secondary sexual characteristics are present or atrophied. Look for the skin signs of AIDS. Enquire about menstruation, but do not be misled by the artificial menstruation caused by oral contraceptives. Enquire for sensitivity to cold and constipation, and check blood pressure and pulse rate. Examine the teeth carefully and look for little pits in the enamel, which are characteristic of frequent vomiting. Check for recurrent sinusitis and parotid gland swelling.

Physical tests, such as haematological and biochemical screening, should be included in your assessment, particularly in those patients who are very emaciated or who are vomiting. Endocrine tests, including the response to stimulatory hormones, may be necessary. A chest X-ray should be arranged and occasionally other radiography, including special X-ray views of the pituitary fossa and CT examination of the brain, may be needed.

Psychological

A full psychiatric history and examination is obviously necessary, particularly to exclude depression and to assess laxative, diuretic, and sometimes alcohol abuse. Then establish the patient's attitude to her current weight, how she feels about putting weight on, and what her perception of her body size is. Does she have an intense wish to be thin or a morbid fear of fatness?

Then assess eating behaviour. Take the patient through an average 'eating day' (if there is one). Does she calorie count? If she binges on one day does she make up for it the next day by saving on calories? How does she feel, physically and emotionally, about eating? Does she feel bloated, guilty, or have some other un-pleasant emotion after eating? Does she eat in secret or alone? Is she uncomfortable eating in front of other people? What habits has she acquired to compensate for what she regards as excess eating (forced vomiting, laxative abuse, excess exercise, etc.)? What are her attitudes to preparing food for others? Does she have food fads?

Investigation of vomiting

In addition to the physical and psychological invest-igations outlined above, a full account of the vomiting behaviour is indicated. Is it true vomiting and if so what is actually brought up? Is it merely retching or waterbrash? Is the vomiting preceded by nausea or by other central nervous system symptoms such as tinnitus? Is the vomiting effortless? Is it preceded or accompanied by headache, visual disturbance, or evidence of gastrointestinal upset? It is most important to rigorously exclude all physical causes for the vomiting before assuming that it is psychogenic. Specialist radiological and endoscopic examination of the gastrointestinal tract may be necessary.

Investigation of weight gain

A careful physical and psychiatric history and examination is necessary, along the lines outlined above, with particular emphasis on eating patterns and attitudes to weight and body shape. Get the patient to keep a diary for a couple of weeks recording exactly what is consumed and when (remember to include alcohol). Is there binge eating, comfort eating, or continual nibbling? What does the patient use for weight control? What is the reason for the failure of previous attempts? Is there chronic hyperphagia, or is it episodic? Is there associated sleep disturbance?

Differential diagnosis
Organic disease

1. delirium (acute brain syndrome)
2. dementia (chronic brain syndrome)
3. physical illness.

Weight loss, anorexia, and vomiting may occur in both delirium and dementia, but rarely weight gain (although there may be spurious weight gain due to fluid retention or congestive cardiac failure). Obesity may occasionally occur in organic brain diseases that cause hyperphagia, such as the Kleine–Levin syndrome or the Kluver–Bucy syndrome.

Anorexia or weight loss may be the result of any acute medical or chronic illness including cardiovascular and respiratory disease, and malignant disease. Weight loss may also occur because of gastrointestinal disease, such as peptic ulcer, malabsorption syndromes, Crohn's disease, or ulcerative colitis. Anorexia may occur in anaemia and is also seen in pernicious anaemia, in which an anaemia-related pica often occurs). Endocrine disorders can also produce anorexia and weight loss. In thyrotoxicosis appetite is usually maintained in the face of loss of weight, whereas in Addison's disease anorexia, weight loss, and vomiting often occur with acute onset. Juvenile diabetes may also be mistaken for anorexia nervosa. Although rare, pituitary cachexia (characterized by pallor, weight loss, loss of secondary sexual characteristics, and anorexia) is still part of the differential diagnosis. Tumours of the hypothalamus and third ventricle often produce weight loss and appetite loss. You should also not forget pregnancy as a cause of anorexia, weight loss, and vomiting. Although tuberculosis is now a rare chronic infection, it produces an anorexia-like picture, and nowadays AIDS is an important cause of weight loss.

Various medical drugs can also produce anorexia and weight loss, particularly CNS stimulants like theophylline, sympathomimetic drugs such as amphetamines and ephedrine, and sometimes beta-2-stimulants used in the treatment of asthma.

Psychotic illness

1. schizophrenia

2. paranoid psychosis.

Some psychotic patients develop delusions about their food or bizarre food fads that lead to rapid weight loss. Weight gain can also occur because of hyperphagia or because of medications like chlorpromazine that the patient is taking.

Affective illness

1. mania
2. depression.

Weight loss is usual with hypomania and is extremely common in depression. Depression is often accompanied by anorexia, and it can be difficult in a young person to distinguish between anorexia nervosa and depression. A significant proportion of patients with anorexia nervosa have depressive symptoms and sleep disturbance. Depressed patients who have lost weight and appetite will, however, not have the typical symptoms and signs of anorexia nervosa, such as a fatness phobia.

Intoxication

Chronic alcoholism often produces weight and appetite loss, and drug intoxication, particularly with amphetamines, may produce a very similar picture.

Acute situational reactions

Under severe stress many people stop eating and lose weight, but will not have the positive symptoms of anorexia nervosa outlined above. Some indulge in comfort eating and may gain weight.

Neurotic disorder

Anxious patients often lose weight and have poor appetites, but they do not have the other characteristic symptoms of anorexia nervosa. Anorexia nervosa is the chief cause of sustained weight loss i.e., below the 25th percentile of expected body weight for height. The syndrome includes amenorrhoea, a fatness phobia, bingeing, vomiting, and a perceptual distortion about body size. It is important to recognize that anorexia nervosa is a syndrome rather than a specific condition, and there are probably several different subgroups. A proportion of anorexics binge and vomit as well as having anorexic symptoms. Some chronic bingers are of normal weight, although they often have amenorrhoea, and a proportion of chronic bingers are actually above the expected weight for their height. Many patients who binge and vomit are ashamed of it, will not readily declare it, and conceal it for a long time. They often have the tell-tale signs of chronic vomiting outlined above, such as pitted tooth enamel. They also disappear mysteriously after meals for short periods of time. Severe bingers need careful medical assessment as they can do themselves much metabolic damage.

Personality disorder

There are no specific syndromes related to appetite, weight, vomiting, and personality.

Management

The management of weight loss, anorexia, vomiting, and weight gain is to make a thorough assessment. If possible keep the patient under observation for a while whilst you gather information. Help the patient to keep a diary of her food intake and the number of binges and vomiting episodes. This is very helpful and interestingly, in its own way, may begin to put the problem right. If the patient has lost a great deal of weight rapidly, hospitalization and intravenous therapy or nasogastric therapy may be necessary, as may correction of metabolic abnormalities in patients who binge and vomit regularly as they may become severely hypokalaemic.

It is imperative to try to develop some kind of working therapeutic relationship or alliance with the patient so that long-term management of the anorexia or bulimia nervosa can be undertaken. Behavioural programmes are very useful for patients who vomit when stressed.

Cognitive therapy also has a place in the treatment of these syndromes. Severe obesity is difficult to treat, but a combination of behavioural and cognitive therapy plus, in extreme cases, gastroplasty is probably best. New drug therapies for obesity, although still experimental, also look promising.

L Patients with problems of sex or sex-related disorders

- Sexual problems are common, but are often difficult to evaluate because of their subjective nature.
- There are few, if any, absolute standards of sexual performance.
- Sexual difficulty is usually self-reinforcing due to secondary anxiety, goal directedness, and 'spectating'.
- Interview both partners separately and then together.
- Look at their sexual development (physical and emotional).
- What sexual knowledge do they have, and when and from where did they get it?
- Is the problem peculiar to this relationship or has it occurred before or elsewhere?
- Take a full history of the problem. Is it intermittent or persistent? Was the onset gradual or sudden?
- Assess the relationship, both weaknesses and strengths.
- Assess goal directedness, spectating, and performance anxiety, and both partners' attitude to the problem.
- Full physical, psychiatric, and drug history.
- Full physical examination (evidence of systemic, endocrine, vascular, central or peripheral neurological disorder). Is there local genital disease?

- Biochemical and haematological screen. Assess for climacteric.
- Special investigations of penile function (for example, blood flow) may be needed. Ask the patient if he is responsive in other sexual situations or to other stimuli, and if waking erections are still occurring.
- Look for signs of alcoholism or depression.

Types of difficulty

1. courtship and bonding disorder
2. hypoactive/hyperactive sexual desire
3. sexual aversion disorder
4. inhibited female sexual arousal
5. male erectile dysfunction
6. inhibited female orgasm
7. inhibited male orgasm
8. premature ejaculation
9. dyspareunia and vaginismus
10. paraphilias
11. gender identity disorder.

Physical causes of sexual difficulty

1. neurological disorders, such as multiple sclerosis;
2. endocrine disorders, such as acromegaly, diabetes;
3. systemic disorders, such as liver disease;
4. vascular disorders, such as hypertension, peripheral vascular disease;
5. drugs, such as antihypertensives, antidepressants, antipsychotics, cigarettes, and alcohol;
6. organic brain disease.

Psychological causes of sexual difficulties

1. depression
2. intoxicants
3. anxiety/obsessional illness
4. personality disorder.

Most patients with sexual difficulties are normal physically and mentally apart from secondary anxiety. Always look for evidence of previous sexual trauma.

Management

- Remove any cause if possible. Stop smoking and alcohol.
- Behavioural/cognitive therapy with specific exercises for specific problems.
- Relationship counselling. Abuse and incest counselling if indicated.

Setting the scene

Sexual difficulties of various kinds are common and may be the presenting feature in the patient's problems, with any unhappiness or anxiety developing secondary to the sexual problem. It may, however, be the other way around, and the patient's unhappiness or anxiety may impinge on his sexuality.

As with sleep, it is often difficult to get an objective account of sexual performance. Many of the measures and goals of human sexuality are subjective and depend on the satisfaction or dissatisfaction of the patient's partner. There are few absolute standards for sexual performance—there is no standard British orgasm! Sexual performance that might disappoint one set of partners may be quite satisfactory for another pair. To a large extent the couple decide if they have a problem or not, although obviously there are certain biological limits. It is most important that the therapist does not set standards, particularly based on his or her own personal experience, which may be highly misleading.

The therapist will carry his or her own attitudes towards sexuality into any consultation about sexual behaviour. It is important that the therapist is aware of these so that they do not intrude too heavily into the consultation or influence its outcome. It is the patient's attitudes that are more important. If there are particular areas of sexuality that make you feel uncomfortable, it is better to avoid counselling in those areas until you are comfortable with them. Society's attitudes towards certain aspects of sexuality are changing rapidly. The recent recognition that AIDS is a sexually transmitted disease has brought many attitudes and ideas about unusual sexual behaviour and sexuality in general into sharp focus and open question.

Like many other problems that you will encounter in psychiatric practice, it is important not to consider sexual problems in isolation. You need to consider the person who has the problem, his previous upbringing, his mental and physical health, the strengths and weaknesses of his relationship, his attitude to sexuality, his previous sexual experiences, his expectations, and his actual physiological constitution.

Sexual difficulty often becomes self-reinforcing because if one or both of the partners perceives a failure within the sexual side of the relationship secondary anxiety occurs, which reinforces failure and also makes the couple, in Masters and Johnson's terms, 'goal directed'. In other words, sexual activity becomes performance orientated and anxiety ridden, and it loses its pleasure. For many sexual problems, relieving the anxiety and the goal directedness and helping the couple to begin to exchange mutual pleasuring is the basis of successful treatment.

There are several stages in a sexual relationship when

problems may occur, and identification of these stages is important in understanding the aetiology of a particular sexual disorder. It is also important to lose the pejorative descriptions of sexual failure (such as impotence or frigidity), which are unhelpful in elucidating a particular problem. Our own classification of sexual difficulty is based, to a large extent, on the DSM III R diagnostic criteria.

1. courtship and bonding difficulty;
2. hypoactive sexual desire (hyperactive sexual desire);
3. sexual aversion disorder;
4. inhibited female sexual arousal;
5. male erectile dysfunction;
6. inhibited female orgasm;
7. inhibited male orgasm;
8. premature ejaculation;
9. dyspareunia and vaginismus;
10. paraphilias (fetishes, transvestite fetishism, and paedophilia);
11. gender identity disorders (such as transsexualism).

Difficulties with courtship and bonding

In some patients, sexual activity never starts because it never has the opportunity to do so. There are such deep-seated difficulties in forming social and courtship relationships as to prevent the development of sufficient intimacy, both physical and emotional, for a sexual relationship to develop. The degree of intimacy and skill in courtship necessary for a sexual relationship to develop is dependent on both psychological and cultural factors. There may be particular difficulty in societies in which cultural taboos and expectations are in the process of rapid change (as in British society).

Difficulties in courtship, bonding, and intimacy are usually caused by deep-seated emotional problems related to childhood relationships or experiences. They need a combination of psychotherapy, behavioural skills, and cognitive skills to put them right.

Hypoactive sexual desire

There is no actual problem with intercourse, except that the patient does not desire it and has a low level of sexual drive. If two partners are equally content with the amount of sexual activity they have, even though it is extremely infrequent by standards of the culture in which they live, then there is no problem. Problems arise when one partner wants more sexual activity than the other one seems inclined to provide. There is probably a normal distribution curve for sexual activity and it is difficult to decide at which point low sexual drive becomes pathological. It is important to make sure that it is the *desire* for sexual activity that is low and not that desire is being inhibited by a particular psychological problem, such as disgust or fear, or that the problem is not related to depression. Rarely, excessive sexual desire is complained of. It is difficult to decide where normal biological limits end and often the problem is that two people with very different levels of normal desire are failing to reach an effective compromise. True excessive sexual desire may be a neurotic defence against boredom or unhappiness. Very rarely is it organic, and it may relate to a personality disorder.

Sexual aversion disorder

Here there is active *avoidance* of sexual intercourse (or its precursor activity) because of a strong inhibiting emotion, particularly anxiety or disgust, which usually relates to previous unpleasant experiences or to strong childhood conditioning of guilt. Such powerful emotions often so inhibit sexual desire that it can appear as though the patient has a biologically low level of desire.

Inhibited female sexual arousal

Normal sexual desire is present, but the woman fails to develop physical sexual excitement, and therefore produces no lubrication during the sexual act. This often makes intercourse painful and the woman watchful and anxious, which therefore inhibits sexual response in subsequent encounters and orgasm will not occur. It is probably the commonest female problem.

Male erectile dysfunction

The patient either fails to achieve an erection at all, achieves one but loses it, or only gets a partial erection insufficient for penetrative intercourse. Occasionally, this is primary in that full erection has never been achieved, but almost invariably it is a secondary phenomenon. Erectile dysfunction in its various forms is the commonest kind of male sexual problem and it becomes increasingly common as age advances, suggesting that organic factors are important. For most patients there is an interplay between organic and psychological factors.

Inhibited female orgasm

Desire is present and sexual arousal occurs both psychologically and physiologically (with full lubrication), but orgasm cannot be achieved. Some women with this problem cannot achieve orgasm at all, others can achieve orgasm by manual stimulation (either by themselves or by their partner), but cannot achieve it during intercourse. This may be because of problems with the partner's technique or because the partner's own orgasm arrives too quickly. Only about one-third of women engaged in sexual activity regularly achieve orgasm during intercourse. Failure to achieve orgasm under any circumstances may be primary or, much more usually, secondary. Inhibited female orgasm is the commonest reason for women to present for treatment, and this is because inhibited female arousal also leads to inhibited orgasm.

Inhibited male orgasm

Some men, no matter how long they try for, cannot achieve ejaculation. In some men this is complete in that ejaculation does not occur during intercourse or during masturbation. In others, ejaculation can occur during masturbation, but not during intercourse. Both problems may be primary or secondary. They are usually due to lack of sufficient stimulation or to inhibitory factors in the man, but occasionally organic factors may be involved. Whether inhibited orgasm is a problem or not depends to some extent on the partner's reaction and how long she takes to reach her own orgasm. Occasionally, retrograde ejaculation occurs into the bladder, or there is *dry ejaculation*—all feeling and no substance. Both are usually related to organic illness or drug therapy, and retrograde ejaculation can be a trick that, once learnt, is difficult to unlearn.

Premature ejaculation

A man has premature ejaculation when he demonstrates persistent lack of ability to control ejaculation during sexual activity. In severe cases ejaculation occurs even before penetration and seems to occur reflexly when a certain level of sexual excitement is reached. The timing of ejaculation obviously depends on several factors, including the partner's response, the novelty of the situation, how frequently the man has intercourse, his age, and on the perceptions (and myths) that the partners have and believe about sexual activity. The problem is often compounded by both partners feeling a sense of failure if ejaculation occurs early so that sexual activity immediately stops. Most men can learn to control ejaculation by recognizing the point in their sexual response cycle (in terms of their own subjective feelings) just before ejaculation is about to occur, and stopping thrusting for a while at that point before resuming thrusting. Men are often reluctant to do so for fear of disappointing their partners, or they use an inappropriate distraction technique that usually reinforces the problem rather than solving it.

Dyspareunia and vaginismus

Pain at the start of, or during, penetration is a common symptom in women. The commonest cause is vaginismus, an involuntary and reflex tightening of the vaginal muscles during attempts at penetration. Pain therefore occurs if penetration is attempted, which reinforces the reflex. It is the commonest cause for the physical non-consummation of a relationship. It may exist with the other female problems outlined above, or may exist in its own right in women who arouse easily, who can be orgasmic, and yet who cannot achieve penetration. It can be due to a fear of pain, to previous sexual trauma, or following a vaginal infection, and therefore may be primary or secondary. Vaginismus may also occur as a result of poor lubrication, which gives rise to painful intercourse.

Deep dyspareunia, in which pain is felt not at the introitus but in the pelvis on deep thrusting, is not uncommon. It is almost invariably organic and relates to pelvic pathology, such as endometriosis, tears in the broad ligament following childbirth, pelvic inflammatory disease, ovarian cysts, etc.

Paraphilias

In some people, usually men, sexual arousal can only occur in response to specific and unusual stimuli or to sexual objects, such as shoes, rubber, leather, etc., or can only occur if the person dresses in the clothing of the opposite sex (transvestite fetishism) or in response to inappropriate sexual objects such as children. Even mild degrees of fetishism may prove a problem for the person's partner (particularly transvestitism), and the person with the condition may have to learn to control his impulses, particularly because indulging in the behaviour reinforces the desire to do it. Antisocial paraphilias, such as paedophilia, are totally unacceptable and both desire and performance need to be suppressed. This is a specialist area of practice that you are unlikely to encounter in your first few months in psychiatry.

Most psychiatrists now accept that homosexuality—the chosen partner being an adult of the same sex—is not a paraphilia but merely a variety of normal experience. The sexual problems outlined above all occur in homosexual as well as heterosexual relationships.

Gender identity disorders

Transsexualism is a condition whereby a person of one biological gender has very strong feelings that he or she actually belongs to the other one and is thus a 'man trapped inside a female body', or vice versa. These feelings are long-standing, usually develop in childhood, and cause much unhappiness and tension within the patient. The current thinking is that if the person can learn to live in his or her chosen sexual gender comfortably for a couple of years (with cross dressing, acceptance at work and socially) then they should be supported by endocrinological and surgical methods. This only applies to people with stable personalities and whose ideas about sexual identity are not clearly related to psychotic illness. This, again, is a specialist area of sexual medicine.

Sexual abuse, sexual trauma, and incest

A number of patients will give a history of previous sexual abuse, trauma, or incest. It is uncertain what the background level of this is in our society, although possibly as many as a tenth of the female population (a much smaller percentage of the male population) will, in childhood or early adolescence, have experienced a sexual relationship with a parent (usually of the opposite sex) or with some other authority figure or relative. It is likely that the prevalence of previous sexual abuse is higher in patients with psychiatric disorder than in the general population, and in many a link exists between the previous abuse and the present psychiatric condition. It used to be taught that women complaining of previous abuse were not telling the truth and were recounting fantasy, but this Freudian idea has now largely been discredited. If you get a history of previous sexual abuse in a patient, you should believe it, unless it is very clearly false.

Many women will not reveal a history of previous abuse until they feel that they can trust the person to whom they are giving the information, and so routine enquiries about abuse whilst you are taking a history will often get a negative reply. Many women, in describing such abuse, do it in a flat, controlled way with little display of emotion, and the inexperienced (who are expecting dramatic emotional responses to the giving of such information) can be misled into thinking that such an unemotional disclosure is therefore false. You should take all histories of abuse seriously and assume that they are true as very few will be false. If the abuse is still continuing, you will need to discuss with your consultant the steps that you should take to help end the abuse. Our experience has shown us that it may be better to discuss this initially with one of the special abuse units set up by most police forces. If a minor is being abused (or is at serious risk) the relevant authorities must be informed despite the risk that ill-judged intervention may have disastrous consequences both for the victim of the abuse and for the family in general. The counselling of abuse victims requires specialist skills and may need many months of intensive therapy.

Investigation of sexual difficulty

Try to interview both members of the partnership separately to start with, and then have a joint interview (see p. 28). You will certainly need to understand the problems of the partner as much as those of the patient. It is not uncommon to find that it is actually the partner who has the problem rather than the person who presents with it.

A full sexual history should be taken looking at sexual development, both physical and emotional, and the acquisition of sexual knowledge. A full history of previous relationships is needed, and you must ascertain whether it is a problem occurring only in this relationship or if it has occurred in every relationship. A full account of the particular problem should be taken, including how long it has occurred, whether it is occurring all the time or only occasionally, whether the patient or the partner has tested out his or her sexual prowess outside the relationship and, if so, what the result was (it is surprising how many members of partnerships do this if they are faced with long-established sexual difficulty, and you will need to enquire in such circumstances about whether the partners are prepared to have full commitment to each other (see p. 29)). If appropriate, you must ask whether the problem presents itself during masturbation, either by the partner or by the individual.

You will also need to assess the quality of the partners' relationship, concentrating particularly on its strengths as well as its weaknesses. Try to assess how much goal directedness, spectating, and anxiety are now contaminating attempts at intercourse. You will need to take a full physical and psychiatric history. Look particularly for any historical evidence of peripheral neuropathy and vascular disorder, look critically at what drugs the patient is taking, and make an assessment of any evidence for alcoholism or depression. If you are assessing a problem of erectile dysfunction, enquire if this only occurs during intercourse, and if it only occurs during intercourse, is it just with one partner? Can the man still masturbate with a satisfactory erection? Does he still respond to erotic stimuli on television, etc.? Does he still wake with a morning erection? Total loss of erectile response and loss of normal morning erections, particularly if it is gradual, is usually indicative of a physical cause, although it can also be seen in a depressive illness.

Full physical examination is usually appropriate looking for evidence of systemic disease, hypertension, other vascular problems, and peripheral neuropathy. The genitalia should also be examined (this examination may well tell you a lot about the attitudes that the individual has to his or her own sexuality and body image, and can also be an educational experience for the patient). If, however, the history tells you that you are dealing with a problem of vaginismus, do not examine the patient vaginally until this can become part of the behavioural treatment of the condition. Specialist neurological or cardiological examination may be necessary. In erectile failure, if organic disease is strongly suspected, measurement of nocturnal penile tumescence, of penile vascular flow and blood pressure, and the response to intracavernosal injections of papaverine, may be necessary.

Particularly in middle-aged men with problems of erectile difficulty, a full blood count, biochemical profile, fasting triglyceride and cholesterol concentration, serum testosterone and prolactin are necessary. In middle-aged women, hormonal and gynaecological assessment of the menopause may be necessary as sometimes appropriate hormone replacement therapy will restore lost sexual arousal. Physical problems that limit the patient's physical mobility or response may also be present (for example, severe arthritis, effort angina).

Differential diagnosis

Organic disease

1. delirium (acute brain syndrome)
2. dementia (chronic brain syndrome)
3. endocrine disorder
4. neurological disorder (particularly peripheral neuropathy)
5. vascular disorder.

Inappropriate sexual responses may be seen both in delirium and in dementia, but particularly in dementia. As the disease progresses it may release previously controlled impulses in the patient, such as paedophilia. In both delirium and dementia, inappropriate masturbation or attempts at intercourse may take place as social inhibitions are lost. Occasionally, these inappropriate sexual behaviours may be the presenting symptom of a dementia.

Men seem much more susceptible to the effects of illness on their sexual function than women. Although local genital disease, particularly if it causes pain or prevents lubrication, can cause sexual dysfunction in women, generalized bodily disorder is less likely to. In men, any condition that reduces circulating levels of testosterone (or increases oestrogen levels), which interferes with the autonomic nervous system or the neurogenic mechanisms of erection, or which interferes with the blood supply to the penis, are likely to cause problems in erectile response. Local genital, urethral, or prostatic disease may occasionally cause premature ejaculation or retrograde ejaculation.

Common medical conditions that may cause problems with erection include multiple sclerosis, Parkinson's disease (sometimes its treatment with levodopa may increase libido), peripheral neuropathies, including diabetic peripheral neuropathy and disease or damage to the spinal cord (including amyotropic lateral sclerosis and tabes dorsalis). Liver disease can cause impotence, particularly if testosterone and oestrogen metabolism are affected, as can pituitary disease (acromegaly often causes impotence). Klinefelter's syndrome causes primary impotence, and in our experience this is not uncommonly diagnosed for the first time when the patient presents with potency problems.

Diabetes mellitus presumably causes problems with potency because of both its vascular and neurogenic effects. Cardiovascular disease, like hypertension and atherosclerosis, that significantly reduces penile blood flow is a very common cause of erectile difficulty in men and is made worse by smoking. Radical prostatectomy may also cause potency problems, as may extensive bowel resection. Alcohol probably causes erectile difficulty through a toxic peripheral neuropathy, which may well be reversible. As immediate first aid for middle-aged men with erectile difficulties, it is well worth suggesting that they stop smoking altogether and abstain from alcohol for six months. Many patients will get a full return of sexual function if they do this.

Antihypertensive drugs, including diuretics and beta-blockers, may cause potency problems. Anticholinergic drugs, cimetidine, tricyclic antidepressants, and mono-amine oxidase inhibitors may also cause erectile difficulty, as may antipsychotic drugs, which rarely may also cause retarded ejaculation or dry ejaculation.

Psychotic illness

1. schizophrenia
2. paranoid psychosis.

Psychotic patients may occasionally show inappropriate or disinhibited sexual behaviour, or more usually they lose interest in sex. Patients may also have bizarre delusions about changing sex, or delusions about external sexual control. Antipsychotic medication may occasionally cause side-effects that are delusionally misinterpreted, such as galactorrhoea or gynaecomastia. Belief that the patient is changing sex is a common psychotic delusion, which is why transsexual patients need to be assessed carefully.

Affective illness

1. hypomania
2. depression.

Manic patients may well show disinhibited or excessive sexual activity, and may embark on sexual adventures that they later regret. They may need to be protected from such exploitation. Depression very commonly leads to loss of sexual interest, sexual aversion, inhibited arousal, and inhibited orgasm, in both sexes. Often these conditions do not resolve once the depression recovers because of secondary reinforcement and therefore may need treatment. Unfortunately, antidepressant drugs have their own complex effects on sexual performance and so it may be necessary to delay treatment of depression-related sexual problems until medication has been withdrawn. Delusional beliefs about sexuality, or of being punished for previous sexual adventures, are also common in depression.

Intoxication

Alcohol, which 'provokes the desire but takes away the performance', is very commonly involved in the aetiology of sexual problems. The effect of alcohol is probably related to its central nervous system effects and also to its toxicity to the peripheral nervous system. Alcohol-related sexual problems are often projected on to the partner, and delusional jealousy may occur. (It also cannot be easy to show enthusiasm for congress with a drink-sodden lover.) Drugs of abuse, such as amphetamines and cocaine, may cause an initial enhancement of sexual activity, but other drugs of addiction, such as barbiturates and the opiates, usually reduce sexual desire and activity.

Acute situational reactions

These usually produce a transient loss of sexual interest and diminish the frequency of, and pleasure in, sexual performance, although occasionally comfort may be found in sexual activity so that it actually increases in frequency. Many sexual problems, particularly in women, relate to previous sexual trauma and this may need specific counselling before the actual problem can be resolved. Immediate counselling after rape or incest is very important.

Neurotic disorder

Anxiety plays a very large part in sexual difficulty. There may be a specific phobic anxiety, as in vaginismus, or there may be a performance anxiety that interferes with sexual activity. In general terms, high levels of anxiety tend to reduce sexual appetite and performance, although very high levels of anxiety and stress may actually produce reflex sexual arousal. Obsessional rituals may become involved in sexual activity, particularly washing and cleanliness rituals after sexual intercourse (which may totally spoil its pleasure), and some women may show a phobic avoidance of contamination with semen (not the same thing as taking a healthy interest in contraception).

Personality disorders

Since both sexual and personality disorders relate to previous experiences, patterns of upbringing, factors of conditioning, and education, it is not surprising that sexual difficulty is common in the personality disordered. Sometimes this manifests itself as excessive or inappropriate sexuality, but often inhibited sexuality occurs.

Management

The first step in the management of sexual difficulty is, if possible, to eliminate or remove any obvious cause of the problem. If an untreatable physical disorder is causing the sexual difficulty, the partners need to be counselled about alternative modes of sexual expression and helped to come to terms with their loss of sexual function. As a general rule men should stop smoking and drinking, and extracurricular sexual activity should cease (otherwise the partner will not show much enthusiasm for putting his own partner's sexual problems right).

Treatment is then an empirical mixture of behavioural and cognitive methods aimed at preventing anxiety, spectating, goal directedness, and helping the couple to eventually re-establish mutually rewarding and reinforcing pleasures so that sexual activity is gradually resumed. There are specific exercises for specific difficulties, such as teaching a man with premature ejaculation that he has to stop before ejaculatory inevitably occurs, masturbatory exercises for men with retarded ejaculation or for women with low sexual arousal or who are non-orgasmic, and for non-orgasmic women the Lo Piccolo 'sexual growth' exercises, which are particularly useful in these patients. Vaginismus is treated by classical deconditioning using a gradual and controlled exposure to penetration. Counselling about previous sexual abuse or trauma, and relationship and marital counselling, may also be necessary.

Very rarely is any medical intervention needed. Occasionally, men with low testosterone levels will only respond to a sexual enhancement programme if they have their testosterone levels artificially enhanced by depot testosterone preparations. There is a growing trend to use intracavernosal injections of papaverine therapeutically for erectile difficulty. This is a technique for the expert, although some patients can learn to inject themselves.

M Patients who have problems with sleep

- Sleep disorder is the commonest symptom of emotional distress.

- To fully assess sleep, a laboratory may be required.

- Assess how well the patient has slept prior to the complaint.

- How long does he sleep?

- Is there difficulty falling asleep, maintaining sleep, or early morning waking?

- How often does he remember waking or dreaming in the night? Does he remember any sexual arousal?

- Any sleep-related events, such as night terror, hypnopompic hallucinations, etc.?

- Is he drowsy or falling asleep in the daytime? Any cataplexy?

- Does he snore? What drugs/intoxicants is he taking?

- Full medical, neurological, and psychiatric history and examination. ENT examination when relevant.
- Biochemical/haematological profile and thyroid function.
- Sleep EEG, blood gases and respiration during sleep, when indicated.
- Multiple sleep latency test.
- Cerebral radiology occasionally.

Specific sleep disorders

1. insomnia (early, middle, and late)
2. sleep walking
3. night terrors
4. sleep anxiety attacks
5. dream anxiety disorder (nightmares)
6. REM sleep disorder
7. sleep apnoea
8. hypersomnia (prolonged true sleep)
9. hypersomnia—episodic (Kleine–Levin syndrome)
10. hypersomnia with sleep drunkenness
11. narcolepsy (plus or minus cataplexy, sleep paralysis, hypnopompic/hypnogogic hallucinations).

Differential diagnosis

1. organic mental states
2. physical illness (pain, asthma, drugs, hyperthyroidism, hypothyroidism, etc.)
3. affective illness
4. intoxicants
5. anxiety (phobic avoidance of sleep)
6. poor sleep hygiene.

Management

- Recognize and remove cause with specific therapy.
- Encourage good sleep hygiene.
- Use hypnotics very sparingly.

Setting the scene

Sleep disturbance of one kind or another is the commonest subjective symptom of emotional distress that you are likely to encounter. It is one that doctors often do not take seriously enough, possibly because one is by and large dealing with a patient's subjective complaints as, without the aid of a laboratory, it is almost impossible to make an objective measure of sleep. This is true even in hospital. A nurse shining a shaded torch on your recumbent patient every half an hour to see if he is asleep is hardly the most effective measure of whether he is having a good night's sleep or not. Like sexual experience, the experience of sleep is subjective, open to personal interpretation, and takes place in private. Clinical analysis, recognition of sleep pathology, and knowledge of sleep physiology is poorly taught in most medical schools. This probably explains why at least one in eight sleeps in this country is induced by some form of medication, whether prescribed or self-medication, and why a substantial portion of the population are regular consumers of hypnotic medication.

People with sleep difficulty may complain of:

1. too little sleep (due to a failure to initiate or to maintain sleep, or to sleep for a length of time that the patient feels is inadequate to maintain his well-being);
2. sleeping for too long a time, or difficulty in waking;
3. unpleasant events occurring during sleep;
4. sleeping at inappropriate times, with difficulty in staying awake;

5. constant fatigue or drowsiness;

6. combinations of the above.

Assessment of sleep disorder

It is important to realize that the patient's own account of his sleep problems and subjective estimate of how long he has slept, how often he woke during the night, and the quality and frequency of his dreams, can be wildly inaccurate. We only remember, for instance, dreams from which we awaken, and may seriously underestimate the amount of dreaming that takes place. To fully analyse and understand sleep the services of a sleep laboratory are needed to record the EEG throughout the night, eye movement, muscle tension (conventionally measured in the facial muscles usually near the chin), and, if necessary, respiration and blood oxygen tension. There are few sleep laboratories in this country, although ambulatory EEG techniques are beginning to allow sleep measurement to be done at home. This is particularly important because measurement in a sleep laboratory is complicated by the fact that the patient needs some nights to adapt to the conditions of the laboratory, but adaptation is much swifter at home.

A careful subjective and, if possible, objective account of the sleep disorder is necessary, followed by a careful medical, neurological, and psychiatric history and examination with special reference to the respiratory and cardiovascular system. The sleep history should concentrate on the patient's previous sleep history and what he regards as normal for him, and compare it with the present. The length of time taken to fall asleep, the duration of sleep, the number of times the patient awakes, the duration of any periods awake, any recollection of dreaming and sexual arousal during sleep, should all be noted. Whereabouts in the sleep cycle such dreaming, sexual arousal, or waking occurs should also be noted. Any sleep-related event, whether the patient feels tired in the daytime or falls asleep in the daytime, whether his partner has noticed him having respiratory difficulty during the night, the strength and duration of any snoring, whether the patient has noticed hypnogogic or hypnopompic hallucinations, and whether he has sleep paralysis or cataplexy, should all be recorded.

A basic EEG followed by a sleep EEG may be necessary, with measurement of respiration and blood gases. In conditions in which the patient falls asleep inappropriately, or is chronically tired, multiple sleep latency tests are also employed. Several times during the day the patient is encouraged to put himself into situations that he usually finds conducive to falling asleep. An EEG monitors the length of time taken for the patient to fall into light sleep, and whether the patient enters dream sleep as soon as he falls asleep. Haematological and biochemical screening is also necessary, and radiological investigation of the brain is sometimes indicated. Drug screening may be needed, as is examination of the ears, nose, and throat, with particular attention to the patency of the nasal passage, the shape of the throat, and investigation of any possible obstruction, particularly with the patient in the recumbent posture.

Insomnia is the commonest sleep problem described by patients, which may be difficulty in initiating sleep, difficulty in staying asleep, frequent waking, early morning waking, or a combination of these problems. Two sleep-related events that may make insomnia worse are **nocturnal myoclonus** (sudden jerking of the limbs), which wakens the patient or prevents him sleeping (it is probably an exaggeration of the normal sudden bodily jerk on falling asleep, although other causes of myoclonus must be excluded), and the **restless leg syndrome**, commoner as age advances, in which there is an inner compulsion to shift and move the legs throughout the night. This is thought to be a possible dystonia (see p. 365).

Narcolepsy, which is rare, is characterized by irresistible attacks of falling asleep in the daytime, usually with a short prodrome of feeling sleepy, but occasionally occurring very suddenly. Such sleep is short and the patient usually awakens refreshed (if allowed to awaken naturally). Of patients who have narcolepsy, three-quarters have another specific symptom as well. A tenth have the full *narcoleptic tetrad* (narcolepsy plus cataplexy plus sleep paralysis plus hypnogogic or hypnopompic hallucinations), and 40 per cent have narcolepsy plus cataplexy (often mild and unrecognized).

Narcolepsy usually starts with sleep attacks and the other features are added later. The patient may have several sleep attacks a day, often in situations conducive to sleep, but may not be able to resist sleep even when highly aroused, such as when driving or swimming. If the patient is prevented from sleeping by external stimulation he may become very irritable or appear confused. Some patients merely have episodic sleep attacks but feel well in between them (type I narcolepsy). Type II narcolepsy is when, in addition to sleep attacks, there is a constant struggle to stay awake. It used to be thought that patients passed rapidly into rapid eye movement sleep (REM or dream sleep) when falling asleep in the daytime, but this may not in fact be true. Brief *microsleeps* may also occur in the daytime. Night-time sleep in people with narcolepsy is characteristically broken and disturbed.

Cataplexy is sudden immobility or loss of muscle tone that may be localized or generalized. The patient may fall and be unable to move or speak although fully alert. He may just have episodes of partial muscle weakness (for example, head dropping, ptosis, or double vision). Cataplexy is precipitated by emotional stimuli, especially laughter, and may, like sleep attacks, seriously curtail the patient's lifestyle. Cataplexy on its own, without narcolepsy, is rare.

Hypnogogic and hypnopompic hallucinations occur as the patient falls asleep or on awakening and are usually auditory but may be visual, are often vivid, and may be terrifying (much more so than in people who experience them but who do not have narcolepsy). These hallucinatory experiences occurring on their own are not thought to represent potential narcolepsy and are common.

Sleep paralysis is a sudden inability to move that is experienced on falling asleep or, more usually, waking, although the patient can move his eyes. It is usually of short duration. The patient usually feels extremely frightened and there may be a terrifying hallucinatory accompaniment. Touching the patient or calling his name will usually stop it. The patient may become very fearful of having attacks so that he develops sleep phobia. Occasional sleep paralysis, occurring on its own, is not uncommon. There is a debate about whether this presages narcolepsy.

The aetiology of narcolepsy is uncertain, but it is almost certainly not a psychogenic disorder. It has a genetic component and is probably a primary sleep disorder. In less than five per cent of patients there may be an organic cause, such as postencephalitis, after head injury, diencephalic tumours, cerebral syphilis, etc. Some patients with severe narcolepsy eventually develop a paranoid illness, although whether this is a direct result of the narcolepsy or the medication taken to treat it is uncertain.

The diagnosis is made by taking a careful history, EEG sleep monitoring, and daytime EEG monitoring. At night there is an early onset of REM, and there is a positive response to the multiple sleep latency test in the daytime, with REM occurring early in attacks (but not if the patient only has narcolepsy). Nocturnal sleep is characteristically disturbed.

The differential diagnosis of narcolepsy includes normal drowsiness, sleep apnoea, anxiety, fatigue, depressive hypersomnia, hypothyroidism, epilepsy (particularly if combined with cataplexy), recurrent hypoglycaemia, hysteria, and myaesthenia gravis.

The treatment of narcolepsy involves counselling so that the patient and his relatives understand the disorder and the patient is helped to adjust at work so that he can perhaps take a lunchtime nap, which may then help him to stay awake, at least until he leaves work. Falling asleep on the way home is a common problem. The second stage of treatment is to try to promote better night-time sleep (clomipramine is particularly useful and may help patients with cataplexy). The third stage, if absolutely necessary, is to use stimulants, and amphetamine taken in small doses morning and midday is by far the best. This should only be used if all else fails.

Sleep apnoea is related to periodic breathing whilst asleep, leading to periods of apnoea lasting 10–30 seconds and occurring at least five times every hour, with consequent waking. There is a profound fall of pO_2 and a rise of pCO_2. Obesity, right heart failure, and polycythaemia may occur in association with sleep apnoea, as does characteristic difficulty in waking, daytime drowsiness with increased accident proneness, a fall in intellectual performance, and sometimes frank mental illness. Sleep apnoea may have a central origin (**Ondine's curse**), but the commonest form relates to airways obstruction due to collapse of the posterior pharyngeal space (preceded and characterized by heavy snoring). Myocardial ischaemia, hypertension, and sudden death may be the outcome of the sleep apnoea syndrome, and therefore it needs to be recognized and treated. Pharyngeal pleating operations, intermittent positive pressure respiration, and, in extreme cases, tracheostomy may be needed.

Hypersomnia (true sleep occurring in excessive amounts with or without drowsiness in the daytime) may be seen in some forms of mental illness, as a withdrawal from reality, may relate to physical disease (including brainstem disease, hypothyroidism, metabolic disorders, and hypothalalmic dsyfunction), or may be an idiopathic disorder such as the rare **Kleine–Levin** syndrome of unknown aetiology.

In this syndrome there is periodic oversleeping lasting for days or weeks, with periods of normality in between. It is associated with intense hunger (megaphagia). It is rare in women and is a disorder almost entirely of young men. When asleep, the patient can be woken, but is then irritable and confused, sometimes with frank delirium. The cause is not known. Hypersomnia can occur with **sleep drunkenness**. There is rapid onset of heavy sleeping on retiring, and prolonged genuine sleep from which the patient can only be woken with extreme difficulty, and if wakening is attempted, the patient is confused and disorientated. It may be triggered off by depression or anxiety, or may be a syndrome in its own right, in which case the patient may need stimulant medication.

Chronic fatigue occurs in patients with type II narcolepsy, sleep apnoea, and insomnia, and such patients feel tired and fatigued in the daytime and have difficulty staying awake and/or arousing in the morning. Other patients with this problem may have depression or anxiety. A chronic feeling of fatigue and exhaustion may occur in respiratory or heart disease, thyrotoxicosis, certain other endocrine or metabolic diseases (for example, renal or hepatic failure), cancer, and in malabsorption states. Exhaustion following mild exercise may be caused by the physical causes listed above, but may also be psychological in origin. A period of fatigue commonly follows a viral illness (such as hepatitis or Epstein–Barr virus infections). Such a fatigue state may become self-perpetuating (the so-called ME syndrome, which, under various names, has been a recognized psychological phenomenon for over a century).

Sleepwalking is not uncommon in children, particularly boys, and tends to occur in the first two or three hours of sleep, often during the first episode of deepest sleep (stage 4) in the night. Walking is usually aimless, although occasionally the patient may show searching activity. Complex activity in sleepwalking is rare and environmental awareness is low, although the patient may fixate on objects or other people with his eyes. Self-injury is rare. The patient often speaks, but the speech is usually incomprehensible. The patient is usually amnesic for the episode and usually does not wake although it is important to note that he can be woken quite safely and shown back to bed. Sleepwalking is uncommon in adults and if it does occur, usually occurs in males. It may be associated with severe psychopathology (some adult sleepwalking may be a dissociative state rather than true sleepwalking). Ambulatory EEG monitoring may be very helpful in distinguishing sleepwalking from other sleep disorders.

Night terrors are common in children and again tend to occur in the first episode of stage 4 sleep of the night, within one or two hours of going to sleep. There is sudden arousal with tachycardia, anxiety, and screaming, and the child cannot be communicated with. Episodes last two to three minutes and the child has no recall of the event. Some medications used for colic or nasal congestion may increase the frequency of the attacks. The effects are much worse for the parents than for the child. The best treatment is to wake the child about an hour after he starts to sleep (i.e., just before the onset of stage 4 sleep), and this often puts the problem right. Night terrors do occur in adults, perhaps more commonly than generally thought, and usually occur in association with severe daytime anxiety.

REM sleep disorder. It is now recognized that very rarely a person, whilst dreaming, may not be paralysed (as most people are when dreaming), and can still move and therefore act out his night-time dreams with potential danger to a sleeping partner. The diagnosis can be confirmed by nocturnal EEG monitoring. Until the attacks are controlled it is probably better if partners sleep apart (as rarely the partner may be severely injured). A drug that suppresses REM sleep may have to be used.

Nocturnal epileptic attacks, usually complex partial or frontal lobe seizures, are often mistaken for the above phenomenon and vice versa. Nocturnal EEG recording may be necessary to establish the diagnosis (see p. 336).

Dream anxiety disorder (nightmares). These are dreams that are frightening or disturbing and which wake the patient from sleep. They are particularly likely to occur during periods of stress, and often the dream content is symbolically related to the stress.

Sleep deprivation. People who are deprived of sleep for long periods of time eventually become somewhat confused, develop memory impairment, cognitive difficulties, and may eventually hallucinate. Hallucinations are often elemental at first, usually auditory but sometimes visual, and resemble those of sensory deprivation. Microsleeps will occur in the daytime and there will be a constant feeling of exhaustion. Many people deprived of sleep for long periods of time are not aware of the often quite severe cognitive impairment that occurs or of the irritability and depression of mood that can accompany it. Such sleep deprivation is, of course, common in young doctors and poses a danger not only to their patients but also to their own health, both physical and mental.

Differential diagnosis

Organic mental states

1. delirium (acute brain syndrome)

2. dementia (chronic brain syndrome).

Sleeplessness (obviously accompanied by other signs and symptoms) is characteristic of delirium, and reversal of sleep rhythm, so that the patient is wakeful during the night and drowsy during the day, is common in dementia. Thus all the causes for the above conditions (see Section 4F, p. 173) may be implicated in sleep disturbance, as may some other physical disorders.

It is important to remember that normal sleep structure and sleep needs change as patients get older. Old people may have naturally occurring early morning waking and may only sleep for four or five hours a night and be perfectly refreshed. It is also important to remember that certain common physical disorders often present with impaired sleep. *Chronic pain* (say from rheumatoid arthritis or some other condition) may profoundly affect sleep (and the right treatment is to treat the pain and not the sleep). *Asthma* often worsens in the night, which may be due to the patient encountering allergens in the bedroom, lack of medication during sleep, or other factors as yet unknown. *Chronic sinusitis* may also cause poor sleep with frequent waking due to coughing. *Sleep apnoea*, described above, causes poor sleep. *Congestive cardiac failure* may cause restless sleep, right heart failure leading to orthopnoea, and left heart failure producing acute attacks of intense breathlessness and fear. Nocturnal asthma and heart failure may be mistaken for epilepsy. Nocturnal seizures may also occur. Hyperthyroidism and hypothyroidism may also cause sleep disorder.

Many medical drugs can produce sleep disturbance.

Some reduce rapid eye movement sleep, which is not usually apparent to the patient but may produce daytime effects like drowsiness or cause rebound drowsiness on their withdrawal. All beta-blocking drugs, for example, whether lipophilic or hydrophilic, will reduce REM sleep. Lipophilic beta-blocking drugs also increase waking during the night and therefore produce an apparent subjective increase in vivid dreaming because the patient wakes out of what dream sleep is left. REM sleep suppression caused by bromocriptine may cause daytime hallucinations, as occasionally occurs with propranolol, levodopa, and amantadine. Beta-2-stimulant drugs may also produce difficulty in sleeping. Monoamine oxidase inhibiting drugs can cause insomnia, and anticholinergic drugs can cause daytime drowsiness. Withdrawal of opiates or barbiturates causes a characteristic insomnia, as does withdrawal of benzodiazepine drugs (and indeed most hypnotics), and so a careful drug history is essential when assessing sleep problems.

Psychotic illness

1. schizophrenia
2. paranoid psychosis.

Occasionally, schizophrenia accompanied by excitement will also be accompanied by wakefulness, and very occasionally patients may develop delusional experiences related to sleep and therefore stay awake. The sleep of most people with schizophrenia appears clinically normal.

Affective illness

1. hypomania
2. depression.

Sleep is characteristically disturbed in affective illness. In hypomania sleep is characteristically broken and short, and many patients with severe mania eventually become totally exhausted.

Sleep is disturbed in depression. In some patients there may be an initial insomnia or difficulty in sustaining sleep, and characteristic early morning waking. Patients wake earlier than their normal waking time and are unable to get back to sleep, and they usually feel particularly low and have morbid thinking about the forthcoming day. Hypersomnia may be symptomatic of milder depression, as may chronic fatigue. Sleep deprivation has been used as a treatment for depression.

Intoxication

Alcohol has a characteristic effect, producing sleep that is broken and disturbed with early morning waking, although heavy indulgence in alcohol may produce a profound stupor with consequent risk of inhalation of gastric contents. Indulgence in stimulant illicit drugs, such as amphetamines, will produce insomnia and difficulty in sleeping, and occasionally drugs may produce such vivid hallucinatory experiences that the patient is unable to sleep. Sedative illicit drugs, such as cannabis, may produce drowsiness and fatigue.

Acute situational reaction

Patients in a crisis, or who are facing disaster, or who have an acute emotional problem, may well have insomnia. Very occasionally you may be justified in treating the insomnia for a night or two as exhaustion increases the patient's inability to cope with the situation threatening him. In such a situation it is often better to use a sedative antidepressant such as trimipramine rather than risk the patient becoming dependent on a benzodiazepine. Occasionally, patients suffering from an acute situational reaction may develop hypersomnia as a withdrawal from reality.

Neurotic disorder

Reactive depression often tends to lead to difficulty in getting off to sleep or to hypersomnia. Patients who are anxious may characteristically have initial insomnia, may have early morning waking, and may develop specific sleep phobias so that they are afraid of falling asleep. They may develop night terrors, develop REM sleep disorder, or have frequent, usually repetitive, nightmares. Insomnia often becomes conditioned in the anxious in that they become anxious about not sleeping and therefore become highly aroused and keep themselves awake. Some patients with obsessional disorder have compulsions and rituals that keep them awake until they become completely exhausted, such as the housewife who cannot rest from her labours and is still hoovering the house at four o'clock in the morning.

Anxiety and depression often present as a chronic fatigue state. Most cases of ME have a predominant psychological basis if they become chronic, whatever the original cause of this condition. It can be seen as a kind of phobic reaction to the pain of becoming fit again after a period of enforced inactivity.

Personality disorders

The personality disordered, who are subject to acute emotional crises, who may use intoxicants, and who are often alcoholic, will often complain bitterly of sleep disturbance so that it is important in assessing a sleep problem to look at the personality of the person who has the problem.

Management

The initial management of a sleep disorder is obviously to make a thorough assessment of what the sleep problem is and of the differential diagnosis, because removing the cause is more important than removing the symptom. The insomnia of depression, for instance, should be treated by treating the depression and not by prescribing hypnotic medication. Almost all anxiety-related insomnia is better treated by behavioural or cognitive management of the anxiety than by giving hypnotic medication. If hypnotic medication is required (see Chapter 5, p. 431), hypnotics should not be prescribed for more than a night or two without a break in between and the patient instructed in better sleep habits as quickly as possible. Do not make the mistake of getting your patient dependent on hypnotic medication, and resist all blandishments to persuade you to prescribe hypnotics. Above all, try to avoid the situation in which the patient is lying in bed wide awake worrying that he is not sleeping. In such circumstances it is better if the patient gets up and does something because lying in bed will merely reinforce his anxiety. Exercise during the day, a warm drink (not coffee or tea) on going to bed, relaxation, and tackling worrying thoughts will usually induce sleep.

N 'Difficult' patients and 'difficult' behaviour

- Patients may be *technically* difficult, or present with chronic difficult or challenging behaviour.
- Behaviour that is particularly difficult to cope with, live with, or tolerate, includes:

1. manipulative behaviour
2. attention-seeking behaviour
3. acting-out behaviour
4. recurrent self-destructive behaviour
5. chronic complaining: fabricated disorder
6. social problems presenting with illness behaviour
7. difficult personalities (irritable, explosive, overly sensitive, or paranoid).

- No matter how difficult the patient, assessment must still be thorough. Difficult behaviour can occur in:

1. organic brain disease
2. psychotic illness
3. affective illness
4. intoxications
5. acute situational reactions
6. neurotic disorder
7. personality disorder.

Management

- Assess thoroughly and carefully.
- Engage the services of other agencies if needed.
- Ensure good cooperation and communication within the therapeutic team.
- Set well defined and sensible limits to behaviour.

Setting the scene

There are two meanings to the word difficult. Some patients are more difficult than others because they are *technically* more difficult, i.e., their complicated problems take more unravelling or understanding, or their treatment is more exacting and personally demanding. Their mental state may baffle diagnostic skills or the way their illness presents is so contaminated by cultural factors as to be assessable only with great effort.

Some patients are technically more difficult to manage because a therapeutic alliance is difficult to create (as with the severely brain impaired), or because of the chillingly alien nature of the patient's behaviour (as in catatonia), or because of acutely challenging behaviour. This may be aggression, verbal or physical, or other behaviour or verbal expressions that threaten the self-esteem or personal integrity of the psychiatrist—the manic patient who unleashes a host of wounding personal remarks, for example.

For most of us, however, after we have gained some experience, such technically difficult patients become a challenge to our skills and, after we have made the correct diagnostic formulation, contained the patient's aggression, seen the patient return to normality, and in some way got the patient *better*, leave us in a state of contentment and even exhilaration. We have won our spurs, or yet again demonstrated that we are worthy of them.

But what happens if the patient does not get better, or does not follow the rules, or presents us with chronically challenging behaviour that will not resolve despite your best efforts? What happens if, despite ourselves, we cannot get on or empathize with the patient? There are the patients who chronically frighten or frustrate us, whom we despair of, who get under our skin, who are irritating or demanding, who never seem satisfied with what we do for them, who ask for things we cannot supply or for an involvement or commitment we are reluctant or uneasy about giving, or who never seem to learn from their experiences or from what we tell them, or who endlessly complain, who present problems we cannot understand or solve.

Patients who present these chronic challenges to us and our colleagues (particularly our nursing colleagues) are particularly likely to be labelled as 'difficult'—using the other meaning of the word as implying chronically difficult or challenging behaviour. Such a label is, of course, pejorative and a value judgement. It is sometimes right and accurately reflects a chronic personality or behavioural defect in the patient that cannot be 'cured', must not be reinforced, and can only be recognized and contained by a 'damage limitation' policy.

But the label is often wrong and merely reflects lack

of skill or understanding on the part of the user, or is used is a means of remaining detached or uninvolved. It is often (like the term personality disorder) a refuge for the incompetent, the cynical, and the burnt out. Use the term 'difficult patient' sparingly and correctly. It is particularly easy when you are starting in psychiatry (and therefore particularly desirous of earning and keeping the approval of fellow staff members) to automatically assume that their attitudes towards a particular patient are right and therefore accept uncritically their dismissal of the patient as a time waster—'he's a psychopath', 'she's just manipulative'. Listen to what they say, but make up your own mind.

There are several types of behaviour that are particularly likely to get a patient labelled as 'difficult'.

Manipulative behaviour

Manipulative behaviour consists of using emotional pressure, blackmail, and bargaining to get one's way. It is particularly seen in people who are still enmeshed in childhood emotional behaviour and in mechanisms like playing mummy off against daddy. They exploit emotional weaknesses and professional anxieties, seek to drive wedges between authority figures, and are adept at playing people off against each other so that they exploit or create tensions within a therapeutic team. Manipulative behaviour can be extremely irritating, but can be countered by good communication within the team (and with the patient) and the setting of clear limits to the patient's behaviour. It is particularly important not to be seduced into making promises that you and your colleagues will not be able to keep. If your patient is forcing you to be a parent, do not be a bad one!

Attention seeking behaviour

Children often behave outrageously in order to gain attention from parents (a smack is better than being ignored completely). Similar behaviour is seen in some adults, particularly the socially impaired and the brain damaged. Through uproar and bad behaviour they achieve notice and may get their own way. True attention-seeking behaviour is rare. A great many legitimate requests for attention from patients, physical symptoms, or complaints of psychological symptoms, are often labelled by the weary or burnt out as attention-seeking behaviour when in fact they are not. When attention-seeking behaviour does occur it is again best countered by better communication and cooperation within the therapeutic team, and by the setting of a clear definition of what is and what is not acceptable behaviour (with the limits spelt out and adhered to) and encouraging the patient to verbalize his needs.

Acting-out behaviour

Some people are incapable of verbalizing their feelings, or have been taught to deny them or ignore them so that when feelings such as anger or despair become overwhelming they are not put into words but into deeds such as assault, window smashing, wrist slashing, etc. Such behaviour can be very disruptive on a ward, particularly if it is repetitive, and can lead to the rejection of the patient. Good communication and support within the therapeutic team, the setting of realistic limits to such behaviour or the provision of better alternatives (such as a 'rumpus room' or punch-bag), and constant encouragement to help the patient verbalize his feelings, is the correct response and often works.

Recurrent self-destructive behaviour

Patients who repeatedly overdose, slash their wrists, get drunk, or abuse drugs, can be particularly irritating and difficult to manage and easily acquire the pejorative label of a difficult or personality disordered patient. Although some patients (particularly those who repeatedly damage themselves with drugs or alcohol) are not seeking help and, indeed, cannot be helped, many patients with such repetitive behaviour patterns are in the grip of forces that they cannot control. If you are patient and tolerant with them, they can eventually learn to curb their behaviour and develop more socially acceptable ways of indicating their distress and seeking help. Rejecting them too early only makes their plight worse and some other doctor's task more difficult.

Chronic complaining/fabricated disorder

Patients who repeatedly present with complaints of physical symptoms for which there appears to be no underlying cause (or who present with emotional symptoms for which there seems to be no justification) are also irritating and are often regarded as difficult and are frequently rejected, particularly if we feel that we are being deliberately misled or deceived. But until we know the patient well, we cannot really judge whether we are being deceived or not. Even if we are, it is more important to find out the motive for the patient's behaviour than just unmask deception and reject the patient. Many doctors and nurses are too suspicious of patient's motives and accept very little of what they are told as genuine. It is, however, better to initially assume that you are being told the truth and to accept as genuine everything that the patient says. If the patient is indeed pulling the wool over your eyes you will eventually discover it and it does not really matter if you have been deceived for a while. It is not a slur on your skills. The patient who presents repeated somatic symptoms needs very careful assessment as much physical illness can masquerade as emotional illness and vice versa.

Social problems

Some people with chronic social problems, such as homelessness, lack of money, or unemployment, etc. will often present to the psychiatric services. They are demoralized and present it in the guise of physical or emotional illness (such things as poverty and home-lessness are stressful and will often produce stress symptoms). Some psychiatrists find such patients dif-ficult and feel that they are a waste of medical re-sources. Often, however, medical services, particularly emergency ones, are the only sources available to the patient to find initial help. Although the patient's needs will not be met by psychiatric treatment or by admission to hospital, the psychiatrist should be in a position to put the patient in contact with the appropriate social or other services and should not feel that his talents are being wasted by so doing. Do not, however, fob the patient off with empty or unrealistic promises about what such services may be able to do just to ease your own feelings of despair. Neither should the psychiatrist be surprised that some patients have learned to milk the system of all its possible advantages in terms of social support and social benefit. Most patients who do this are only obtaining what they are actually entitled to (a great deal of social benefit never gets paid to people who are entitled to it because they are unaware of their rights). Only rarely, in our experience, is false-hood used to obtain benefits. This, of course, cannot be condoned or supported.

Difficult personalities

Patients who are continually querulous, irritable, ex-plosive, overly sensitive, paranoid, or suspicious, are very difficult to support and help and you may have to set limited and long-term goals in terms of helping them to change their behaviour.

Assessment

Difficult patients are often poorly assessed and prematurely rejected. In assessing such a patient you should ignore the dismissal and prejudice of others and make your own full assessment, including physical, social, behavioural, and psychiatric components, before deciding on the best means of disposal and treatment. This means that you must get as much information about the patient as possible, not only from himself and his relatives but also from his general practitioner and any other services that the patient may be involved with. Do not make rushed judgements or hasty decisions, and always try not to let your pride prevent you from really understanding what is going on in the patient's life circumstances that may be making him behave in the way that he is.

Differential diagnosis

Organic disease

1. delirium (acute brain syndrome)
2. dementia (chronic brain syndrome).

Organic brain disease can make some patients very difficult, not just because they are potentially assaultive but often because one has to constantly repeat what one has said as attention and memory span is so short. Dementia often releases unpleasant and previously hidden personality traits so that the patient's behaviour becomes difficult to tolerate. Many doctors also find managing dementia difficult because success in management is so limited and depends often more on social factors than on medical treatment. Relatives may drag the patient from one useless consultation to another, and often want to secure inappropriate admissions of the patient to hospital as they cannot deal with the burden of looking after him.

Psychotic illness

1. schizophrenia
2. paranoid psychosis.

Some psychotic patients are difficult if they are aggressive, mute, or otherwise difficult to communicate with, or if they are severely thought disordered. Patients with chronic schizophrenia who have lost their volition and have many of the negative symptoms of schizophrenia can also become difficult patients with whom it is difficult to keep one's patience. If you try to concentrate purely on the patient's symptoms and not on the person himself, this can increase your own difficulties. Patients who do not respond to treatment can also become irritating. Chronic schizophrenic patients that are constantly demanding help, the need for and nature of which they cannot actually formulate, also need a great deal of patience. Remember that if you find the patient difficult, so will the relatives and they will need a chance to ventilate their feelings and grieve for the person they have lost.

Affective illness

1. mania
2. depression.

Hypomanic patients can be very difficult, partly because they are exhausting, as it is impossible to keep up with their energy, partly because as they feel so well that they resent control and containment bitterly, and partly because they are extremely good at making pointed, perceptive, and accurate personal remarks about their attendants, which increases tensions within the therapeutic team.

Depressed patients, who seek constant reassurance that they are going to get well, who have persistent somatic symptoms, or who need constant support, can also be very trying and are perceived as being difficult. Such patients, because their behaviour irritates their attendants, are often not assessed properly and their degree of depression not fully understood, which therefore either increases suicidal risk or causes a physical illness to be overlooked.

Intoxication

As mentioned earlier, patients who seem to deliberately and repeatedly intoxicate themselves either with alcohol or other substances can be very difficult patients indeed, and it is often difficult to find much empathy or understanding for them. It is particularly difficult to deal effectively with alcoholic patients who 'break the rules' about not drinking. They may very swiftly be rejected, but the policy of 'I will only treat you if you stay sober' can be very short-sighted and unproductive. Remember that drink brings out the worst in all of us, and your patient may be very different when he has dried out.

Acute situational reactions

Depending on what our own personal tradition is of dealing with crises, we may find that some patients, particularly those from other cultures, whose response to acute situations is apparently unexpected, overloud, overdemonstrative, or overindulgent, may also be classed as difficult. Our native culture is one in which overt displays of emotion, including tears, are rather frowned upon, and we may wrongly judge patients, who in our terms 'overreact', as lacking moral fibre, when their behaviour is perfectly acceptable within their own culture and probably more healthy than our emotional constipation.

Neurotic disorder

If we do not understand the distress that much neurotic illness brings with it, we will be at a loss to understand our patients and therefore may find their behaviour difficult. Likewise, many patients with neurotic disorders do resort to 'childish' methods of coping with them, such as manipulation. It is most important to ask when confronted with a patient who appears to be exhibiting blatantly manipulating behaviour, 'Why is this person doing this now?' Patients who are anxious but who do not show much somatic manifestation of it are particularly difficult to assess, and it is therefore often difficult to understand how anxious they are actually feeling. Patients with multiple somatic complaints may be seen as difficult. The behaviour of the severely obsessional patient may be difficult for others to tolerate or to understand.

Personality disorder

People with severe personality disorders may be very difficult to understand or to tolerate, particularly if their behaviour makes them consistently collide with authority, society, or with other people. Luckily, some psychiatrists are much more tolerant of the personality disordered than others and do feel that treatment, although goals are limited and very long-term, is justified and warranted (see Chapter 6, p. 536). The lazy, the incompetent, and the cynical amongst us, however, often label any behaviour we do not like as 'personality disorder', and since the majority of psychiatric professionals, whether medical or nursing, see personality disorder as something that is untreatable and best avoided, a very good way of dodging responsibility for treating patients is to label those patients as having a personality disorder. Be careful therefore before accepting other professionals' diagnoses of personality disorder in patients who are about to see you, and do remember that the diagnosis of personality disorder requires an in-depth knowledge of the patient, of his behaviour over a long period of time, and information from other people who know the patient well. It is not based on a snap diagnosis.

Management

The management of the difficult patient involves swallowing your pride (but accentuating your pride in your craft), and assessing the patient carefully and thoroughly, both physically and mentally. Try to get the patient to cooperate with you in setting realistic treatment goals, and engage the services of other agencies if they are more appropriate to your patient's care, but do not be pushed into accepting the patient into psychiatric care if psychiatric care is unlikely to do much for him. Have a thorough discussion of the patient's needs with other members of the therapeutic team and, particularly with manipulative or acting out behaviour, have carefully defined (and sensible) limits in terms of containing the patient's behaviour. If you do this you will find that many difficult patients stop being difficult, as most difficulties are in fact related to failures in communication and failure to understand the patient in front of you. This does not imply that you should be 'little goody two shoes', but you should, at all times, try to think about the interests of the person who has presented to you for help.

It is also important, if you always seem to be the victim of attention-seeking or manipulative behaviour, to ask yourself if there is something within you that encourages it. Look critically at your ward (or community) milieu as well. Have you set up rules that are just asking to be broken, flouted, or misunderstood? Have you set up a parental ambience in the staff that will encourage childlike dependence and rebellion in the patients?

Finally, most difficult patients stop being difficult once you have got to know them well enough to understand the reasons for their behaviour, usually rooted in their past experiences. You may still not be able to do much about the patient's behaviour, but it will not irritate you so much.

O Patients with abnormal movements

- Teach yourself to notice them.
- Look at videotaped examples.
- Be alert to movement disorders.
- In cases of doubt, videotape the patient and study at leisure.

Classification

1. Dyskinesias

    (a) myotonia
    (b) fasciculation
    (c) myoclonus (focal or generalized)
    (d) tics
    (e) chorea
    (f) hemiballism
    (g) athetosis.

2. Dystonias

    (a) generalized dystonias
    (b) focal dystonia
    (c) hemiplegic dystonia
    (d) tremor (resting, postural, and intention).

3. Akinetic syndromes

4. Manneristic movements

5. Stereotypy

6. Perseveration

7. Echopraxia.

Differential diagnosis

1. organic brain disease
2. encephalopathies
3. lipid storage disease
4. Huntington's chorea
5. Creutzfeldt–Jakob disease
6. Wilson's disease
7. Parkinson's disease
8. drug-induced parkinsonism
9. other drug-induced movement disorders (such as phenytoin)
10. brain damage/infarcts/tumours
11. intoxicants (heavy metals, illicit drugs)
12. alcoholism
13. epilepsy
14. metabolic disorders (such as uraemia).

Management

- Recognize the disorder.
- Remove the cause.
- Specific treatments (for example, levodopa).
- Many movement disorders are helped by anxiety management and counselling.

Setting the scene

Abnormal movements of various kinds are common in psychiatry. Like some of the other topics in this chapter, such as sleep disorders and seizure behaviour, movement disorder is not well taught, and often movements are not even noticed or, if they are, the psychiatrist runs away from them in a panic calling for the nearest neurologist. It is most important, first of all, to recognize that the patient has an abnormal movement and to be able to classify it. It is no use saying 'the patient was a bit twitchy' or, as sometimes happens, fail to recognize the import of abnormal movement because the patient is known to be psychotic or disturbed and, since disturbed people move oddly, one does not remark on it.

Teach yourself to look critically at the way in which the patient is moving and at any abnormalities of posture that he has. Try to accurately recognize what the movement disorder is. You need to be able to analyse movement and also to visually recognize abnormality. For this purpose, as with seizures, it is important that you review at least one of the several excellent videotapes on movement disorder that should be present in your postgraduate library as soon as possible.

Having noticed that the patient has an abnormal movement, and having classified it, you can then begin to think about a differential diagnosis and possible management. Be very alert to movement disorder because so often in psychiatry it is iatrogenic, and it is easy to blame subtle changes in movement on the patient's mental state so that you accept them without recognizing the early signs of tardive dyskinesia induced by your medication. Remember, too, that dyskinesia and bradykinesia are equally important movement disorders. Patients who are aware of their movement disorder will often try to conceal movements by making them look semi-purposive, and may be able to suppress them for short periods. Find out what the movements are like when the patient is off-guard, asleep, or alone. Severe movement disorder is also disturbing to relatives and friends, and you may be embarrassed to look at the patient critically (make a video record of the patient if you are).

Assessment of movement disorders

First ask yourself if you are looking at the twitching of an isolated muscle group or of several muscle groups working together. Is it always the same muscle group that is involved, or does the disorder flit from side to side and from limb to limb? Are you seeing a repetitive, recognizable movement, or at least some elements of movement? Does the patient seem aware of it? If so, what is his attitude to it and how does he explain it? If you draw the patient's attention to the movement can he stop it or modify it? During the movement does anything else obvious go on in the patient? Does he make a noise, for instance?

A careful account of the movement disorder and careful observation should be followed by a formal medical, neurological, and psychiatric history, and a full examination of the patient is mandatory. Occasionally, special investigations, such as lumbar puncture, electromyography, EEG, CT, and MRI scanning, may be indicated. A full family history and assessment for evidence of cognitive impairment is also important.

Types of abnormal movement

Dyskinesias

1. Muscle twitching

Myokymia Repetitive twitching of a small group of individual fibres, which is not strong enough to move the affected part. It commonly occurs in the face, is of little diagnostic import if it remains confined to the original focus, and suggests fatigue or tension. Patients often find it subjectively distressing and it may continue for a long time.

Fasciculation Repetitive twitching of individual fibres, but more widespread (although only one muscle or limb may be affected and there is no muscle movement).

Patients may not be aware of it. Of more sinister import, it may be seen in local muscle disease, motor neuron disease, demyelination, occasionally in thyrotoxicosis, and other conditions that cause partial denervation of the muscle.

2. Muscle jerking

Single shock-like jerks of a muscle, which may be local, irregular, repetitive, generalized, or rhythmic.

Segmental (focal) myoclonus This may be due to local spinal disease (tumour, infarct, etc.), or to midbrain disease (as in palatal myoclonus). It is usually rhythmic. Occasionally, epilepsia partialis continuans may resemble it, and reflex myoclonus of a muscle group may occur.

Myoclonus associated with epilepsy This includes:

- myoclonic absences (patient may be unaware)
- Lennox–Gastaut syndrome
- infantile spasms.

Myoclonus with encephalopathy (progressive) For example, Lafora body disease, Batten's disease, familial myoclonic epilepsy, and other leucodystrophies.

Myoclonus with cerebral disease For example, Creutzfeldt–Jakob disease, Alzheimer's disease, subacute sclerosing leucoencephalitis, and post-traumatic.

Myoclonus with systemic disease For example, uraemia, hypocalcaemia, hepatic coma, CO_2 retention.

Idiopathic—usually benign, often familial.

3. Muscle jerking—tics

These are stereotyped, irregularly repetitive jerking movements of a single muscle group. The patient is aware of them and can often, for a time, suppress them.

They are common and usually disappear in childhood. They may occur as an isolated condition in adult life, often in association with tension. They can be symptomatic of encephalitis, may follow trauma, and may be drug induced. They also occur in Gilles de la Tourette syndrome.

4. Muscle jerking—chorea

In this disorder, jerking movements occur, which are a little like tics, but which are widely distributed (although may be unilateral), can be partially suppressed, or made semi-purposive. They include:

Huntington's chorea (see Section 6D, p. 487)   Other hereditary choreas can occur, but they are usually benign.

Sydenham's chorea   This occurs following rheumatic fever and recovers. It does not cause intellectual impairment and is not associated with a positive family history. It occurs in the young.

Chorea gravidarum   This is probably Sydenham's chorea that is reactivated by pregnancy (or the pill).

Symptomatic chorea (cerebral)   This can be caused by cerebrovascular disease with thalamic damage, cerebral birth injury, tumours, trauma (usually unilateral), and encephalitis lethargica.

Symptomatic chorea (systemic disorder)   Thyrotoxicosis, hyponatraemia, hypoparathyroidism, polycythaemia rubra vera, neuroleptic drugs, phenytoin, and alcohol, can all cause symptomatic chorea.

5. Muscle jerking—hemiballism

This is sudden occasional gross jerks of a limb or limbs, which fling the limb away from the body. It is due to thalamic damage often caused by cerebral birth injury, and occasionally by tumour or infarct (particularly in the elderly).

6. Involuntary muscle movements—athetosis (paroxysmal dystonia)

Writhing movements of a limb or limbs that can be continuous or intermittent, which start distally and move proximally, and over which the patient has no control. They are seen in cerebral palsy.

7. Involuntary muscle movements—dystonias

Dystonic movements are sustained rather than jerking in character, and produce a prolonged change in posture or position. They include:

Generalized dystonia   This may occur for no known cause or may be genetic (there are several forms). It may be symptomatic of various leucodystrophies and lipid storage diseases, cerebral palsy, Wilson's disease, and the juvenile form of Huntington's chorea. It may also be drug induced (neuroleptics) and may then be acute or chronic. Paroxysmal forms occur and some forms have a marked diurnal fluctuation.

Focal dystonia   There are various forms of focal dystonia including spasmodic torticollis and blepharospasm, which are now thought to be organic in nature. Dystonias associated with occupation (writer's cramp, musician's cramp) are thought by some to be organic (although organic treatment is usually unhelpful), but most psychiatrists see them as related to tension and they often respond well to specific muscular relaxation treatments, such as biofeedback, massage, etc.

Hemiplegic dystonia   Dystonia is occasionally found in just one limb or unilaterally, and is often associated with weakness. It is usually due to a stroke, tumours, chronic focal infection, or develops following trauma.

8. Tremor

Tremor involves the rhythmic oscillation of part of the body. It includes:

Resting tremor This is seen only in extrapyramidal disease, particularly Parkinson's disease, postencephalitic parkinsonism, and in other rare extrapyramidal disorders. It can be neuroleptic drug induced.

Postural tremor This may be physiological, and may occur in both anxiety and in thyrotoxicosis, heavy metal poisoning, following treatment with sympathomimetics, antidepressants, and lithium. Severe postural tremor occurs in cerebellar disease, Wilson's disease, and, rarely now, neurosyphilis. Benign essential tremor is seen in the absence of precipitating causes and tends to be familial. It is made worse by anxiety.

Intention tremor This is seen in brainstem or cerebellar disease due to multiple sclerosis, vascular damage, occasionally tumours, and the rare spinocerebellar degenerations.

9. Akinetic syndromes

These are characterized by slowness of voluntary movement and rigidity, which give rise to the characteristic postural and locomotion abnormalities so typical of Parkinson's disease. There is increased tone in response to passive movement, which may be continuous (*lead pipe*) or interrupted (*cogwheel*). Resting tremor is common. Patients have a characteristic gait—they do not swing their arms and they shuffle with small steps and a festinant gait. Patients may be unable to move, be slow to move, or have a reduced amplitude of movement (all may occur in the same patient). There is poverty of facial expression and sometimes unpleasant restlessness of the legs (akathisia). Tardive dyskinesia involves repetitive movement of the mouth, tongue, sometimes of the facial muscles, the shoulders, neck or abdomen. It is usually drug induced, but may be postencephalic or occur spontaneously.

Parkinson's disease is the commonest cause of the

akinetic rigidity syndrome (including drug-induced parkinsonism and postencephalic parkinsonism). Akinetic rigidity syndromes also occur in association with other brain degenerations, such as progressive supranuclear palsy, progressive autonomic failure (Shy–Drager syndrome), other multiple-system atrophies, cerebrovascular disease, and disorder of the basal ganglia.

A degree of the akinetic rigidity syndrome may also occur in Alzheimer's disease, Binswanger's disease, following brain damage, in Pick's disease, Creutzfeldt–Jakob disease, neurosyphilis, and in some intoxications (such as manganese). There are certain hereditary causes of the syndrome including Wilson's disease, juvenile Huntington's chorea, Lesch–Nyhan disease, and other rare disorders.

10. Manneristic movements
A mannerism is an apparently purposeful act (like shaking hands), but which is consistently carried out in an odd or unusual way.

11. Stereotypy
An apparently purposeful act but performed out of context in a repetitive, stereotyped, and meaningless way.

12. Perseveration
A requested command is carried out and is then endlessly repeated without further request or need.

13. Echopraxia
An apparently purposeless copying of another's movements or gestures without being asked to do so (for example, clapping hands). It often occurs with echolalia.

Differential diagnosis
Organic brain disease
1. delirium (acute brain syndrome)
2. dementia (chronic brain syndrome).

368 | Practical Psychiatry

The importance of movement disorders in organic brain disease should be obvious from the list of disorders described above. Huntington's chorea or Creutzfeldt–Jakob disease are typical examples of the need for the psychiatrist to be able to recognize and assess movement disorders. The occupational dystonias are also a legitimate part of psychiatric practice and should not be abandoned to the neurologists.

Psychotic illness

As indicated elsewhere (p. 469) all patients presenting with psychotic illness should be carefully examined for evidence of movement disorder because so much movement disorder is iatrogenic. It should be remembered, however, that schizophrenics, even untreated, may occasionally develop movement disorder, particularly the akinetic syndrome, and drug treatment may merely awaken something prematurely that would have developed anyway. Some primary disorders of movement (for example, Huntington's chorea, Creudzfeldt–Jakob disease, encephalitis) may initially present with a psychotic illness. Catatonia (see p. 377) may also be the presenting sign of a psychotic illness or of an underlying physical illness.

Affective illness

Apart from muteness and stupor (p. 377), movement disorders are rare in affective illness, although tremor is an extremely common side-effect of antidepressant treatment, particularly tricyclic antidepressants and lithium.

Intoxication

Tremor is common in alcoholism and with abuse of sympathomimetic drugs. A parkinsonian syndrome is sometimes the result of indulgence in contaminated street drugs. This is not uncommon in the United States, but so far is rare in this country.

Acute situational reactions

These may exacerbate or reawaken previous movement disorders, such as tics, Sydenham's chorea, etc., or may make an existing disorder a great deal worse.

Neurotic disorder

Anxiety commonly causes tremor of a postural type (occasionally resting) and will again make a pre-existing movement disorder worse. Very occasionally hysterical tremor or hysterical movement disorder (usually associated with gait) may be seen.

Personality disorder

Since many patients with personality disorders become transiently anxious or indulge in illicit substances, a secondary movement disorder may occur in the personality disordered.

Management

The management of movement disorder involves recognizing the kind of disorder that you are seeing and making the necessary investigations related to the differential diagnosis. Particularly with psychiatric patients, carefully enquire as to what drugs, both licit and illicit, the patient is taking, and then remove the cause if possible. The management of organic movement disorders is outwith the scope of this book, except to say that patients with movement disorders that are organic are often faced with lifelong disability and will therefore often develop secondary psychological phenomena. Many movement disorders are made worse by stress and anxiety, and treating this will often make the movement disorder a great deal better. The various drug treatments for movement disorder (for example, levodopa) often have profound secondary psychological effects including affective disorder and hallucinations. The management of many chronic movement disorders is therefore an example of when cooperation between neurologist and psychiatrist is particularly important.

P The mute patient

- Such patients are difficult to assess—you have to do all the work!
- Do not rush into treatment until assessment is complete, unless the patient needs immediate first aid.
- Always be tactful and polite. Assume that the patient can hear you, understand you, and will remember what you are doing.

Assessment

- Is the mutism complete, partial, or selective?
- Is anything else obviously wrong (mental or physical disorder)?
- What kind of communication and rapport can you establish?
- Assess conscious level.
- Assess posture (fixed? resistance to movement? waxy flexibility?).
- What is the patient's response to you and others?
- Is there negativism or obedience?
- Retardation?
- Is he continent or incontinent?
- Does he eat or drink?
- Can be dress himself?

- What is his facial expression?
- Eyes open or closed?
- Any emotional response to questions?
- Perform a physical examination including:

  General medical examination
  What is the muscle tone like?
  Any echopraxia/echolalia?
  Any sensory response?
  Any eye movement to command (or following)?
  Any eye blinking (spontaneous or following treatment)?
  Do pupils dilate if you squeeze neck?
  Are pupillary reflexes present?

- Assess communication:

  Is the patient mouthing, muttering, or whispering?
  Will the patient write if he cannot speak?

- Perform necessary physical investigations:

  Haematology and biochemistry, blood gases, syphilitic
  serology.
  EEG is often indicated, and cerebral radiography is
  sometimes necessary.

Differential diagnosis

1. akinetic mutism
2. organic mutism; causes include brainstem infarct or tumour, colloid cyst of third ventricle, widespread demyelination, water intoxication, liver failure, Cushing's syndrome, Addisonian crisis, hyponatraemia, epileptic twilight state, typhoid, and typhus
3. catatonic schizophrenia
4. depressive stupor
5. intoxication
6. hysteria
7. malingering.

Management

- Investigate thoroughly (many are organic)
- Abreact
- Treat the cause.

Setting the scene

Although the problem is comparatively rare, mute patients (whether they have attendant behaviour disturbance or not) pose particular difficulty in assessment because the main means of communication with the patient have been lost and he is often (although not invariably) uncooperative, so that the assessing psychiatrist has to rely on the scraps of information obtained from a truncated mental and physical state examination (with often a rising state of frustration). Such frustration and lack of communication often lead to impetuously taken decisions about what is wrong with the patient, and ill conceived action plans.

In managing the mute or unresponsive patient, be careful not to rush into making a diagnosis or starting to treat the patient until you have made a thorough unhurried assessment, unless the patient is clearly severely physically ill, for example, with advanced dehydration, or is cyanosed or has respiratory difficulties. It is important to remember that florid hysterical symptoms may be masking an underlying organic or psychotic disorder. It has certainly been our impression during the last few years that nowadays muteness or unresponsiveness in a patient usually suggests an underlying organic disorder rather than a psychotic illness.

Assessment

In communicating with a mute, unresponsive or apparently comatose patient, always be tactful and polite and assume that the patient, although unresponsive, can both hear you and will remember everything that you say and do. Talk to the patient as you examine him, never take him by surprise, tell him everything you are going to do, and why you are doing it. Do not startle or frighten him, and stop if you detect signs of irritation or rising tension within the patient.

In the old days, mute patients were divided into those who were 'mute of malice' and those who were 'mute by the visitation of God'. In other words, those patients who were choosing not to speak and those who, because of illness, were unable to. It is still a useful working diagnostic distinction. Mutism may be pure (in other words the patient is mute but everything else is normal). It may be intermittent or partial, it may be selective, and is usually accompanied by other symptoms and signs of physical or mental illness, and may be accompanied by clouding of consciousness.

If you can, take a full history from a friend or relative before seeing the patient. How did the mutism start? Was is sudden or was it gradual? What other symptoms accompanied it? Were there any recent physical or mental symptoms preceding this mute episode? Have there been significant life events?

Then approach the patient, introduce yourself, and explain what you are going to do and why. Try to gain an unhurried first impression, and make a cool, thorough assessment of the patient. Have a plan of assessment in your mind before you start. Try to answer these general questions:

1. Is this mutism complete or partial? Is it intermittent? Is it selective?

2. Apart from the mutism, is there anything else obviously wrong with the patient?

3. What kind of rapport can you develop with this patient?

4. How well can you communicate with the patient without speaking?

5. What is the conscious level of the patient and does it flucuate? Is there clouding of consciousness?

6. Are there other signs and symptoms of mental illness?

7. Is there evidence of physical disease?

Then make a systematic examination looking at the following topics:

1. *Conscious level*   Is the patient stuporose but alert, drowsy but rousable, drowsy but only partly rousable? Is there evidence of clouding of consciousness? Are there short-term fluctuations in his consciousness level?

2. *Posture*   Is it fixed (such as a psychic pillow)? Is it comfortable or not? What does the patient do if you move him? Is there resistance to passive movement? If you passively move the patient's limbs and leave them, do they return to their original position or remain immobile in the position you moved them to (waxy flexibility)?

3. *Response to examiner and others*   Is it consistent? Is it different to the examiner than it is to nurses or relatives? Does the patient show resistance to commands, or apathetic compliance, or automatic obedience (i.e., when asked to do something potentially painful like the conventional 'stick out your tongue and let me put a pin in it', does he respond positively)? Is the patient completely non-responsive?

Does he show any spontaneous actions (stereotyped or manneristic behaviour in particular)? Is he playful, mischievous, irritable, or assaultive (do not persist with the examination if you detect rising tension or hostility)? Is there retardation of movement (if movement exists)? Is it only in the initial part of the movement?

Does the patient indicate his toileting needs and, if so, how? Is he continent or incontinent? If he is incontinent, does he notice and show any emotional reaction? (If the patient is restless, always remember to check the bladder to see if there is retention of urine).

Does the patient drink or eat if offered sustenance? If you actually put a glass to the patient's lips, is there automatic swallowing or does nothing happen? Can the patient dress himself?

What is the patient's facial expression (is it vacant, sulky, smiling, or perplexed)? Are the eyes open or closed? Are there any emotional expressions such as tears? Does the patient respond with any show of emotion when sensitive subjects, such as friends or relatives, are discussed?

4. *Physical examination* In the unresponsive, resistant patient this is difficult. A general medical examination is necessary, looking particularly for signs of cardiac and respiratory failure, liver failure, and severe dehydration. As full a neurological examination as possible should also be made, looking particularly for evidence of raised intracranial pressure or focal cortical abnormality.

Is there echopraxia or echolalia? Examine muscle tone. Can you elicit any sensory response?

If the eyes are closed, can they be opened? Do the eyes move to command, do they look away from the speaker, or look at the speaker? Can the patient follow your finger with his eyes? Is there an unblinking stare, or is there spontaneous blinking or blinking on approach of a hand or finger? Is there eyelid flickering? Do the pupils dilate following a painful squeeze of the neck (if not this suggests a lesion of the third ventricle or midbrain)? Are there the usual pupillary responses?

5. *Communication* Is the patient mute but trying to communicate by facial gesture, mouthing, whispering,

or muttering (see Section 4E, p. 165)? Make sure that you give the retarded patient time to respond. Occasionally, the patient will only speak when your back is turned (characteristic of catatonia).

6. *Physical investigation* Blood chemistry (electrolytes, liver and renal function, thyroid function) and haematology. Blood gases (when indicated). Syphilitic serology. An EEG is often helpful (as is occasionally a CT scan of the brain). The EEG in psychotic or simulated mutism is usually normal, although it may reflect, particularly in catatonic schizophrenia, a marked degree of tension. There may be EEG evidence of generalized brain disturbance, evidence of a focal disturbance, or continuous epileptic activity.

7. *Psychological investigation* Abreaction using intravenous barbiturates or benzodiazepines is a very effective diagnostic measure (see p. 411).

Differential diagnosis

Organic brain disease

1. delirium (acute brain syndrome)
2. dementia (chronic brain syndrome).

Stupor, with or without other behavioural changes, may occur in both acute brain syndromes and in chronic brain syndromes.

Akinetic mutism is a stupor (usually due to lesions of the midbrain or the third ventricle) in which the patient appears to be quietly asleep with relaxed breathing. He can be wakened, but very rapidly falls asleep again and sometimes may fall asleep whilst talking. He may at times, when awoken, appear confused or confabulate. Patients who recover are usually totally amnesic for the event. If it is accompanied by headache and vomiting, it usually indicates raised intracranial pressure (look for papilloedema). If there are recurrent short-lived attacks of akinetic mutism, particularly if they appear to occur when the patient changes position, suspect a colloid cyst of the third ventricle.

Organic muteness in which the patient is apparently alert but expressionless and unresponsive, usually indicates widespread disturbance of cortical function. Catatonic features (see p. 378) are common in organic mutism and are certainly not confined to catatonic schizophrenia.

The causes of akinetic mutism and the organic mute state are many. For example, trauma, brainstem infarct, widespread metabolic disturbance in the brain, or widespread demyelination, water intoxication, advanced liver disease (in advanced liver disease stupor is fluctuating and proceeds from delirium into stupor and then into coma, and there is often a characteristic foetor hepaticus with a flapping tremor, liver palms, and, in men, gynaecomastia and soft testes), Cushing's syndrome, Addisonian crisis (often preceded by emotional symptoms), hyponatraemia, epileptic twilight state, rheumatic chorea, typhoid, and typhus (in typhus the stupor is often called *coma vigile* and is accompanied by both catatonic and extrapyramidal symptoms).

Psychotic illness

Occasionally, schizophrenic patients may remain still and unresponsive in response to command hallucinations, but the characteristic stupor of schizophrenia is a catatonic stupor. This varies in depth and duration. There is usually a fixed and often bizarre posture (i.e., the psychic pillow, in which the patient's head remains six inches off the real pillow as though supported by an imaginary one). Even if he is standing the patient can remain immobile and have a bizarre posture for long periods of time. Any movements are not retarded, although the initial component may be, but

378 | Practical Psychiatry

there may be marked negativism and a resistance to passive movement. There may be grimacing and manneristic gestures, including characteristic pursing and pouting of the lips. The patient often looks perplexed or terrified.

The patient is characteristically unresponsive to stimulation and command, is rigid when touched, but may show automatic obedience. His eyes usually follow movement, but not if he is asked to. Usually there is food and drink refusal, waxy flexibility, and often echopraxia and echolalia. The patient may speak if the examiner turns his back. He is usually incontinent or may have retention of urine and faeces without soiling. Rarely, there is sudden and extreme overactivity and aggression (so called catatonic excitement).

Catatonic stupor (and particularly catatonic excitement) is now rare, presumably because schizophrenia is treated with appropriate medication at an early stage of onset. It should be particularly remembered that catatonic stupor is not characteristic of schizophrenia and is common in organic disease. Occasionally, patients with schizophrenia and with paranoid psychoses may show extreme withdrawal (often because they are preoccupied with their own hallucinatory experiences) without true catatonic symptoms. Neuroleptic medication may *cause* catatonic stupor.

Affective illness

1. mania
2. depression.

Very rarely, patients with an extreme degree of mania may become mute because their thoughts are occurring so rapidly that they do not have time to express them. It is usually extremely obvious that the patient has been manic before this stuporous state occurs, although mutism interspersed with wild excitement may initially be mistaken for catatonic schizophrenia (although in the mute state the patient will not have any of the characteristic features of the catatonic state).

A patient with severe, retarded depression may slip slowly into stupor. Characteristically his movements and thoughts become slower and slower, often with fluctuations, until he appears stuporose (usually the patient is never completely in stupor). If any speech or movement does occur, there is obvious gross retardation throughout both. Facial expression is one of distress and despair. The other features of depression, such as early morning waking, previously expressed depressive delusions, and weight loss, will usually be apparent in the history.

Intoxication

Occasionally, intoxication with barbiturates may give rise to a stuporose state. Transient psychotic states induced by LSD, PCP, etc. may include mutism. Patients grossly intoxicated with alcohol may also be stuporose, but this is usually obvious (it will briefly respond to intravenous naloxone if you are uncertain what you are dealing with).

Acute situational reactions

Occasionally, people overwhelmed by emotional stress or disaster may pass through a transient mute and stuporose state. This can often be seen as an extreme degree of denial, 'She pined in thought, And with a green and yellow melancholy she sat like Patience on a monument, Smiling at grief.'

Neurotic disorder

Mutism and stupor may occur as part of an hysterical reaction. The patient only rarely shows catatonic symptoms or negativism and is usually responsive, except for total (and obviously non-organic) aphonia.

The patient can usually be encouraged to whisper and gradually regain speech. Abreaction may be helpful. The mutism is often symbolic of the underlying conflict in the patient's life (like something the patient cannot talk about). It is important in managing the condition to discover the underlying reason, otherwise symptom substitution may occur, or the patient may be left defenceless and as a result attempt or succeed at suicide. Hysterical mutism is often selective, there is often a clear secondary gain, and the patient often shows characteristic *belle indifférence*. Patients with hysterical mutism are often easily communicated with, will obey commands, and will write if given instruments to write with.

Personality disorder

Elective mutism may occasionally occur in patients with a personality disorder. Clinically the patient is clearly choosing not to speak, but in other respects can be communicated with. Occasionally, unconsciousness is consciously simulated with the patient lying inert and unresponsive (but not usually showing negativism) and making no attempt to communicate. Unconsciousness can sometimes be imitated with great skill, and may not respond to abreaction. Usually consciousness is regained if some fairly drastic neurosurgical procedure is suggested.

Management

The management of the mute patient involves making an accurate diagnosis, although if abreaction is employed often diagnosis and treatment go hand in hand. Intravenous amylobarbitone or diazepam given slowly (see p. 411) is often very helpful. Patients in organic stupor do not usually respond to abreaction, although very occasionally some speech is regained. Patients in catatonic stupor may relax sufficiently for thought disorder or hallucinatory experiences to be revealed under abreaction. The severely depressed will often be able to express depressive ideas. Patients with hysterical mutism almost invariably begin to speak and reveal their problems. It should be remembered, however, that both barbiturates and diazepam may release previously controlled aggressive behaviour or induce an explosive outburst of psychotic experience, so that sufficient staff must be available to control the patient if he does explode. Under the influence of both barbiturates and diazepam, it is possible for the patient to fabricate and dissociate further, and this investigation should not be done lightly.

The treatment of organic stupor depends on the cause. Since the stupor will usually last for a long time, even if recovery occurs, the patient will need careful nursing to prevent hypostatic pneumonia, bed sores, etc. Catatonic stupor is best treated with intravenous neuroleptics, such as haloperidol or droperidol, and, if this fails, with electroconvulsive therapy (which can be life-saving). If the stupor is long maintained, the patient will need rehydration and good nursing care. Patients in a depressive stupor need ECT, again with careful nursing because of the physical problems that may arise from dehydration or hypostatic pneumonia. Careful observation is also needed because often, as retardation lifts, suicidal feelings can be acted upon. Patients with hysterical mutism need to be helped to regain their powers of speech and communication, and need both supportive psychotherapy to deal with the underlying problems that have caused the hysterical symptoms and also a careful behavioural regimen to avoid secondary reinforcement of the underlying symptoms. Patients who are clearly malingering need firm discouragement.

Future management

Patients with recurrent schizophrenic episodes or recurrent depression need educating (as do their relatives) about the early symptoms of schizophrenia or depression so that potentially life-threatening episodes of stupor can be avoided in future by prompt and early treatment.

CHAPTER 5

Treatment

A General principles (*primum non nocere*)

In psychiatry treatment involves much more than just giving a prescription (either for a drug or for a course of some psychological therapy). It also involves the *management* of the patient both in terms of his understanding of the illness and his daily life, plus the daily lives and relationships of those people to whom he is close and even of people who stand in less close but equally meaningful relationships, such as colleagues at work or his peer group. It is impossible to treat psychiatric illness in isolation. Most psychiatric 'illness' also shows a conspicuous tendency to get better, and it is important to make sure that your treatment and management do not get in the way of this recovery process, and that the treatment is not worse than the condition itself (substituting a lifelong dependence on benzodiazepines for a mild and transient anxiety, for instance). The medical adage *primum non nocere* is important in psychiatry. Most treatment should be aimed at hastening recovery, preventing handicap, developing insight, and developing the patient's own skills in dealing with his problems and preventing recurrence, or at least helping the patient and his family to recognize relapse quickly if it should occur, and to equip them to deal with it.

Very few treatments in psychiatry are specific. Antipsychotic drugs do not cure schizophrenia, nor antidepressants depression. They contain and control unpleasant symptoms and help to make the unbearable

bearable until natural recovery occurs. About the only specific treatment in psychiatry is penicillin for neurosyphilis, and even this treatment does not offer a cure for the damage already done, but merely prevents further damage from occurring. Most drug treatments in psychiatry are good at removing positive symptoms (hallucinations, altered mood, etc.), but are of little use for negative symptoms, such as lethargy, loss of fighting spirit, boredom, and institutionalization, for which psychological treatments are much more appropriate.

When starting psychiatry it is important to beware of the seduction of the illness model that you have been assiduously taught in medical school. There are few real illnesses in psychiatry—most illnesses are reactions (understandable or not) to circumstances rather than illnesses, and even the few conditions that do follow the illness model need as much psychological treatment and management as physical treatment (for example, depression, epilepsy, etc.). Illnesses that recur need support, explanation, and the development of the patient's own skills in coping with them, rather than medication. Because you are medically trained you will tend to think in terms of treatment by drugs or other medical intervention (as, sadly, will your examiners). You need to be able to develop the skill to see people, their lives, their 'illness', and their situation as a whole, and begin to recognize how much you can do for people by helping them to alter their situation or the reactions of other people to them, and also how much your own personality and optimism is involved in getting people better, or helping them to endure the unalterable.

When planning treatment you need first of all to ask yourself 'What is it I am treating?' This does not mean just trying to identify the 'illness' you are treating but also the various elements in the patient's life that may also need to be managed if one is to have a successful treatment outcome. You do need, of course, to be good at diagnostics and not, for instance, treat an excited, deluded, hallucinated man for schizophrenia when in fact he is manic, or call confusion thought disorder or vice versa. Except in an emergency, it is wise to accumulate enough medical, social, and psychological evidence about a particular person before embarking on a treatment plan. For this reason it is often best if you admit somebody to hospital, even if they are acutely ill, to wait for two or three days if you can to see if the condition spontaneously resolves once the patient has been withdrawn from the stressful environment that may have precipitated the illness, and to learn a little more about the illness and the person who has the illness, before you start treatment. The art of psychiatry is to keep a balance between overreaction and inaction.

It is also useful to ask yourself the question 'What am I trying to do?' Try to be systematic about your treatment aims, have a clear idea of what treatment goals you are trying to reach, and ask yourself what key symptoms you are trying to alter. In particular, identify key symptoms that you should monitor so that you can detect whether or not the treatment has worked (for example, weight or sleep in depression, or the encapsulation and disappearance of delusional ideas in schizophrenia). Some symptoms are much easier to monitor than others. There are even problems with monitoring such apparently clear-cut entities as weight or sleep, but determining if a patient has really stopped having delusions or has lost his hallucinations can be difficult. Patients who retain insight are only too well aware that if they go on declaring their odd ideas they will remain under treatment.

Do not concentrate on the 10 per cent of the person that is 'ill' and ignore the other 90 per cent of the patient that is well, so that you concentrate on reducing symptoms without ever looking at the resources and the skills that the patient already has, although he may not be putting them to good use. These must be put into your treatment plan; concentrating wholly on illness reinforces sickness behaviour.

In a treatment plan it is important, if you can, to change one variable at a time. Do not introduce two treatments at the same time so that you cannot recognize the effect of either. It is also important that you consider both the possible benefits of the treatment and its possible toxicity (this does not just apply to medical or drug treatment). Psychological treatments also have their side-effects (for example, dependency or unpleasant transference effects in psychotherapy). If the patient is embarking on a course of formal psychotherapy, you have to be certain (as does he) that he can commit the necessary time to it and endure the possible emotional turmoil it will produce.

It is best to treat your patient as a colleague with whom you should discuss the planned treatment as much as possible. This certainly increases compliance. It may be possible to do this even with a severely psychotic person, although occasionally you will have to override the patient's wishes if you consider him dangerous to himself or to other people. In order to enhance compliance it is important to avoid complex treatment regimens. Any necessary drug treatments should be kept as simple as possible, and you must avoid trying to treat the patient with different classes of drugs at the same time unless it is absolutely necessary. In behavioural and cognitive treatments, and in psychotherapy, you will discover the value of explaining, reviewing, and rehearsing your treatment programme with the patient and always trying to answer his questions honestly.

Be eclectic—one hopes that as you gain experience you will tend to become eclectic and you will draw from all the various treatment methods and disciplines techniques and ideas that you can apply to the particular individual in front of you, rather than sticking rigidly to one model of psychotherapy or to one model of behaviour therapy. As you gain in experience, and as you gain in confidence in using these techniques, you will find that more and more problems in psychiatry are amenable to psychological therapy without needing recourse to drugs or to other physical treatments. This is what makes psychiatry worthwhile and enjoyable.

When you feel insecure professionally you are likely to become unduly rejecting of other models or approaches, or overly accepting of them. Discovering the role of different treatment models in managing the same symptoms in the same patient is a rewarding and maturing process.

B The therapeutic team

Psychiatric 'illness' is multifactorial and medical treatment forms only a small part of what should be offered to the patient. Medical treatment may be totally inappropriate for what is a reaction to circumstances rather than an illness, and most of the therapeutic effort should be directed towards helping the patient to take stock of himself, to look at the stresses and uncertainties in his life, to make decisions about how to manage them, or to change his circumstances. To do this one has to make a social and psychological assessment of the patient as well as a physical and a psychiatric one. Although as you grow in experience in psychiatry you will develop these skills, at first you will be inexpert and greatly hampered by the medical model that you are taking into psychiatry. You therefore need the help and support of other disciplines who are more used to assessing these aspects of the patient than you are. You will learn a great deal from them.

Some of them use methods of assessing the patient similar to your own, but others use very different methods and very different models. It is useful to take a holistic and wide-ranging view of the patient, to have several models to operate, and to take a multifactorial approach. The medical needs of the patient may be important, but you may also need to help him change his beliefs, his thinking, and his social circumstances as well as the beliefs, thinking, and social circumstances of his family and significant others. This is best done by a therapeutic team—a collection of professional people with different skills who join together to plan the overall management of the patient, bringing to the team their separate skills.

Teams work both in hospital and in the community, although at present you are more likely to encounter one when you work in the community. There is a *team leader* (who is usually the senior medical member of the team, because of his or her overall clinical and legal responsibilities), but the leader of the team does not have to be medical, and there may be times when it is better if he is not. The team usually assigns a *key worker* to be the active liaison worker with and advocate for the patient, who reports back regularly to the other members of the team. To be effective, multidisciplinary teams should be small with no more than four to five members, and composed of people from no more than three disciplines. Too many disciplines and too many members lead to sterile arguments. There are also problems if individual members of the team are responsible to line managers outwith the team. For instance, the psychologist or social worker in a team is not primarily responsible to the team but to his or her own manager. Such divided loyalties can present insuperable problems. The team that is entirely responsible to itself does need some outside supervision, as some teams can become very inward looking and lose perspective.

The team should hold regular meetings in which views can be freely exchanged and treatment plans worked out. A good team with high morale can be extremely exciting to work in. A poor team with low morale and with cynical burnt-out members who spend most of their time discussing their own problems and giving themselves therapy, can be very destructive. The morale of a team is partly dependent on the leader, upon whom a great deal of responsibility lies, but often unfortunately is outwith the remedy of members of the team because it is dependent on external forces like workload and finance.

Poor morale and too heavy a workload with lack of support leads to burn out. Burnt-out therapists are weary, cynical, and jaded, and find everyday clinical problems and the problems of their patients apparently insurmountable. They lose their sense of perspective and sense of humour and optimism. Groups can avoid this by having a good leader, by having some control over their workload, and by individuals within the group having a life outside it.

The role of the junior doctor within the group is to learn from others, to be prepared to admit ignorance, to recognize the limitations of the medical model, and to begin to acquire counselling, psychotherapeutic, behavioural, and cognitive skills from others, to apply them, and to use his medical knowledge wisely (as one of the perspectives that the group has in assessing and managing a particular patient).

The team may be composed of people from several different disciplines, and it is important for you to recognize the contribution that each can make and also the contribution that people from other disciplines, who may not be part of the team, can provide to the management of the patient.

Nurses

Psychiatric nursing has a long history and tradition, but it is presently undergoing painful changes in the way it sees itself and its role. Nurses, for a long time, were regarded purely as medical handmaidens, keepers, and containers of the disturbed and purveyors of medication. All this is slowly changing. You will still meet nurses, particularly in hospital, who are all for a quiet life (particularly on night duty), but you will also meet nurses who see their role as counsellors, psychotherapists, or cognitive and behavioural therapists, and who work hard to provide a good therapeutic atmosphere on the ward. Some nurses are now recognized *nurse therapists* and are particularly skilled in behavioural and cognitive techniques.

Community psychiatric nurses may work as part of a therapeutic team providing community care or home treatment, or may have a semi-independent role working particularly in primary care. Trained psychiatric nurses may be nurses on the general register who have done postgraduate psychiatric training, or may be nurses who have undergone psychiatric nurse training (some of whom then take general training). Some nurses specialize in the management of the mentally handicapped and impaired, either in hospital or in the community. A nurse who is skilled in counselling, behavioural and cognitive therapy, who can also touch, clean, and physically comfort patients, as well as being adept in physical procedures such as injections, is a very valuable colleague who can teach you a lot.

Occupational therapists

The traditional medical view of the occupational therapist is a totally inaccurate stereotype of the purveyor of jolly games and distraction for patients until they get better (providing genteel physical exercise, pottery, and knitting woolly bunny rabbits), which is unfortunately the traditional nursing view as well. Nothing could be further from the truth. In psychiatric practice, occupational therapists are concerned with counselling, behavioural and cognitive therapy, teaching living and social skills, and rehabilitation (both physical and psychiatric). In some hospitals they are still unfortunately employed to amuse the inmates until they get better. This is becoming very unusual. Many occupational therapists in psychiatry now work in the community as part of a therapeutic team. Like nurses, they are the most valued of colleagues, providing that you genuinely accept them as equals.

Clinical psychologists

Clinical psychology is a young discipline that is still engaged in finding its particular role. It is having something of a power battle with psychiatrists and so there is often an unfortunate and unnecessary degree of mutual antagonism between the two disciplines. Many experienced clinical psychologists can work well in a psychiatrist-led team, both psychiatrist and psychologist each giving of their skills without denigrating those of the other. Unhappily, in many services there is too wide a gulf between psychiatrists and clinical psychologists, each failing to recognize the role and unique skills of the other and neither recognizing that they cannot cure everybody. Clinical psychologists also (quite rightly) are irritated by psychiatrists' views of them as mere testers of intelligence (usually a futile pursuit), or merely as treaters of socially embarrassing phobias.

Clinical psychologists are scientifically trained, are excellent at evaluating the results of therapy, and are usually extremely well trained in behavioural and cognitive techniques. A few are trained in psychotherapy. Some are learning to retreat into management, so that the stereotype of the clinical psychologist as a person who gives you well argued reasons why he

cannot possibly treat your patient because of lack of resources and his time commitment to important mana-
gerial work, is sadly sometimes true. If they cannot
settle into the therapeutic team they make excellent
outside consultants and have a lot to teach the young
psychiatrist.

Social workers

Social work is another comparatively young profession
that is also painfully finding its role and value. Social
workers rightfully resent the image of 'lady bountifuls'
and solver of welfare problems that other disciplines
tend to have of them, although they are often more
knowledgeable about welfare rights than the rest of
us. Many are excellent psychotherapists and are truly
eclectic in their treatment practices. Some remain
wedded to a concept of 'casework' that is now obsolete,
and some are so strident for 'patients' rights' that they
see the other professions in a conspiracy against their
clients. Some social workers work happily in a multidisciplinary team, but most, like clinical psychologists,
work most effectively as outside consultants.

The role of the social worker in the Mental Health
Act and the ability of a social worker to block what the
psychiatrist feels as a necessary compulsory admission
without providing a viable alternative, can produce
much tension between the two disciplines. Good social
workers, however, provide a very valuable different
perspective of the patient and his problems that is both
refreshing and very necessary, and a good social worker,
particularly one who is prepared to recognize the inter-
dependence of therapists within a team, is an extremely
valuable member of that team. Because social workers
have statutory rights to remove children from home,
as well as having powers to incarcerate, mentally ill
patients are often frightened of them.

Physiotherapists

Physiotherapists are very rarely part of a multidisciplinary team, except perhaps in psychogeriatrics. They have many of the skills of the occupational therapist (there is unfortunately often tension between the two disciplines), but rarely have behavioural or cognitive skills. Like the occupational therapist, they are particularly valuable in planning rehabilitation, particularly physical rehabilitation. The increasing interest in 'body work', both in rehabilitation and in the management of anxiety, may make their role more valuable in the future.

Art therapists

Art therapists are a rare breed. They may work in hospital, or work attached to a day centre or mental-health treatment centre. Art therapists are often trained in behavioural or cognitive therapy, or have psychotherapeutic skills. They use the medium of art (in all its forms) to help patients look at their feelings and at their particular life situation. For some patients this can be extremely valuable and can not only free the patient from clogging emotions but also help his therapist to understand him a great deal better.

The same is true for *music therapy*, which works best when applied to an individual in terms of helping him or her to free his emotions and understand them rather than as a general means of relaxation.

Some therapists also employ *drama therapy* and *role play*, which can not only lead to abreaction of feelings but also to the patient's better understanding of his relationships with others, particularly within his family, and this can be most valuable. One or two centres have trained drama or music therapists, but you will be lucky if you meet one.

C Counselling

A great deal of your time (often without you realizing it) will be spent in counselling your patients. It is therefore important to have a good idea of what counselling actually is and how it differs from other therapeutic techniques. You need to remind yourself from time to time that you are counselling the patient rather than just talking to him. This helps you to think about and plan what you are doing in your interactions with the patient. The word counselling has bad connotations for both the medical profession and laymen. 'Counselling' may have slightly sinister overtones (don't administrators 'counsel' employees before they sack them?). The traditional British image of the counsellor is of a pruriently curious and totally inept man, or of a rather silly woman in a funny hat and tweed suit with odd ideas. Announcing to the average British patient that he needs to be counselled will cause him to draw back in alarm, and you will have to convince both the patient and yourself that counselling is necessary. Doctors find non-directive counselling hard as they are used to telling people what to do. That is the antithesis of counselling, and you will need to learn to be non-directive to be an effective counsellor.

You will also need good interviewing and communication skills. You need to be able to draw the patient out, to delineate his problems, and put his life circumstances and previous experiences into perspective. You will need to be able to communicate information. Patients cannot be expected to deal with life problems unless they have adequate information. A good example of this is pregnancy counselling; a woman cannot decide what to do about her potentially unwanted pregnancy until she is armed with all the facts about alternative strategies. But remember that people can assimilate only a small amount of information at any one time, and even less if they are disturbed or upset. You may have to repeat information several times, check that it has been received and understood, and plan your strategy of information so that the most important bits are rapidly retained. You also need to develop the skill of reflecting back to the patient the impression you have of him, or that you are picking up some emotion that he is not expressing ('You tell me you are fine, but there is a lot of sadness in what you are saying'). Some schools of counselling use reflecting back to an extreme degree (for example, the Rogerian school). This can be an effective technique, but can also become a ridiculous caricature of itself. The beginner is advised to use it only in small doses.

Having reflected and explored the patient's problems, the next thing to do is review solutions to them and to help the patient make his own choice. At this stage it is very important for the eager young doctor in you to take a back seat and help the patient really make up his own mind about what he is going to do and what solutions are available. If the patient cannot see any solutions you may have to suggest some, but do it with an even weighting so that you do not bias the patient into taking the solution that you think is most appropriate. If you hear yourself saying, 'if I were you' bite off your words! You must allow the patient to make his own decision even though, to you, it seems not to be the best solution. The only way that the patient is going to learn is by making his own mistakes (in the same way that adolescents only learn by making their own mistakes; they never learn from the precepts of their parents, however well-meaning).

You will often need to help the patient to implement his decision by assisting the patient to mobilize the appropriate resources or by rehearsing with the patient

how he is going to announce that decision to significant others, or to develop the necessary assertive skills
to deal with reluctant purveyors of welfare rights.

To be an effective counsellor you therefore need to
drop the medical model and your desire to control
what your patients are doing, and you will need training
in, and feedback of, your counselling skills as it is not
something that necessarily comes naturally. You will
need the personal qualities of warmth, empathy, and
genuineness (you should have these anyway or you
would not be going into psychiatry). Make sure that
these personality traits have not been covered up by a
grubby patina of paternalism or maternalism. You will
also need to know something about yourself. You need
to develop the ability to accept a person for what he is,
even if you do not like him very much. You may well
be helping him to change from what he is, but unless
the patient feels that he is accepted and that his existing
feelings and wishes have some value, he will not want
to change. This acceptance of other people obviously
has its limits. You may accept that the pederast is a
person, but do not get so laid back that you accept his
behaviour.

This does not mean that you have to become a goody
two shoes and cease to have your own values and
opinions, nor that you should not acknowledge your
feelings about patients. If Mrs Jones irritates you profoundly, do not suppress your irritation with Mrs Jones
with the thought that it is a bad feeling to have, but ask
yourself where that feeling of irritation is coming from.
It may well be due to some behaviour in Mrs Jones.
You may need to reflect back to her that she has this
effect on other people as she may wish to change the
behaviour. When you have thought about it, you may
also have learnt something about yourself. Your feelings
may not be rationally based on Mrs Jones's behaviour,
but on how much she reminds you of a former girl-

friend, or of your mother, or of a previous teacher at school. You will learn a lot about yourself as you practise and train in counselling, and you will not always like what you learn about yourself, but, just as you have to learn to be accepting of your patients as individuals, you have to learn to accept yourself.

Specific aspects of counselling

You will often find yourself being asked to give a patient *support*, and sometimes your consultant may even talk about *supportive psychotherapy*. This is a very important task, but very few people are prepared to explain to you exactly what support is meant to be. We take it to mean helping the patient through a bad time or through a treatment experience so that he has some idea of what is going on and has a chance of asking questions. We hope that he will be able to draw some emotional strength from you (but not too much and only temporarily) and come out of the experience not sadder but wiser, so that if he goes through the experience again he will have better insight into what is happening and will know that the experience will eventually pass. As a result of learning how to cope with the experience, you hope that he will be able to pass this skill on to other people. You will certainly use support in helping people through grief, through a bad depression, or a schizophrenic episode, and will also, of course, support relatives and friends.

Support, although often never formalized and its effectiveness often forgotten, is one of the most important things that you can do, since most psychiatric conditions are self-limiting. It consists of talking the patient through the experience, finding out how he is feeling, how he sees the situation, and allowing him to discharge emotion. You need to be seen as someone who is prepared both to accept the patient's feelings and to talk about them, and to use the interviewing skills outlined in Chapter 1 to help the patient to see that his experience is being understood by another human being. Support also means helping the patient to develop perspective on the way that he is feeling and what is happening to him, and giving him information about what is happening. Although a patient's illness is unique to him, you will have seen many other people suffering from the same condition and can therefore pass on insights and information gleaned from your knowledge of other people in the same situation. Patients going through intensive behavioural or psychotherapeutic treatment, being administered by somebody else, need support so that they can understand what is happening to them and understand the very strong emotions that such treatment may unleash so that they do not run away from these emotions and therefore run away from a necessary treatment process.

You will need the ability to handle *grief*, and must know how to *break bad news*. This means talking with the patient about what has currently been happening to him, allowing him to express his fears and anxieties about what may be happening to him, and giving his own idea of what is wrong with him. Having reviewed this, it involves telling the patient as directly and as bluntly as possible what the problem is (this also applies to breaking bad news to relatives).

So for the last few months, then, some very strange things have been happening to you. You have had very strong feelings that your thoughts are not your own and that other people are reading them, and you have been troubled by unpleasant voices that seem to be talking about you and telling you to do things that you don't want to do but find very difficult to resist. You were very worried that you were going mad and therefore haven't told anybody about this until very recently. You have been in hospital for a few days now and we have had a chance of getting to know you and have done some tests and have given you some medication, which already seems to have reduced the intensity of your voices, and you feel that your mind and your thinking are coming back to your control, but you still want to know what is wrong with you. We feel that you have a condition called schizophrenia. (Pause.) What does that mean to you?

When you break bad news the patient is unlikely to retain much of what you have told him. Immediately after the breaking of bad news he will be preoccupied with his own thoughts and feelings and may hear very little of what you subsequently say. It is important to think about what you want this patient to particularly remember from the interview, and to think about the timing of any reassurances that you are able to give.

Notice in the example just given (which is obviously time compressed as you would not normally do it as quickly as that) that you point out to the patient that he is getting better before you tell him that he has got schizophrenia. Having told him that he has schizophrenia you try to draw him out so that you can understand what his own beliefs are about the condition so that eventually (but probably not in this interview) you can correct them if necessary. You had better sort out in your own mind what you mean by schizophrenia and ask yourself what your image of it is. If it is of the shambling wrecks in the back ward of your mental hospital, you are not going to be very positive with your patient, but if your image of schizophrenia is (as indeed it should be) of somebody who, with the right support, counselling, and judicious use of medication, can return to live in society and still be a fruitful member of it, you are much more likely to give your patients a positive image of the condition.

Having broken the bad news you must then help the patient to express his grief, verbally and emotionally, and you must therefore learn to be tolerant of emotional displays in others. The traditional response of a doctor to somebody crying is to try to suppress it, but you must learn to encourage it and to allow the patient, through crying, to discharge his feelings. In addition to breaking bad news and allowing expression of grief, you may have to try to explain the natural processes of grief. We live in a society in which grief is rare and often not encountered until quite late in life, so that most people are unacquainted with emotional and physiological consequences of grief. It is important in grief counselling not to expect the person to recover from his grief too soon, and to recognize that he will have to rehearse and talk through his grief on many occasions and that full recovery from grief does not take place for months, and nor does adjustment to loss.

Behavioural counselling aims to help people to change their habits or behaviour, even though at first they have some resistance to doing so (for example, counselling people who are addicted to smoking or to alcohol). Sometimes small changes in behaviour lead to lasting changes in emotion and feelings. Practising a behaviour that is incompatible with a particular feeling (such as guilt) often leads to the eventual disappearance of that feeling. For example, in sex therapy the patient who feels guilty every time she touches her private parts is encouraged to keep on practising a behaviour that is perfectly natural. If she continues to do this the guilt feeling will gradually disappear. Behavioural counselling also encourages the patient to *specify behaviours and feelings* (to look at what he is actually doing and to be prepared to say how he is actually feeling). This often helps the patient develop new perspectives on both his behaviour and on his relationships with other people.

Counselling may also contain elements of cognitive change (see p. 409), which is particularly useful in helping people to break entrenched habits and negative patterns of thinking that may prevent people from achieving their full potential at work or in education.

D Psychotherapy

Although you will be counselling patients from the day you start psychiatry, it is unlikely that initially you will be engaged in formal psychotherapy except of a very limited kind. It is, however, an essential part of your later training. It is also essential, as you start to engage in psychotherapy, that you have proper instruction and have a supervisor with whom you meet regularly and who gives you feedback on your performance. Psychotherapy can be frightening at first, and is doubly so if you are unsupported and alone. Psychotherapy is potentially disturbing because, even more than counselling, it may reawaken or bring into focus your own previous life experiences or emotional feelings that may, for a while, be quite troublesome, and once again you will need to come to terms with yourself.

Psychotherapy contains all the counselling principles described previously, but in addition it emphasizes the therapeutic use of the relationship that develops between the psychotherapist and the patient, in particular the recognition and use of **transference** and **counter transference** relationships. Transference means the development in the patient of emotional feelings towards the therapist. These feelings can be strong, may be painful, and often seem irrational or bizarre. They may be uncomfortable for the young therapist who does not have the experience to realize that the feelings, although intense and real, are not related to the therapist as a person, but are related to what the therapist represents to the patient. They are usually re-enactments of previously strongly held feelings for another person, the therapist being invested with the attributes of that other person. It is important to ask both yourself and the patient, 'Who do I represent?' If the patient who has strong feelings for the therapist (usually either of love or of hate) can learn to understand where the feelings come from, and that they can be contained within the therapeutic relationship (so that the patient does not have to run away from them or act on them), it can be extremely valuable. In individual psychotherapy the development of transference is therefore fostered and encouraged, and then interpreted.

Counter transference refers to a similar process occurring between therapist and patient. Such feelings, of course, are likely to arise in any intimate relationship and, as a young therapist, you must not be surprised that such things happen and must not be taken unawares. You must not act on the feelings, but learn to recognize that they arise from previous experiences you have had. It is useful to ask yourself what is it in the patient that encourages such feelings in you, and also who the patient might represent to you. You should not conceal or suppress such feelings, but acknowledge them to yourself and always discuss them with your supervisor.

Psychotherapy is also concerned with helping people to verbalize feelings rather than acting them out. This is often a long and painful process, particularly in people who have spent most of their lives bottling up their feelings or concealing them from others, and requires a great deal of skill, particularly if you are containing the accompanying acting-out behaviour at the same time.

Psychotherapy is also involved in *interpreting* the patient's behaviour. Interpretation shows the patient the roots of his behaviour and the unconscious meaning of his acts, which are usually related to previous incidents in the patient's life or the way he grew up in childhood. Beginners often overdo interpretation, often interpret too quickly without really understanding the patient, and make the cardinal mistake of not letting the patient make his own interpretations. Do this by offering the patient an observation and seeing what he makes of it by saying something like, 'You indicate that you feel very angry with me. I wonder if you can relate that to any other relationship that you have had?', or 'I wonder if that reminds you of anything that has happened to you in the past?'

Psychotherapy means seeing the patient regularly, at least weekly, and being prepared to spend at least an hour with the patient per session. It should therefore not be undertaken unless you have a sufficient time commitment to it. Many beginners start with **group therapy** in which a group of people with similar problems meet and look at their own and at each other's experiences with the help of a group leader. There are often two group leaders, one of whom can be a trainee. Groups can be very successful. It is possible to learn a great deal about how people interact together in groups, and also a lot about psychodynamics, particularly if you learn under an experienced therapist. Badly run groups can be destructive, sap your morale, and are a very negative experience. You need good supervision to extract maximum learning and information out of the experience. Some hospitals run experiential groups in which trainees work together in a group and experience group dynamics for themselves. With a good leader, providing the rules are carefully followed, such experience can be valuable, but if the leader is poor and things get out of control, the experience can be very destructive.

Co-therapy is when two therapists, usually of similar experience (occasionally a trainer and a trainee), of opposite sex, and from different disciplines, work together, usually with a couple. This is usually in sex therapy or marital therapy, and can be an extremely good learning experience. Two inexperienced therapists working together can draw much support from each other. Co-therapy also gives you a chance of being an active therapist whilst your co-therapist adopts a passive role and observes the interaction between you and the two people you are counselling. Switching roles between active and passive gives you a chance of observing exactly what is happening in the treatment sessions. Inexperienced co-therapists need regular supervision.

Psychotherapy is a necessary part of the training, experience, and practice of all psychiatrists, although some psychiatrists are more suited to psychotherapy and some will eventually spend all their time doing it. There are problems in psychotherapy. Many trainers and practitioners use rigid inflexible models of human behaviour, thought, and emotion, which take no account of the patient's culture or even of common sense. Models of psychotherapy are often believed in with a conviction approaching that of religious zeal. The unfortunate consequence of this holier-than-thou attitude is that people who do not believe what the psychotherapist professes are cast into the outer darkness or are seen as enemies. Psychotherapists, more than in any other branch of the profession, can always be right (since so many of their concepts are extremely nebulous and untestable). If you disagree with them, then you are 'showing resistance' to their ideas. The hypotheses and working models of psychotherapy should be open to change in the light of experience, but unfortunately many adherents of psychotherapy treat their beliefs like tablets of stone.

E Behaviour/cognitive therapy

Behavioural therapy

If psychotherapy is based on the premise that the patient needs to find out the roots and causes of his present symptoms, then behaviour therapy takes the opposite view that it is often better to learn how to lose a set of symptoms than to discover how one acquired them.

Learning how to get out of a situation will often tell you how you got into it. Behaviour therapists therefore concentrate on helping the patient to make small, but lasting changes in his behaviour. Making small changes in behaviour is often possible when making a big change is not. If enough small changes are made at a pace that the patient can accept and at the price of only a small degree of anxiety, then often much progress can be made. When you have carried out a few behavioural programmes you will learn that the more progress a patient makes the more confident the patient becomes about taking larger steps. If you can help a patient to make behavioural changes then emotional changes will also follow, as practising a behaviour incompatible with an emotion leads to extinction of that emotion.

Behaviour therapy is perhaps best known in the management of anxiety for which it is extremely suitable, but all kinds of behaviour are amenable to treatment programmes, with or without anxiety management. In anxiety management, the behaviour therapist teaches the patient self-control skills of anxiety symptoms, and also (this is often extremely important) teaches the patient the ability to discriminate between being anxious and not anxious, and to label anxiety symptoms correctly. The therapist therefore teaches a way of helping the patient to break the vicious circle of terrifying anxiety symptoms increasing the patient's fear, which further increases his anxiety symptoms. Once the patient feels that he can recognize and have some control over his symptoms, anxiety levels often fall. Although behaviour therapy was originally used largely for phobic or situational anxiety, it is equally suitable for patients with chronic tension or with apparently spontaneous panic attacks.

An important part of behaviour therapy is the initial analysis of the patient's feelings and behaviour, and accurately recording their frequency. In difficult or complicated cases this behavioural analysis is extremely important, and since you will have had little experience of this, the advice and help of an experienced behaviour therapist will be important and should be obtained. In a therapeutic programme, as the patient is slowly altering his behaviour, feedback on his performance (particularly the analysis of any blocks or difficulties the patient has in the treatment programme) is extremely important. It is often in looking at and analysing the blocks to progress, that the patient begins to learn how his symptoms originated.

The techniques of behaviour therapy include anxiety reduction methods such as relaxation. Relaxation is a positive treatment and a technique that the patient has to learn, and there are several techniques available depending on the wishes and skills of the patient. Most therapists start off with the patient practising alternate tensing and relaxing of the muscles, which teaches the patient to recognize the difference between tension and relaxation—**discrimination**. This technique only works if the patient cooperates, does not feel anxious about being relaxed, is prepared to practise, and is taught properly (intensive relaxation, for instance, cannot be taught in groups but has to be taught individually). For patients who cannot use this method to learn to relax, then various breathing control methods are available including Benson's method. Biofeedback may be employed, as occasionally may hypnosis or some kind of massage technique such as aromatherapy. Some very tense people have to learn what being relaxed feels like and the latter techniques are very useful for teaching this discrimination.

In phobic anxiety, once good relaxation skills have been acquired, formal desensitization to the feared object is carried out. Having established a hierarchy of fears related to the particular object, the patient is encouraged to expose himself (either in imagination or in reality) to the least-feared stimulus, whilst practising relaxation. If this is done a few times the fear disappears and the patient can then move up the hierarchy. Such desensitization, which usually is very successful, is the basis of much behaviour therapy and has an innate common sense to it. If desensitization is initially done in imagination, then eventually it should, if possible, also be carried out in actuality, although this can be difficult until the patient has sufficient control over his anxiety.

The patient can be exposed directly to the most-feared stimulus, either in imagination or in actuality, without a previous hierarchy of exposure. This is called **flooding** or implosion. Providing the patient is well supported during the experience (sometimes intravenous diazepam is used), it can be an effective method, particularly if the patient learns that the expected and feared consequences of high anxiety (that he will either die or go permanently mad) do not happen. After a short while, extreme levels of anxiety disappear and are followed by a feeling of calmness. This is an empirical observation, but its mechanism is now better understood because of the increased understanding of the benzodiazepine receptor.

Other ways of dealing with anxiety are to use **distraction**, so that the person's mind is occupied with something else whilst the feared stimulus is being presented, or to use **modelling**, in which the patient observes someone else handling the situation calmly and then models the desired behaviour. This is particularly effective in children.

Behaviour therapy principles are also used in *assertiveness training* and *social skills training* for people who find difficulty in expressing their wishes to others, or who suffer from severe anxiety in social situations. Behavioural treatments can also be applied to other behaviours (either reinforcing or extinguishing them) by using **operant conditioning** in which desired responses by the patient are praised and reinforced, and unwanted responses are either ignored or 'punished' (by withdrawal of praise or support or by criticism). Even difficult forms of behaviour (including psychotic symptoms) will sometimes respond to this. A *token economy* can be set up in which desired behaviour is rewarded by tokens, which can be exchanged for goods or services. The rewarding of wanted behaviour is more likely to be successful than the punishment of unwanted behaviour. Another technique practised by behaviour therapists is **thought stopping**, which is particularly useful for obsessional thinking (but which can be used in other situations) in which the patient is taught to use either cognitive means or some kind of physical stimulus to stop unwanted or disturbing thoughts as soon as they emerge.

Behavioural techniques are widely practised in psychiatry and have an established place. Patients with difficult behaviour or who have complicated problems need a full behavioural analysis and a properly planned programme (it is here that clinical psychologists can be very helpful), but simpler problems respond to a common sense 'seat of the pants' behaviour therapy. Although very successful, used in the wrong hands behaviour therapy can become too mechanical and can concentrate too much on the behaviour and not enough on the person who is exhibiting the behaviour. It is possible to ignore the person with the problem altogether, and thus the feelings, doubts, and anxieties that he has about the treatment and about himself. Anybody who practises behaviour therapy will learn that some of the phenomena seen in psychotherapy, such as the transference reaction, will occur, and therapist–patient interaction cannot be ignored. The therapist's personality and optimism is also very important in supporting the patient through the treatment. The therapist is often a role model for the patient. To see behaviour therapy as merely changing behaviour and not also as a therapeutic interaction between two individuals is to ignore its greatest strength.

Cognitive therapy

Like behaviour therapy, a great deal of cognitive therapy is common sense and practitioners have used its principles for years. Recently, however, the underlying principles of cognitive therapy have been codified and a more formal scheme of practice has been established, which is of particular importance in difficult or resistant cases. Both research and clinical experience shows that many maladaptive behaviours are initiated, accompanied by, or reinforced by negative thoughts. The patient, often without realizing it, has his mind filled with thoughts predicting failure, lack of success, or unpleasant consequences. Cognitive therapy basically teaches the patient to recognize these thoughts, to learn to stop them, and to eventually substitute them with positive thoughts. This is not the same as a behavioural thought stopping technique for obsessional illness. The cognitive therapist gets the patient to actually write down his thoughts, teaches him to become aware of his thoughts, and then works to substitute negative thoughts with positive ones. Even if you are not practising formal cognitive therapy it is important to ask a patient going through any form of treatment or who is dealing with any difficult situation to actually look at what he is thinking about and, if necessary, to help him to think more positively. Cognitive therapy is also important in rehabilitation. A patient who has been through a depressive illness, for instance, may have lost the biological symptoms of the depression, but will continue to think in the negative way that comes with depression and will go on being filled with thoughts of failure unless you help him to change. Advocates of cognitive therapy say that it may be successful in treating depression on its own without the use of antidepressant medication, and there is some evidence that this may sometimes be true. In rehabilitation after depression, practising behaviours that are incompatible with feeling depressed coupled with cognitive therapy can be a very powerful restorative, and these techniques are not used enough.

Cognitive therapists also teach the patient to recognize how irrational his negative thoughts are (and to substitute more rational thoughts).

F Other therapies

Hypnosis

Hypnosis has a reputation of being dangerous and difficult to practice. This is not true. Hypnosis is easy to learn and to use providing that you know both its limitations and your own. It is not a panacea for all ills but is useful sometimes in relaxation, occasionally in abreaction, and in temporarily aiding patients to break habits such as smoking. Confined to these uses, and if it is not used in the severely personality disordered (particularly those with dissociative personality disorders) or the psychotic, it is not dangerous. Greater experience is needed for its use in regressive therapies or for psychotherapy. Not all people are easy to hypnotize. Hypnosis has nothing to do with the personality of the therapist but everything to do with the intensity of the concentration of the person being hypnotized. Before hypnotizing a patient it is necessary to talk through the fact that he remains in control of himself at all times and will be aware of what is going on.

A light hypnotic state is an excellent form of relaxation, particularly if you can teach the patient an autoinduction technique so that he can induce relaxation when he needs it. Hypnosis is a useful technique to have in your armamentarium of therapies. Practice with someone versed in the technique is needed to learn how to do it as it is not something that you learn from a book. It is also useful to experience it yourself so that you are better able to instruct and reassure your patients.

Abreaction

Abreaction is a technique whereby either using hypnotic suggestion or intravenously injected medication (usually a barbiturate plus amphetamine, or diazepam on its own) the patient is encouraged to relive a painful experience and to discharge the emotion related to this experience, or to recall an event or a memory that has been long suppressed, or to face a feared situation as in 'flooding'. In acute traumatic stress disorder, reliving the painful experience can be extremely helpful and abreaction may occasionally be helpful in psychotherapy to help people remember unpleasant events that they would much rather forget. Often, of course, this can be done just by talking through the experience, particularly when you have built up trust and rapport with the patient. Unfortunately, some doctors use abreaction as an unnecessary short cut. Some patients, too, get rather addicted to abreaction and demand more and more of the experience.

If you are asked to abreact a patient you need to find out a great deal about him before you do the abreaction. The actual abreaction must be recorded so that it can be played back to the patient and the content of what he said discussed later. Diazepam in particular may make him forget what he has said. If you have used chemical means for the abreaction remember that the patient will be somewhat disinhibited and garrulous for some hours after the experience (in fact the patient often says more *after* the actual abreaction than during the experience itself), and nursing staff or other people looking after the person who has been abreacted need to go on recording what is being said, but also need to prevent the patient from 'spilling the beans' too widely or too freely. Give enough of the intravenous medication, slowly (using a 'butterfly' or flexible cannula) so that the patient is slightly 'drunk', but not fast asleep. You can 'top up' the drug from time to time if needed. The patient needs (as with hypnosis) to be reassured that he will remain in control, but will be relaxed enough to say what he really wants to say but has been afraid to. When he is relaxed, talk him through the event and his memory of it as you would normally, but concentrate on getting him to relive his feelings.

G Physical treatments—electroconvulsive therapy

The Royal College of Psychiatrists recommends that within your hospital or unit there should be one consultant who is directly responsible for supervising electroconvulsive therapy (ECT) and also responsible for training young doctors in the technique. Do not allow yourself to be put on the rota for carrying out ECT until you have been taught the practical aspects of the technique, are familiar with local procedures, have had training in the use of the particular apparatus used for inducing therapeutic convulsions in your hospital, and are aware of for how long you should stimulate the patient and with what wave form.

Most units have reverted to using bilateral placement of the electrodes, which should be firmly placed at a point four inches above the mid-point of a line joining the lateral angle of the eye to the external auditory meatus. Make sure that you have been shown how to find this point and have been instructed in the proper use of the electrodes in terms of using firm pressure and enough (but not too much) electrode solution. If your hospital still uses unilateral electrode placements, get instruction in assessing handedness and the precise placing of the electrodes. We are emphasizing *practical instruction* because you cannot learn ECT procedures from a book, and the thought of you doing your first ECT with this book in one hand and the patient in the other fills us with dread!

Do not carry out ECT single-handed. There must be an anaesthetist present who is responsible for the anaesthetic, muscle relaxant, and resuscitation aspects of the procedure, although you should also be competent in resuscitation techniques before taking part in ECT. Excellent guidelines on the use of ECT have been published by the ECT subcommittee of the research committee of the Royal College of Psychiatrists. Your hospital must have a copy of this and be following its procedures, and if not, you should seriously consider whether you should be working there. You should certainly insist that you do not take part in ECT treatments unless the guidelines are followed. Do not administer ECT until you have personally checked that the patient has consented, is physically fit for the procedure, has the right indications for it, that resuscitative apparatus is available *and working*, that the supervising nurses know what to do, and that the patient is properly supported until recovery. Never assume that someone else will have checked this—do it yourself.

The use of ECT is now reserved for patients with moderate or severe depressive illness that has not responded to antidepressant medication, or for patients who are suffering from life-threatening side-effects of severe depression (such as retardation or dehydration), or who are actively suicidal. Occasionally ECT may be useful in catatonic stupor, but its use otherwise in schizophrenia can only be justified very rarely. It is a lifesaving and very effective treatment for depression, particularly if psychotic symptoms are present, but it is only useful in speeding up recovery from the depression and will not prevent its recurrence—antidepressants are also needed.

Before the patient has his first ECT it is important that the procedure is explained to him. In particular it should be stressed that he will be both anaesthetized and will have muscle relaxation during the procedure so that he will remember nothing of it and will be protected, as far as possible, from harmful consequences. He is likely to have a mild headache on recovery, and may notice some mild confusion and transient memory impairment after the procedure. It is important that the patient understands that he is having an electrically induced convulsion and, although the precise mechanism of this treatment is unknown, there is no doubt that it is effective in relieving depression and that this form of treatment has been chosen because the medical team feel that if the patient continues in his depressed state there is risk of suicide or prolonged psychological suffering. The patient should be encouraged to ask questions about the procedure and the reason for giving it. You may have to repeat these explanations from time to time. You should make a note that you have given the patient this explanation and that the patient appeared to understand, and a consent form should be signed. If the patient refuses consent and it is believed that the ECT is necessary, he will have to be detained under the Mental Health Act and a second opinion about the need for it obtained from another consultant. The need for a second opinion also applies to the patient who is deemed to be incapable (because of his mental state) of giving valid consent. The consultant who gives a second opinion (or an appointed doctor under the Mental Health Act (Section 58 (3: B) and 58 (4))) may suggest alternative forms of treatment for the patient. If so, take it as a positive suggestion and not as questioning your clinical judgement.

Patients who are to have ECT will need support beforehand and should be starved for at least six hours before the procedure. There should be a pleasant waiting area, a separate treatment room, which should also be as pleasant and as non-clinical as possible (but containing adequate resuscitation equipment), and a completely separate recovery area where patients can recover from the procedure in dignity and quietness, but well supervised by competent nurses. If patients are having out-patient ECT they should be reviewed before being allowed to go home (in terms of recovery from minor side-effects and confusion), and should not go home on their own.

Before having ECT the patient needs a thorough physical examination to exclude, particularly, raised intracranial pressure, cardiovascular disease, and respiratory disease. If the patient is taking certain drugs, such as benzodiazepines or carbamazepine, you may not be able to induce a seizure and the use of such medication should be reviewed. The anaesthetist should be aware of any problems that the patient has, such as hypertension, and should also know what drugs the patient is taking, and, with you, must be responsible for checking that sufficient resuscitation equipment exists and is in working order. If the patient does not have a convulsion after the passage of the current, keep him oxygenated and give a second shock either of a slightly higher intensity or slightly longer duration, depending on the stimulus and machine you are using. If this fails to produce a modified convulsion (sometimes it is very difficult to tell) abandon the procedure and discuss it with your consultant. The patient's mental state should be reviewed before each treatment. If depressed patients become elated during a course of

ECT, this is usually taken to indicate that subsequent treatment should be delayed or cancelled.

There is no such thing as a course of ECT. Patients should be assessed after each treatment. Most patients have about half a dozen treatments. If there has been no response at all after a dozen, then there is little point in continuing with the treatment. There is no point in giving it more frequently than two or three times a week, and some patients may need only once-weekly treatment if they become particularly confused afterwards. Anybody having ECT for depression should be prescribed concomitant antidepressants to prevent relapse after the ECT has been successful.

ECT should not be given to patients with raised intracranial pressure, cerebral aneurysms, a previous cerebral haemorrhage, previous aortic aneurysm, or current respiratory infection, and nor should it be given to a patient within three months of a myocardial infarction. It can be given to patients who are pregnant, although particular anaesthetic care is needed and, in late pregnancy, ECT may induce premature labour. It can also be given to patients with epilepsy (spontaneous seizures may occur after ECT in people who have a low convulsive threshold). Old age is not a contra-indication to ECT. Reserpine and ECT should not be used together.

If you are giving ECT you are personally responsible for the patient and for anything that goes wrong, and so you are only being fair to yourself and to your patient if you learn the procedure thoroughly before you start and always personally check the patient and the ap-paratus before you begin. Hospitals in which ECT becomes part of a production line process without much thought being given to whether the treatment is needed or being carried out humanely and safely, are usually unpleasant places to work in. You may think our emphasis on taking personal responsibility reflects personal experience of what happens if things go wrong—you would be right!

H Physical treatments—drug therapy

When you start psychiatry you will be faced with a bewildering variety of drugs, mostly powerful and poisonous, and there will be great pressure on you to use them. This pressure will come from patients and their relatives, from nurses who want patients' behaviour controlled quickly, and not least from polite men in business suits who will take you out for lunch to extol the virtues of their particular product. Drugs are not, however, a panacea, although for the right patient at the right time they can be immensely beneficial. They are undoubtedly overused, frequently abused, and cause a great deal of iatrogenic illness. Whenever you are writing a prescription for a drug, particularly if it is at somebody else's request or it is a routine repeat prescription, ask yourself the important question, 'Could I justify this prescription in a coroner's court?' You will be surprised how often the answer to this question is no. If you cannot justify the prescription, do not write it. Likewise, think very carefully before prescribing a new preparation. Occasionally these can be justified, but it is better to get to know a small group of drugs well and really know how to prescribe them before reaching for every new preparation that comes along.

Drug treatment in psychiatry is changing all the time and we are more concerned here with the principles of the use of drugs rather than providing lists of possible drugs you could use with their doses; information that would very rapidly become out of date. Keep up to date with the British National Formulary, which is revised constantly, and always have it with you. Look up the doses and side-effects of the drugs that you use and their interactions, and remember that in psychiatric practice many symptoms are iatrogenic. Be especially careful not to use drug combinations, but try to stick to monotherapy. We have merely listed brief details and the names of the more commonly used drugs. The skilled use of drugs is an art as well as a science, and comes with experience and a wide knowledge base.

Psychotic illness

Drug treatment is essential in psychotic illness, although it will only remove the positive symptoms of the psychosis, such as delusions and hallucinations, or control agitated and disturbed behaviour. Neuroleptic drugs that block dopaminergic receptors are used for treating psychosis. The more powerful the neuroleptic effect, the less the sedative effect of the drug. Brief sedation may be necessary at the start of treatment, but it is the neuroleptic effect that actually controls psychotic symptoms. Powerful neuroleptic drugs can often be used in small doses, and taken just once a day. Neuroleptic drugs are often used in depot injection form. The patient has an injection every two or three weeks and the drug is gradually discharged from the oil-based depot into the bloodstream. Depot injections are overused. If there is clear evidence that firstly, your patient is non-compliant with therapy, and secondly, that he actually needs the drug, then a depot injection can be justified. Always use a test dose first and wait two weeks before commencing regular depot injections. Do not prescribe injections closer than intervals of two weeks unless there is a compelling reason to do so. If you are having to use very large doses of the depot neuroleptic, consider trying one of a different type.

Many patients can be maintained on oral medication if you are prepared to prescribe it in a dose that minimizes side-effects, and it is taken just once a day and the task of making sure the patient takes his medication is undertaken by a responsible person. Many people who have recovered from a psychotic illness are unlikely to break down again and do not need continued medication. In many patients, continual medication will not prevent relapse, and attention to their social circumstances and the emotional atmosphere in which they live is much more important in terms of preventing breakdown.

Antipsychotic drugs

The original antipsychotic drugs were the **phenothiazines**, of which chlorpromazine was the first and has therefore been given an arbitrary neuroleptic potential of '1' so that other drugs can be compared with it. There are three classes of phenothiazines, **aliphatic** (low neuroleptic potential, fairly sedative with moderate extrapyramidal and autonomic effects), **piperidines** (moderately sedative, low extrapyramidal potential, but likely to have autonomic effects, such as hypotension), and **piperazines** (less sedative, more neuroleptic, and therefore more extrapyramidal effects).

Other commonly used antipsychotic drugs are **butyrophenones, diphenylbutylpiperidines**, and **thioxanthenes** (more powerful neuroleptics), and **substituted benzamides**. New compounds, whose place in the therapeutic armoury is still uncertain, are the **tricyclic dibenzoxazepines** and a **dibenzodiazepine**, clozapine (effective but toxic).

Chlorpromazine (an aliphatic phenothiazine) is still widely used, but is sedative and commonly causes weight gain, hypotension, and an irritating photosensitive rash, and so, apart from short-term use in an emergency to control and sedate the excited and restless, we would not recommend it for use in treating psychotic illness. You will be surprised how commonly it is used by psychiatrists who perhaps think that obesity and lethargy are symptoms of the psychosis and not side-effects of the drug used to control it. There is a syrup form, useful in emergencies, as it is not unpalatable and will act rapidly—certainly more quickly than the intramuscular injection. Like most antipsychotics it should be used cautiously in patients with liver disease, brain damage (particularly extrapyramidal disorders), and epilepsy.

Thioridazine (a piperidine) is sedative and less neuroleptic than chlorpromazine. It is useful in small doses for short-term control of agitation or overactivity. Large doses (over 800 mg daily) may cause pigmentary retinopathy and must be avoided. It has no place in the long-term management of schizophrenia.

Fluphenazine (a piperazine). An oral preparation is available, but little used. There are two depot forms, the decanoate, which is very widely used, and the enanthate. Test doses of both, by deep intramuscular gluteal injection, are recommended before maintenance therapy is commenced.

Trifluoperazine (a piperazine). There is no depot form of this drug. It is widely used as it is quite strongly neuroleptic and has little in the way of sedative effects, particularly if introduced in small doses that are gradually increased. It has the advantage that once-daily oral maintenance therapy is possible, and patients remain reasonably alert whilst taking it.

Haloperidol (a butyrophenone) is a powerful neuroleptic that has little in the way of sedative effects, and is widely used. There is a useful liquid form of the drug and an intramuscular injection which can be used intravenously, which is particularly useful in emergencies. Large doses of the drug can be used for short-term control of extreme excitement, and the drug also has the advantage that once-daily oral maintenance therapy is possible. There is also a depot form. **Droperidol** is an alternative for emergency use.

Flupenthixol (a thioxanthene) is a powerful neuroleptic with only weak sedative properties. There is an oral form that is little used in psychosis, but is used in small doses as an antidepressant. The depot form is widely used and effective. This drug should not be used in patients who are grossly overexcited as it may have alerting properties. It is only weakly sedative.

Pimozide (a diphenylbutylpiperidine) is a powerful neuroleptic that has little in the way of sedative properties. It is often used in a large loading dose, dropping down rapidly to maintenance oral therapy. There is no depot form. Maintenance therapy need only be given once a day, and the drug is often well tolerated. Patients with abnormal electrocardiograms should not be given the drug (all patients should have this test before the drug is used—we think this is unnecessary but it is a recommendation you cannot ignore).

Sulpiride (a substituted benzamide) is a powerful neuroleptic with little in the way of sedative properties. It is possibly slightly excitatory, and certainly should not be used in hypomania. Once-daily dosage for maintenance therapy is possible with this drug. There is no depot form.

Other depot preparations (such as zuclopenthixol, pipothiazine, and fluspirilene) and oral drugs (for example promazine, triperidol, and oxypertine) exist, but we have covered the main ones that are in common use. Before prescribing a drug, we would urge you to look it up in the British National Formulary and to carefully study its contraindications, its side-effects, and its dosage. Doses given in the British National Formulary are likely to be slightly conservative and there will be times, particularly in acute emergencies with extremely disturbed patients, when you will have to exceed the stated dose. Get advice before you do so, and get to know the use of one or two of these drugs intimately. You will obviously have to take note of local prescribing policies which will be based to some extent on the cost of the various preparations. One antipsychotic drug may be more expensive than another, but if it helps the patient to be free of psychosis and yet remain alert so that he can work, rather than be dull and sleepy and, although not very psychotic, totally incapable of doing anything for himself, then the increased cost is more than justified. Do not give more than one antipsychotic drug at a time; sometimes very large doses are needed to control symptoms, but use a single drug.

Side-effects of antipsychotic drugs

Apart from some autonomic and cholinergic side-effects and side-effects related to dopamine blockade, such as inappropriate lactation, the main side-effects of all antipsychotic drugs are extrapyramidal. *Parkinsonian side-effects* are common, tend to be dose-related, are often subtle, and may, unfortunately, be mistaken for the condition that the drug is treating rather than as a side-effect of the drug itself. A shuffling gait, a mask-like face, hypokinesia, and a lack of spontaneous movement, can look like retardation or even incipient catatonia. If you know the patient well and see him every day, you may get so used to his mild bradyphrenia and hypokinesia that you fail to notice it. Likewise, *akathisia* may be mistaken for psychotic restlessness or for made movements, as can *dystonic reactions*, which may also be mistaken for, and mislabelled as, hysteria or attention-seeking behaviour.

Tardive dyskinesia (oral–buccal–lingual facial dyskinesia) is unfortunately so common that in its milder forms it may easily be overlooked or you may merely think the patient is chewing gum or has ill-fitting false teeth. You therefore need to be continually on the alert for these extrapyramidal side-effects as they are unpleasant for the patient (for example, dystonic reactions)

and will interfere with drug compliance or may interfere with rehabilitation (as in akathisia, bradyphrenia,
and hypokinesia), and are potentially irreversible (as
in tardive dyskinesia).

Parkinsonian side-effects and akathisia are best
treated by reducing the dose of the drug. Only rarely
should antiparkinsonian medication be given as most
antiparkinsonian drugs have their own muddling
effect on mental state. If you have to use such a drug,
use it for two or three weeks and then withdraw it
again. On no account prescribe antiparkinsonian drugs
routinely to prevent parkinsonian side-effects, and do
not be persuaded to do so by nursing staff or even by
your consultant. There is absolutely no need for it.

Dystonic reactions should be treated by an intravenous injection of an antiparkinsonian drug such as
procyclidine, which may have to be repeated once or
twice until the blood level of the drug that has caused
the dystonic reaction has fallen. If continued antipsychotic treatment is needed, use a lower dose of the
antipsychotic drug or consider switching to a different
one with a lower neuroleptic potential.

Once it has appeared, tardive dyskinesia is almost
impossible to treat, although you should consider very
seriously withdrawing the antipsychotic drug responsible for causing it. The management of tardive dyskinesia is aimed at prevention by making sure that only
those patients that have demonstrated a clear need for
continual antipsychotic therapy actually get it, by using
as small a dose of the appropriate drug as possible
compatible with patient safety (many patients take far
too high a dose of maintenance antipsychotic drug),
and by, if at all possible, giving your patient drug 'holidays' during which the antipsychotic drug is withdrawn
for two or three months (or even longer if you can
manage it) before the drug is restarted. Possibly about
a fifth of patients who take long-term maintenance

antipsychotic therapy (either orally or by depot injection) will develop some degree of tardive dyskinesia, and you should therefore always be doing your best to try to prevent it, although it must be remembered that some patients with chronic schizophrenia who have never had a neuroleptic drug will eventually develop the condition.

Neuroleptic malignant syndrome

This is one very rare but important side-effect of neuroleptic therapy that all psychiatrists must be able to recognize as it can occur in patients taking any phenothiazine or butyrophenone and is potentially rapidly fatal. Early signs are unexplained fever (with a neutrophil leucocytosis) and dysphagia, followed by diminution in consciousness and severe muscle rigidity. There is often urinary incontinence. It usually occurs either shortly after the patient has been placed on neuroleptic medication or when there has been a dose increase. There is usually a raised plasma urea and sodium concentration, raised liver enzymes, and a characteristic rise in creatinine kinase. Renal failure due to myoglobinuria may occur, and death may be due to this or to respiratory or cardiac failure.

If the condition occurs, admit the patient to an intensive therapy unit, stop the neuroleptic, cool and rehydrate the patient, check blood gases, pH, and bicarbonate frequently, and give intravenous dantrolene. Nasogastric levodopa or bromocriptine may help the severe rigidity.

Affective disorders

Depression

Most psychiatrists would agree that patients with moderate to severe depressive illnesses need and usually respond to antidepressant drugs, of which there is a large variety. It is best to learn how to use perhaps no more than three or four antidepressants, each having different properties. For most patients, it is still best to use the older tricyclic antidepressants (despite their drawbacks in terms of side-effects) as at least these are proven in efficacy and do work as antidepressants. Most antidepressants can be given in a once-daily dosage, usually at night (with some antidepressants most of the total daily dose can be given at night with a small supplement in the morning). There is no need for complicated dose regimens as the more complicated the regimen the worse the compliance. Many patients who need antidepressants are either suicidal and therefore are at risk from an overdose of the medication, or their illness makes them unreliable in terms of taking it. They may, for instance, feel so hopeless that they feel it is not worth taking medication as they are certain that they will not get better. Supervision of the patient by a responsible person is necessary. It is wise to prescribe no more than a week's supply of medication at a time. Make sure that somebody keeps it secure from the patient. In severe depression start with a large dose of your chosen drug (at least half the final expected dose). In moderate depression start with a smaller dose (about one-quarter of the expected dose), and slowly increase it.

Antidepressant drugs are often prescribed in too small a dose and for too short a length of time, particularly on an out-patient basis. After recovery from a severe depressive illness, antidepressants should be maintained in full dosage for at least six months and the drug then slowly withdrawn. If it is the second or subsequent depression then it is often advisable to maintain antidepressant medication in full dosage for up to a year. A small proportion of patients seem to need to take antidepressants (usually in half the initial therapeutic dose) for very long periods of time. These are patients who are subject to frequent relapses; continued use of a tricyclic antidepressant for several years may be preferable to taking lithium.

Before prescribing any antidepressant it is necessary to take a full medical history and to perform an appropriate physical examination, in particular to assess the cardiovascular system, the visual system (looking for early glaucoma), and the genitourinary system. Avoid the use of tricyclic drugs, if at all possible, in people who have early glaucoma, urinary retention, or obvious cardiovascular disease. If you do prescribe a tricyclic make sure that the benefits outweight the potential side-effects and dangers. Antidepressants should also be prescribed cautiously in patients with early autonomic failure, epilepsy, brain damage, or who have a family history of a low convulsive threshold.

There are several types of antidepressant:

Tricyclic antidepressants, which are the oldest, most widely used, and probably the most effective of the antidepressant drugs. These block the reuptake of noradrenaline and serotonin from the synaptic space. Down regulation of transmitters may also occur. Tricyclic antidepressants, like most antidepressants, take at least ten days to show much effect, and the patient may actually feel worse for at least the first week of the drug being taken and needs to be supported through this period. One should not assume that the antidepressant is ineffective until the patient has been taking the maximum tolerated dose for at least three weeks. Some tricyclic antidepressants (amitriptyline, trimipramine) are more sedative than others (protriptyline, imipramine) and are probably best used in patients who have a degree of anxiety or agitation contaminating their depression.

Imipramine is the prototype tricyclic antidepressant and is still widely used. It has some alerting and arousing properties, and tends to increase insomnia, and is best avoided in patients who are also anxious or agitated or have severe insomnia. It is best to give a twice-daily dose.

Amitriptyline is the most widely used tricyclic antidepressant and the yardstick against which others are judged. It is more sedative than imipramine and is therefore particularly useful in agitated patients. It is best given in a single daily dose at night.

Trimipramine is even more sedative than amitriptyline and is particularly useful for patients with severe insomnia. It need only be given in a single dose at night, but even given in this way it may cause daytime sedation.

Clomipramine is less sedating than amitriptyline or trimipramine and is said to be particularly useful in patients with obsessional or phobic symptoms, particularly if they also have depressive symptoms.

Nortriptyline (a derivative of amitriptyline), amoxapine, protriptyline, dothiepin, and lofepramine are also used as antidepressants, and you may find that these are the drugs favoured in the hospital in which you work.

Tetracyclic antidepressants are structurally different from tricyclics and may work by enhancing noradrenaline release. They have fewer anticholinergic side-effects than the tricyclic antidepressants and are probably less poisonous, but may not be as effective. They should be considered in the elderly and in patients who are likely to suffer from cholinergic side-effects. Mianserin and maprotiline are two in common use. With mianserin, it is recommended that full blood counts are performed every four weeks during the first three months of taking the drug, particularly if patients develop signs of infection.

Trazodone (a triazolopyridine) is another antidepressant that is not chemically related to any of the others. It tends to be sedative, but is also less anticholinergic than tricyclics and, although expensive, may be used as an alternative. It has been known to cause priapism because it has alpha-receptor antagonistic properties.

Viloxazine (an oxazine) is also occasionally useful and probably works by inhibiting reuptake of noradrenaline, but is not anticholinergic. It can be an extremely effective antidepressant, but a proportion of patients who take it suffer from severe nausea and vomiting that limits its usefulness.

5HT reuptake inhibitors have recently been introduced as antidepressants. They are virtually free of noradrenergic and cholinergic side-effects and may prove to be useful alternatives to the tricyclics. Two in current use are fluvoxamine and fluoxetine. Nausea may be an unacceptable side-effect of both. They interact with lithium and monoamine oxidase inhibitors.

Monoamine oxidase inhibitors prevent breakdown of monoamine neurotransmitters in the synaptic cleft thereby prolonging their action. They are little used nowadays, although they still have a place in atypical or resistant depression and in severe anxiety states, including agoraphobia. They have severe potential dangers because of dietary and drug interactions. They potentiate several drugs, particularly opiate analgesics and tricyclic antidepressants and some antihypertensive agents. Patients must avoid cheese, Bovril, Oxo, or other meat extracts, broad bean pods, Marmite or other yeast extracts, red wine, some beers (including low alcohol beers), and pickled herrings. A period of at least 14 days must elapse after the patient has taken the last dose of a monoamine oxidase inhibitor before he can stop taking the precautions, both in terms of other drugs or foodstuffs, otherwise severe hypertensive reactions may occur. Phenelzine is the most commonly used monoamine oxidase inhibitor, but occasionally tranylcypromine is used. Although they can be useful, you should certainly not consider prescribing these drugs without first discussing it with your consultant. You must take care to ensure that any patient in your charge who is taking these drugs is fully versed in the drugs that they must not take and in the foodstuffs that they must avoid. It is best to get a list from the pharmacy and make sure that the patient understands it. The patient should carry a warning card.

Mania and hypomania

The treatment of this condition falls into two stages. The first stage involves immediate control of the over-activity and excitement with a powerful neuroleptic, usually haloperidol. It may be necessary to start with an intravenous dose, and large doses (up to 100 mg a day) may be needed for several days. It is better to use a non-sedating neuroleptic such as haloperidol (as manic patients struggle wildly against feelings of se-dation), but this is one of the rare occasions when two neuroleptics can be used, a dose of thioridazine or chlorpromazine being used at night to provide some much-needed sleep.

As soon as excitement subsides, lower the dose of haloperidol to a maintenance level, watch for the onset of depression, and try to withdraw the haloperidol as soon as you can. If the excitement and overactivity is life-threatening, ECT can be used, but this is rare and you will need your consultant's advice before attempting it.

When the episode is over, consider if it is likely to recur and, if so, consider lithium prophylaxis. This also applies to patients who swing between mania and depression (bipolar illness) and some patients with recurrent unipolar illness. Remember, however, that prophylaxis is only rarely indicated for first episodes and that lithium is a poison, the long-term taking of which has to be carefully justified. Do not give large doses of haloperidol and lithium together as severe extrapyramidal symptoms may occur and the risk of precipitating the neuroleptic malignant sydrome might be increased.

Lithium. Although occasionally used as an antidepressant in resistant depression, its main use is in long-term prophylaxis of affective disorder. Its mode of action is uncertain, although there are several persuasive theories. Before prescribing it, check your patient's cardiovascular, renal, hepatic, and thyroid function (i.e., history, examination, biochemical profile, serum T3, T4, and TSH concentrations, ECG, urinalysis, and creatinine clearance). Repeat the biochemical profile, creatinine, and TSH concentration every six months. Be alert to the toxic side-effects of overdosage.

Mild side-effects include tremor, nausea, polydipsia, and polyuria. Check lithium level and reduce the dose if necessary.

Severe side-effects include diarrhoea, vomiting, drowsiness, weakness, incoordination, ataxia, tinnitus, blurred vision, muscle twitching, fasciculation, cogwheel rigidity, dysphasia, and focal neurological signs. Stop the drug and do blood concentration.

Very severe side-effects are delirium, seizures, hyperpyrexia, and coma. Stop the drug and admit the patient to an intensive therapy unit. Consider dialysis.

There are several preparations of lithium, both short-acting and sustained release. Local practice will determine which one you use. The aim is to keep blood levels between 0.6–1.2 mEq/l for maintenance therapy. Once the patient is stable, check lithium levels every three months. Tremor and polydipsia/polyuria are common side-effects of a normal dose, as are weight gain and hypothyroidism (if the patient needs lithium then thyroxine supplements are acceptable). Severe side-effects appear at blood levels over 2 mEq/l, and potentially fatal ones at levels above 2.5 mEq/l.

Thus the decision to use lithium should not be made lightly. Even if a patient cycles in mood frequently, if he can recognize the prodromal signs of a change in mood, has insight, is cooperative, and responds well to conventional treatment, it may be best not to use lithium.

Carbamazepine has its advocates as a substitute for lithium, but in our experience its use has been disappointing.

Anxiety and sleep disturbance

Hypnotics and anxiolytics

Never write a prescription for a hypnotic or anxiolytic drug without thinking twice (or even three times) about it. If you do prescribe one, make sure that the prescription is for no more than two weeks' supply for an anxiolytic and no more than a few days' supply for an hypnotic, preferably given on alternate nights. Almost all anxiety and sleep problems can be solved by means other than medication, and there is an ever-present risk of causing dependence with any agent that you use. At the moment the concerns about dependency are focused on benzodiazepines. Recently introduced medication, said to be effective for anxiety (buspirone) or inducing sleep (zoplicone), has not yet been shown to cause dependence, but we would urge you not to use it until its potential for causing habituation and dependence has been more thoroughly assessed. One of us can remember benzodiazepines being introduced as a remedy for the dependency problems that barbiturates were causing in the sixties.

If you are dealing with a patient who is psychotic and therefore agitated or sleepless as a result, then phenothiazines or other neuroleptics are more preferable for controlling the anxiety or sleeplessness than an anxiolytic drug. If sleeplessness or anxiety are due to depression, then an antidepressant used at night, particularly a more sedating one, is all that is needed. You should not prescribe an anxiolytic and an antidepressant together.

In uncomplicated anxiety, if you can teach the patient what anxiety is, support him whilst he is anxious, and teach him ways of reducing his own anxiety, there will be no need for an anxiolytic drug. We have to recognize that occasionally some patients are so frightened or so overwhelmed by their anxiety that behavioural and counselling methods will not immediately work, and for them a short course of diminishing doses of a long-acting benzodiazepine (such as diazepam) for no more than a couple of weeks can be justified. It is important to make sure that the medication is withdrawn at the end of a couple of weeks and not thoughtlessly represcribed. You will often find that you are prescribing diazepam for your own or the nurses' anxiety about the patient rather than for the patient's real needs. Do not prescribe short-acting benzodiazepines such as lorazepam for anxiety as their dependency potential is much higher.

The occasional use of a hypnotic benzodiazepine for one or two nights (or two or three times a week for no more than two weeks) can also be justified for symptomatic sleeplessness if in the meantime you are doing something about the reasons for the patient's insomnia. Use a short-acting benzodiazepine like temazepam. Above all, avoid routine prescriptions of hypnotic drugs and do not allow nurses to bully you into prescribing hypnotics for patients at night in case they cannot sleep. If the patient is sleepless and restless at night, the night staff should talk to and support the patient. You should not prescribe hypnotics so that the night sister can have a quiet night. Counselling and support is not just a daytime occupation.

Benzodiazepine dependence

Patients who have been taking benzodiazepines for a long time may become dependent on them. Reducing the dose leads to definite benzodiazepine withdrawal symptoms, which look so much like the original anxiety that the drug was prescribed for that they are often mistaken for it. If benzodiazepine hypnotics are stopped suddenly after the patient has taken them continually for more than a few days, there is often a long withdrawal period in which the patient is sleepless, restless, and dreams frequently.

Withdrawing a patient from benzodiazepines, particularly if he is severely dependent, will take a long time. If he is dependent on a short-acting benzodiazepine like lorazepam, then substitute a long-acting one like diazepam (5 mg of diazepam for every 1 mg of lorazepam). When the substitution has been achieved, slowly withdraw the diazepam by no more than 2 mg a fortnight and give the patient a great deal of support and help as you do so. Encourage the patient to join a group of former benzodiazepine dependent patients, from which he will get a great deal of support. He will need anxiety management and cognitive therapy.

The real answer to benzodiazepine dependence is, of course, not to prescribe the drug in the first place. Except for delirium tremens (and then only for a short time in diminishing doses), do not prescribe benzodiazepines to people with alcohol or drug dependence problems and do not prescribe them for people with epilepsy unless you want to use their anticonvulsant effect. Other people's anxiety is unpleasant, but often you are tempted to prescribe to relieve your own feelings of inadequacy and helplessness, and this is not a good reason for doing so.

I Administration

You will notice, as you develop experience in psychiatry, that there are happy wards and unhappy ones, happy hospitals and unhappy ones (just as in the community there are happy homes and unhappy ones). Such happy places are good to work in for the staff and therapeutic for the patients. They do not occur just by happy accident, but have to be worked at, and largely arise out of good administration. The real purpose of administration (seen as a treatment) is to try to encourage good confiding and trusting relationships between members of staff working in a unit and between their patients to create a warm, comfortable, and nurturing atmosphere, which, however, must achieve the difficult balance of at the same time preventing dependency and encouraging independence in the patient and fostering his desire to return to the real world.

As a newcomer you will probably work as a ward doctor and will be very much involved in trying to help to create a good therapeutic atmosphere on the ward. This is achieved by making sure that there are effective channels of communication between staff members, that joint decisions are made about the management of patients, and that attempts are made to recognize and defuse tension between staff members, between members of staff and patients, and between patients themselves. This is why it is important for you to get to know the roles, responsibilities, and skills of other members of the therapeutic team (and not assume that you know what they are), and for regular meetings to take place between both members of the ward team and the patients, and also between members of the ward team themselves, during which tensions and disagreements can be aired and resolved, and during which staff can be supportive to each other and acknowledge the work that each is doing. Support of each other is particularly needed during times of tension.

These goals are achieved by holding regular staff meetings, which should be interdisciplinary and have a leader who should preferably be neither the nurse nor the doctor in charge of the ward, but someone who should have some experience of running a group. The leader should facilitate the making of group decisions, should help to defuse tensions, should make sure that praise is given when it is due, and in particular should guard against one member of the ward team being scapegoated during times of tension.

Because you only visit the ward occasionally and nurses are there all the time, it is particularly important during times of tension when you are dealing with a difficult patient (for instance, a patient who is very manipulative and who tries to drive emotional wedges between the staff, or a patient who is extremely manic and therefore exhausting), that you should make sure that you are supportive to other staff members on the ward, visit the ward frequently, talk through the problems, respond quickly to calls for help, and are empathic with (but do not immediately respond to) appeals for the patient's discharge or transfer elsewhere.

A particular difficulty occurs when a patient is admitted with a puzzling psychiatric condition that you need to observe for a few days before treating, and yet the patient's behaviour is such as to throw stress on the nursing staff who cannot understand why you do not do something and give the patient some medication. Often you will have to strike an effective compromise between scientific curiosity and practical help to the nursing staff, and you should remember that observing behaviour in the context of a very artificial situation like a ward may reveal very little useful information. If you do have to delay treatment to perhaps get a special investigation done like an EEG, it is very important to tell the staff why you are waiting and for them to understand the need for an accurate diagnosis to be made before treating the patient.

Therapeutic community

Some units (and occasionally whole hospitals) work as a therapeutic community. Both patients and staff meet regularly for group discussions that are run along psychodynamic lines. Decisions about ward policy and procedures are decided by consensus, and use of medication is kept to a minimum. Providing that there are checks and balances within the system, that there is some outside supervision, and that the unit has some control over who is admitted, a therapeutic community can be extremely exciting and stimulating to work in. Unfortunately, they often go wrong because unsuitable patients are admitted or because pathological relationships develop between members of staff. It is unlikely that you will start work in a therapeutic community (particularly as they seem to be disappearing), but the experience can be valuable, although at times uncomfortable.

Record keeping

It is important to keep accurate and up-to-date records of your interaction with patients, and a very good record of decisions made about patient care. You should, as a matter of routine, make a note of any interview with a patient, every encounter with his relatives, summarize decisions made at ward rounds, and record the gist of telephone conversations about him. Medical records in hospital are, however, not your property (technically they belong to the Secretary of State) and, of course, are open to anyone working on the ward, or visiting it, who has a need to review the history and management of the patient. Occasionally therefore, you may feel that very confidential material should not be recorded in the patient's notes but kept separately (discuss this with your consultant). This particularly applies to patients in psychotherapy, when you need to keep accurate notes of what has been said, but for good reason, do not want the rest of the ward staff to know what has been disclosed. Under such circumstances you may consider keeping separate records on paper that you have purchased yourself. If you do this it should be with the consent of your consultant and you should keep such records secure.

The patient's case record is a legal record, a management tool and a measure for audit; it may also be a valuable research source. Case records should therefore be kept to a high standard and follow an acceptable plan since the performance of yourself, your hospital, and your consultant will be judged by them. In the middle of the night, in want of sleep and sustenance and besieged by several conflicting demands at once, this may seem to you very unfair, but you will have to wryly accept that if the late-Victorian psychiatrists were preoccupied by the effects of excessive masturbation, we late-Elizabethan ones are preoccupied by performance indices and audit. How this preoccupation will be viewed in an hundred years' time remains to be seen.

The Court of Electors of the Royal College of Psychiatrists' in their document relating to statement of approval of training schemes for general psychiatric training for the membership of the Royal College published in April 1989, outlined guidelines for the standard of case records in approved training schemes. You should read the whole of this statement early in your training. Your tutor should have a copy, which is available from the College. The following is an extract from this document.

The organization of the record

There are several acceptable ways of organizing a case record, including:

1. Organization by successive admissions, with all information relevant to that admission (correspondence, nursing observations, investigations, reports by social workers, psychologists, and occupational therapists, and out-patient follow-up notes), compiled in the same compartment as the in-patient medical notes.

2. Organization by data source, with separate compartments for in-patient admissions, out-patient care, nursing observations, correspondence, and investigations.

3. Organization as a consecutive record, all sources being compiled in chronological sequence.

4. Organization in problem-orientated form.

The College would not wish to express a preference for one method of organization, but rather to stipulate the elements that should always be present in a case record of teaching standards.

Case records should be typed or written legibly.

The contents of case records of teaching standard

1. The *reason for referral* (or admission) should be stated, with an account of the circumstances and events leading to it.

2. The clinical state should be documented by an exploration of symptoms and an examination of the physical and mental state.

The *exploration of symptoms* includes verbatim statements made by the patient about the main complaints together with the answers to clarifying questions about these and related symptoms. It also includes an account of the development of the illness and of the psychiatric history.

The *mental state examination* includes:

(a) an exploration of the patient's preoccupations and concerns, including his/her self-esteem (self-image), hopes, griefs, and fears;

(b) the review of major psychiatric symptoms, such as morbid ideas (content and form), perceptual anomalies, and mood disorders;

(c) observations about appearance, behaviour, affect, speech, and rapport with the interviewer;

(d) the testing of cognitive functions including orientation, intelligence, concentration, memory, and (in appropriate patients) neuropsychiatric testing.

3. The patient's account of the personal history and clinical state is amplified by *corroborative accounts*, especially from relatives and (for in-patients) nursing staff, who observe behaviour in a variety of settings, and other members of the multidisciplinary team. If the patient has had psychiatric treatment before, the case records are obtained, studied, and summarized.

4. There is an account of the *personal history*, including the family background, childhood and schooling, work record, psychosexual and marital history, health, lifestyle (including deviant behaviour), and present circumstances. If this has already been explored at a previous referral, it is not always necessary to start afresh at the beginning. It may be acceptable and even preferable to update the earlier account by further clarification and exploration of recent events. The personal history pays particular attention to the nature and quality of relationships, especially with the family of origin, partner, and children.

5. There must be a consideration by the trainee of *diagnosis* (assessment), including the differential diagnosis, and *treatment* (management). The diagnosis should not be limited to the clinical state, but should include an assessment of personality and social circumstances, with an attempt to clarify the interaction of past and present factors in producing the recent situation. In the best teaching units this discussion will often include the results of reading in the library about the salient features of the patient's illness. The discussion of management should include a plan of further investigation if necessary, and an account of the style and role of psychotherapy and social treatment, as well as pharmaceutical treatment, with details of the part to be played by each member of the team.

6. The patient's *progress* in hospital, out-patients, or at home is documented by frequent, legible, and concise notes. Changes in clinical state and treatment plan are clearly recorded. At the time of discharge, a note is made of the clinical state (comparing it with that present at the height of the episode), and of recommendations for future treatment.

7. Major episodes, whether treated in hospital or at home, are drawn together by a typewritten *summary* for ease of reference. These summaries may be organized episode by episode *or* in the form of an overall summary of the whole course of the illness. For patients treated in the out-patient clinic, letters to the general practitioner serve as summaries.

Make sure that the ward notes are kept secure on the ward and are not on open access. New members of staff, such as trainee nurses and medical students, must understand the need for confidentiality and that both you and they must not discuss patients outside the ward in such a way that the patient can be identified. However tempting, do not indulge in telling lurid tales of a patient's exploits to people who may be able to identify the patient.

In general terms, if a patient tells you something in confidence you should keep that confidence, although occasionally you may need to decide whether, in the interests of public safety, the information should be shared. You should always tell the patient that anything he tells you must be reported to your consultant, although it will not go further.

At the end of the patient's stay in hospital, or at the end of out-patient treatment, you will probably be responsible for informing the patient's general practitioner of what has happened during this period, and also for informing relevant members of the community team such as the community psychiatric nurses. Although you may keep a long summary of the patient's previous history, mental state, treatment, and progress in the hospital records, it is usually recommended that the summary you send to the general practitioner is short and to the point, and does not contain confidential information. The reason for this is that you do not know and have no control over who will see the discharge summary when it is sent to the general practitioner, nor how such a summary will be stored in the patient's notes. Some general practitioners show their patients all letters and other information that has been sent to them by the hospital. This is a perfectly acceptable practice, although unfortunately, some general practitioners who do this do not have the courtesy to inform other doctors that they do so. It is therefore better to assume that all general practitioners do this. If there is information of an extremely confidential nature that you feel it is vitally important for the general practitioner to know, it is probably better to speak to him personally. If you do this, make sure you record that it has been done in the notes.

Patients now have the right to see everything written about them after November 1, 1991, subject to certain safeguards. This means that anything you record about a patient should be accurate, should be fair, and should be capable of being substantiated. Your own personal reactions or personal comments about the patient that are recorded in the notes should also be capable of being substantiated and should be relevant to the patient's treatment and care.

A particularly vulnerable point for many patients is the transition between the protected world of the hospital and the cold realities of living in the community. This is why weekend leave, trial leave, and formal rehabilitation is so important, and why home treatment is so valuable. The most vulnerable and damaged patients are often the ones most rapidly lost to follow-up and who, because of their illness or personality defects, are least appreciative of efforts to help them. For such patients, special care must be taken and a systematic record kept and used. There should be a formal mechanism to review patients who have been lost to follow-up, and everything done to find what has happened to the lost patient. Your consultant will have particular responsibility for this. We recommend that you read the *Guidelines for good medical practice in discharge and aftercare procedures for patients discharged from in-patient psychiatric treatment* published by the Royal College of Psychiatrists (Council Report CR 8), a copy of which should be held by your tutor or hospital library.

Compulsory treatment

A few patients that you encounter will be obviously mentally ill and clearly in need of treatment, but will have no insight into this and will refuse your help, or their delusional or hallucinatory experiences will direct them to reject any offer of help or alternative explanation as to what is happening to them. People who are mentally ill may be a direct threat to their own health or safety, either because they harbour intense suicidal feelings that they are likely to act upon, or because they have destructive command hallucinations (for example, the patient with schizophrenia whose voices are telling him to cut off his own genitalia), or seriously neglect themselves. People who are severely mentally ill may be a risk to others, either because they directly seek the life of other people in response to command hallucinations, or feel compelled to assault other people, or their mental illness leads them to neglect children who may be in their charge. Mental illness may also have made them temporarily irresponsible so that they give away all their money or spend it foolishly. Likewise, people who are mentally impaired may be at risk to themselves either because of self-destructive acts, lack of care of themselves, or lack of ability to comprehend and cope with their environment. They may be unable to control their aggressive impulses towards other people.

Under these circumstances, compulsory detention in hospital may be justified, either so that the patient can be observed for a while while the diagnosis is worked out, or a treatment plan developed for treatment and implemented. The powers to do this (with the necessary safeguards) are contained in the 1983 Mental Health Act. As you progress in your psychiatric training you will need to develop a full understanding of the Act and of all its sections. For this the relevant books should be consulted. We merely append here some practical details of the Act that you will need to know in your first few months in psychiatry, and cover what your own particular duties are under the Act.

People may be detained under this Act if they are suffering from 'mental disorder'. This means mental illness (which is not otherwise defined), arrested or incomplete development of mind (severe mental impairment, mental impairment), psychopathic disorder, and 'any other disorder or disability of mind'. People cannot be detained or described as suffering from mental disorder purely by reason of promiscuity or other immoral conduct, sexual deviancy, or dependence on alcohol or drugs. In other words, society allows people to drink themselves to death without trying to stop them; you can only admit an alcoholic compulsorily if he develops delirium tremens or a psychotic illness related to the alcoholism. You may sometimes feel as you look at the degradation, misery, and suffering that alcoholism causes, that it is liberalism gone mad.

The majority of detained patients you initially meet will be compulsorily detained because of mental illness. The Act does not define what it means by mental illness, but you can take it to mean, by and large, any clinically definable mental illness. Most will be psychotic, but under certain circumstances patients with what are normally regarded 'neurotic' illnesses may be detained (for instance, the patient with a severe obsessional illness whose rituals have become so compelling and all embracing that he has taken to neglecting to eat, or the patient with anorexia nervosa whose life is in jeopardy may occasionally be detained under the Act).

Patients may be detained for *observation* (Section 2), and such detention lasts for 28 days. It requires an application from the nearest relative or, more usually, an approved social worker and the supporting recommendation of two medical practitioners, one of whom must be approved as having special experience in psychiatry under Section 12 of the Act (you are unlikely to be approved under this section of the Act, at least until you have your membership of the Royal College of Psychiatrists). Patients detained for observation may also be treated, but patients may also be detained for *treatment* (Section 3). Applications for admission under this section of the Act are again made by the nearest relative or by an approved social worker, and the application must be supported by two medical recommendations, one of the certifying doctors being recognized under Section 12 of the Mental Health Act. The patient is initially detained for six months, detention may then be renewed for a further six months and then subsequently for one year at a time. Applications for renewal of the detention are made by the responsible medical officer (who will usually be your consultant).

Patients may be admitted as an emergency for 72 hours (Section 4) on application by the nearest relative or an approved social worker (who must have seen the patient within the past 24 hours) and one medical recommendation. This doctor does not have to be recognized under Section 12 of the Act, but, if possible, must be a doctor who has previously known the patient.

The patient must be admitted within 24 hours of the examination by the doctor, or of the application being made if it was earlier, and the patient must be discharged after 72 hours unless a second medical recommendation is received so that the requirements for detention under Section 2 are then complied with.

Patients detained under Section 2 may be discharged by the responsible medical officer, by the hospital managers, or by application from the nearest relative, but the nearest relative's request may be blocked if the doctor in charge of the case certifies that the patient is dangerous. The nearest relative can then apply to a Mental Health Review Tribunal, as may the patient, who can appeal to the tribunal within 14 days of admission. Mental Health Review Tribunals have the power to discharge patients. Patients detained under Section 3 may be discharged by the responsible medical officer, by the managers of the hospital, or by application from the nearest relative (providing 72 hours' notice has been given and only if the responsible medical officer has not certified that the patient is dangerous). The nearest relative may apply to a Mental Health Tribunal on the patient's behalf within 28 days after his application for discharge has been refused, and the patient may appeal to a Mental Health Review Tribunal within six months of his admission under Section 3. If he does not apply and is further detained, the managers of the hospital must automatically refer his case to the Tribunal for review. It is important that the patient knows his rights, and you will need to make sure that the patient has been informed of his rights of appeal to a Review Tribunal and that he has understood it, particularly if he comes from another culture.

Patients already in hospital on an informal voluntary basis may also be detained if they seek to leave if they are suffering from one of the mental disorders defined in the Act and it is felt that they should be detained in the interests of their own health and safety or for the safety of others. Under the Mental Health Act registered mental nurses have the power to detain the patient on the ward formally for six hours whilst a medical opinion is obtained. This only applies to psychiatric nurses in a psychiatric hospital or unit. On a general medical or surgical ward nurses, however, have a common-law duty to detain a patient if it can be shown that to let the patient go might be dangerous for him or others.

The nurse's holding power only lasts for six hours and is terminated when the doctor in charge of the case or his nominated deputy has signed a medical recommendation under Section 5 of the Act that will then detain the patient for 72 hours. At the end of 72 hours the patient must be discharged unless another doctor recommends further detention (and there is an application from the nearest relative or an approved social worker so that the patient then becomes detained under Section 2 or 3 of the Act). The nominated deputy of the responsible medical officer should be a senior doctor who has some experience in psychiatry (usually the senior doctor on-call). You can only act as a designated deputy for the purposes of the Mental Health Act if you have been formally nominated as such by your consultant. It would be rather against the spirit of the Act if a very junior doctor was so nominated.

Other sections of the Act apply to the admission and detention of patients from the courts and from prison; they will become more important for you in your later training.

If a patient is detained in hospital or is admitted from outside and detained under the Act, you must make a careful note of the date and of the time that the patient was detained or admitted. You should also record in the notes the time and date when any leave of absence for the detained patient started and finished. For patients held under Section 4 or 5, if the patient is to be further detained after 72 hours, steps should have been taken to do this long before the section expires. The 72-hour period takes no notice of bank holidays or weekends when senior doctors may not be around. You will also need to remind your consultant when the patient has been in hospital for four months after admission under Section 3 so that a decision can be made about whether or not the section should be renewed.

Only very rarely will you be required to sign a medical application for a Section 2, 3, 4, or 5 when you are a very junior doctor. You will not be allowed to sign a medical recommendation for detention when your consultant is co-signatory. Two doctors from the same hospital can only rarely be co-signatories (occasionally you may be a co-signatory for another consultant within the hospital, providing that you are not working directly for that consultant). The usual signatories will be your consultant and the patient's general practitioner, or the general practitioner and another doctor recognized under Section 12 (occasionally a fully registered medical practitioner from a general hospital may sign if the patient was previously a patient under his care). Together with other members of the ward team, you must expect, from time to time, to be interviewed by a doctor from the Mental Health Commission about a patient and your treatment plan for him.

Consent to treatment

Most consent to treatment is implied by the informed patient voluntarily putting himself in a position in which treatment can occur. At times, however, you should formalize consent by getting the patient to acknowledge in writing both that he has understood the procedure to be applied and the need for it, and that he consents to it (as with ECT).

Problems arise either when the patient refuses consent and you feel that he needs the treatment (and you feel his refusal is determined by his mental state), or when his mental state is such that he is clearly incapable of giving consent because he is not in his right mind and therefore cannot understand what he is being told (he may have agreed to the treatment, but you know that he does not know what he is saying).

If a patient, who is clearly sane and whose illness has not affected his judgement, refuses treatment there is nothing you can do (except consult his relatives) unless your proposed treatment is lifesaving when your duties under common law may apply.

If the patient is mentally ill and his judgement is clearly impaired, it will be necessary to detain him under Section 3 of the Mental Health Act in order to carry out the treatment unless it is a grave emergency and you need to save his life, in which case your common-law duties apply. If he is so detained and you want to give ECT then you will need a second opinion on the necessity for such treatment, by a doctor approved by the Mental Health Act Commission. This doctor will have access to the patient's records, will want to discuss the patient with you and other ward staff, and will want to be acquainted with your treatment plan. He may well suggest an alternative line of treatment. Patients detained under Section 3 cannot be given psychotropic medication for more than three months without either the patient's consent (written certification of his competence to do so is needed), or a certificate from a commission-appointed doctor that such treatment is necessary and that the patient has not consented because of his mental illness. It is therefore important to record when medication was first started.

If urgent treatment is needed, it can be given even if the patient refuses providing that it *is* urgent and needed to save the patient's life or to prevent a serious deterioration in his condition, to prevent serious suffering, or to prevent the patient being a danger to himself or others: this does not apply to Section 4 patients. The treatment should not be irreversible (for example, leucotomy). The foregoing does not absolve you from any responsibility under common law, and only applies to mental illness. Common law covers you for treating physical illness if the patient refuses to give his consent.

In all cases like this it is mandatory that you discuss the matter, before acting, with your consultant or with a senior doctor. Do not make these decisions yourself, and always record reasons for so acting in writing.

Note that if you are working in Scotland, Northern Ireland, or the Republic of Ireland, you will find that the spirit and purpose of mental health legislation is the same, but that there will be technical differences (in terms of the numbering of sections, etc.) that you will need to be aware of.

J Home treatment

A developing trend in psychiatry, which is to be welcomed, is to question the value of taking patients out of their own environment, putting them into the strange environment of a hospital, only to have to eventually return to the environment that probably caused the problem in the first place. For many years psychiatrists have seen the need for a better transition between hospital and home by using day hospitals. A further extension of this is the development of home treatment programmes in which even very seriously disturbed and psychotic patients are not admitted to hospital at all, but are treated by a team that comes from the hospital into the patient's own home.

It is possible that in your training, perhaps even early on, you will become part of such a team. Home treatment does not mean the occasional visit of a therapist to the patient's home. It means that therapists are in the patient's home night and day until recovery has occurred, giving medication, giving support to the family and patient, and containing the patient's behaviour. Home treatment only works if there is excellent information exchange between the various members of the team and a trusting relationship between them. Record keeping is as important as it is in hospital, and the nursing and other staff involved in home treatment need a highly visible medical presence at all times. The need to physically examine patients and to prescribe for them is just as important as it is in hospital. There is no doubt that in a well run home treatment service, recovery of the patient is often more rapid than it would be in hospital. This technique is particularly useful when cultural problems would make in-patient treatment difficult. Because recovery is more rapid, and because there is some evidence that relapse is less common because the family have been taught ways of coping with the patient's behaviour, it is a very cost-effective form of treatment and may become the preferred mode of practice for psychiatry in the future.

At the moment home treatment is not fully established and makes many psychiatrists and nurses feel anxious. Because it is threatening to the established order, it has its vociferous critics. Such critics are often only waiting for the first suicide or first serious assault or homicide to occur during home treatment to initiate a rush back into hospital treatment (forgetting that homicide and suicide are not unknown in psychiatric hospitals). Home treatment units have already shown that almost all psychiatric conditions can be treated in the community and that the need for hospital admission is small. Most of us would also recognize, however, that a period of 'asylum' away from the stresses of home may be appropriate for some patients, and that a few patients are so dangerous that they will need secure accommodation. We also need to build up and reinforce community tolerance of the mentally ill.

K Family therapy

Just as it may be very appropriate to treat the patient in his home, so it may be appropriate to treat the entire family unit with a modification of group psychotherapy. This is usually done in the clinic or in out-patients, and one-way mirrors or video may be used to record the sessions, as detailed analysis of what went on during a session is often very useful but difficult to do whilst the session is in progress, particularly if undertaken by the participating therapists. As with marital therapy (which, in a sense, family therapy is an extension of) there are usually two co-therapists.

The aim of family therapy is to try to involve the whole family in the treatment process, and it recognizes that only changing family attitudes and behaviour is likely to lead to changes in the attitudes and behaviour of an individual family member. Often a family's re-action to a patient's behaviour (as in anorexia nervosa) will reinforce that behaviour. Sometimes the patient is not the sickest member of the family and his behaviour is merely the result of pathological elements in the family, or he is being scapegoated and forced into the sick role.

Family therapy is widely used in child psychiatry, although it is useful in adolescent and adult psychiatry as well. It needs a great deal of experience and skill to practise it well, but is a valuable technique to acquire during your training. It should be distinguished from family *counselling* when, usually in the home, the whole family is seen for information giving, breaking bad news, and simple behavioural/cognitive counselling. This is useful and you should try to get some experience of such home visits during your training. General practitioners are increasingly practising it.

CHAPTER 6

Psychiatric conditions

A Introduction

We are including here a brief summary of the common
psychiatric conditions that you are bound to encounter
in your first few months in psychiatry to remind you
of facts you need to know (but may have forgotten) so
that you can communicate information to your patients
and their relatives and prepare workable treatment
plans. This chapter is meant to be brief, and appears at
the end of the book deliberately as a reference section
to an otherwise practical manual.

Patients and their relatives will want to know what
is wrong, why it happened, what the treatment will be
(and whether it will have any side-effects—they will
assume that it will, and will also assume that chemotherapy will be more powerful than psychotherapy, but
may not want either), how long the condition will last,
whether it will resolve completely, and whether it
will happen again. There will also be a hidden list of
questions related to blame for things going wrong,
scapegoating, and reflections on 'weakness', sanity, and
silliness, which you may need to uncover, confront,
and address.

What should you say and how much should you
reveal? The obvious answer is the truth as you see it
and as you know it, but always be prepared to admit
ignorance and take care not to mislead the patient.
Obviously the patient's mental state must modify some
of your answers so that you are, for instance, optimistic
and reassuring with someone who is severely depressed,
and guarded in your replies with someone who has

schizophrenia until his mental state is sufficiently recovered for him to be able to understand you. Remember
also that medical terms have one meaning for you and
another for the lay-person. For instance, we know that
when we say that there is a genetic factor involved in
the occurrence of major affective disorder or schizophrenia, it does not mean that everyone in the family
is going to get it, but the family who receives that
information may think so unless you explain carefully
what you mean (that it is the inheritance of a *vulnerability* toward the condition, which can be modified by
other factors, social, medical, and psychological). If a
condition is genetically determined, it does mean,
however, that a biochemical mechanism must lie behind
it (since that is how genes express themselves), and
that is a useful concept to get across to the patient.

Likewise, use names carefully. Schizophrenia will
mean one thing to you, but another to the relatives.
Define what you mean first (and explore the patient's
and relatives' ideas about what is wrong) before you
use names. Avoid terms like 'neurotic' altogether; they
have become too debased and pejorative in common
use. Try to be positive in giving information, look to
what can be done to change things, correct gloomy
misapprehensions that the relatives or patient may have,
but be realistic about future potential if it is likely to
be impaired. Explain psychodynamic and 'psychohistoric' concepts simply, and remember that the media
may have already filled your audience's heads with ill
digested facts about the condition you are talking about.
The girl with anorexia may tell you that she is 'denying
her sexuality', or the alcoholic may tell you that 'alcoholism is an illness'. Reflect such statements back,
'Is that how you see it?' 'How much do you think that
applies to you?' 'That may be true for some people, but
I would have to know you a great deal better before I
could say if it was true for you or not.'

It is helpful to use two 'psychohistoric' concepts. Firstly, if unpleasant things have happened to a person in the past, and if that person did not have a chance of grieving properly or talking it through and discharging the emotion he felt at the time, then similar feelings will often return during times of stress or if something awakens the memory of the experience. Secondly, we learn about relationships by example from our childhood relationships, and if something happened to distort that learning experience (a parent dying, rejection, the ridiculing of feelings, or a lack of warmth or trust) then such difficulties may unconsciously be reflected in our adult relationships. Learning the roots of our relationship difficulties may help us to change the bits that we do not like. See Section 4J (p. 291) for an example of a 'common sense' explanation of why some people are aggressive, which we have found useful in discussions with patients and relatives.

B Affective disorders

Definition

These are disorders characterized by mood disturbance, an inappropriate elation or depression, that is often associated with abnormalities of thinking and perception. Not included here are disorders such as anxiety or obsessive–compulsive disorders.

Classification

There is no universal agreement on classification. At various times, mood disorders have been classified by aetiology (reactive or endogenous, primary or secondary), by symptoms (neurotic or psychotic), or on the course of the illness (unipolar or bipolar). The only classification that does stand up to testing is the distinction between unipolar and bipolar types, although there is some overlap between the two and you cannot tell which is which in a first episode. A widely adopted practice is to describe an episode under each of the categories set out below.

1. (a) episode severity—mild, moderate, or severe;

   (b) type—depressive, manic, or mixed;

   (c) associated symptoms:
      (i) neurotic
      (ii) psychotic
      (iii) agitated
      (iv) retarded;

2. course—unipolar, bipolar;

3. aetiology—predominantly reactive, predominantly endogenous.

Epidemiology

Symptoms of depression are common (with a point prevalence of 13–20 per cent in a recent study). They are more common in women of low social class, and in divorced or separated people. *Full* depressive syndromes are, however, less common in such people. These can be divided into bipolar and unipolar.

Bipolar

Pathological swings in mood occur in both directions (i.e., both depression and mania). Onset tends to be in the mid-twenties, and there is an increased incidence in social classes 1 and 2. Lifetime risk of bipolar illness is 1 per cent, the distribution being roughly equal between men and women.

Unipolar

Mood alteration is always in the same direction (i.e., always depressed or always manic). The mean age of onset is the early thirties, and it is evenly distributed among the social classes. It carries a lifetime risk of 6 per cent. It is twice as common in women as in men, for reasons that are unclear.

Clinical features of depression

1. Appearance and behaviour

The patient often has characteristically depressed features (for example, furrowed brow, tearfulness, or a hunched posture). Movement is often limited, although there may be fidgeting and agitation. In severe depression the patient often neglects personal hygiene and his normal standard of dress. Some severely depressed patients maintain a calm exterior that belies their mental state—so-called masked or smiling depression.

2. Speech

Speech tends to be hesitant, monotonal, and slow.

3. Mood

Subjectively, mood is one of sadness or misery that is independent from external events (for example, an act that would usually please the patient or cheer him up has no effect on him). It is often said that the sadness is qualitatively different from a normal appropriate feeling of sadness, for example, following loss. The patient may also have associated feelings of anxiety or irritability. Objective measures of mood are sleep, weight, appetite, and libido. Sleep may be disrupted in one of three ways. There may be complaints of early morning waking; the mental state on waking is usually one of intense depression and anxiety. The patient will often lie awake for hours thinking about the things that he is most anxious about (anxious ruminations). Similarly, another common disturbance is onset insomnia when the patient will lie awake pondering on negative aspects of his life. Both may also be seen in patients with anxiety. Alternatively, some patients (especially in milder depression) complain of hypersomnia, but despite the fact that they sleep excessively, they complain that they wake unrefreshed as if they had had no sleep.

Changes in appetite (decreased appetite and weight loss that is usually more than can be accounted for by the decrease in appetite alone) also accompany depression. In mild forms of depression patients sometimes report a carbohydrate craving, and may increase their food intake and even put on weight. Libido is usually decreased or lost in depression. Depression is often worse on waking and gradually lightens as the day goes on, although in mild depression the reverse is sometimes true. Changes in psychomotor activity (agitation or retardation) are also seen. Interest in work, energy, and motivation are also characteristically reduced. There may be changes in bodily function, for example, constipation, and in women, amenorrhoea.

4. Thoughts

There may be preoccupations, overvalued ideas, ruminations, or delusional thinking. Morbid thinking generally covers three areas. Firstly, the past, when there may be excessive guilt over past trivial misdemeanours. Secondly, concern with the present—loss of self-confidence and self-esteem. Thirdly, the future, which the patient often sees as hopeless, and in which suicidal thoughts and plans are common and must be assessed fully (see Section 4H, p. 215). Delusions are often persecutory, but are mood congruent. (The depressed patient may feel that persecution is what he deserves for his past deeds.) Other delusions are concerned with guilt, worthlessness, poverty, and bodily functions (hypochrondriacal delusions of ill-health that may take the extreme form of nihilistic delusions).

5. Perception

There may auditory hallucinations. These are often simple and mood congruent, for example, voices in the second person telling the patient that he is wicked, evil, or worthless. The patient usually is distressed by their content and agrees with the assessment of himself. There may also be visual hallucinations (usually pseudohallucinations) of scenes of death and destruction, but these are more unusual. Olfactory hallucinations, usually unpleasant, may also occur.

6. Cognitive function

There is usually a subjective complaint of lack of concentration and attention, although in mild depression this may not always be supported by formal testing. In severe depression there may be a clinical picture similar to the cognitive deficits of dementia ('depressive pseudodementia').

7. Other associated symptoms

The patient may complain of physical symptoms, particularly pain or gastrointestinal symptoms, or an apparent increase in any existing physical disability that he has. Other psychiatric symptoms, such as anxiety, obsessions, dissociation, may also be part of this clinical picture and may, as with physical symptoms, be the presenting complaint with the depression hidden behind.

Clinical features of mania

1. Appearance and behaviour

The patient appears intensely overactive both in body and mind. He will often neglect hygiene and appear dishevelled. Clothing is commonly mood congruent, that is brightly coloured and often mismatching. The patient may be socially disinhibited.

2. Speech

Pressure of speech is frequent, even in hypomania, and there may be sudden changes of subject with clang associations and flight of ideas, indicating speeding thoughts and loosening of association.

3. Mood

Mood can be one of elation and euphoria, but is often interspersed with irritability and anger, which can turn to aggression. The objective parameters of mood indicate overactivity. There is a decreased need for sleep, increased energy (which is often accompanied by increased appetite and the patient will often show a disregard for the social niceties of eating), but weight is still lost due to overactivity. Energy and motivation is abundant, but concentration is often impaired so that whilst many ambitious plans are attempted, few, if any, are carried through. The increased energy and drive is accompanied by an increased libido. This is often expressed in a disinhibited way, and in women, unwanted pregnancy is a risk.

4. Thoughts

These become increasingly muddled as mania becomes more severe, with extreme pressure of thought and flight of ideas leading to incoherence. Secondary delusions are common and tend to be grandiose, paranoid, or religious, and mood congruent.

5. Perceptions

Hallucinations are common and tend to be mood congruent, for example, voices telling the patient how wonderful he is. Rarely, mood congruent visual hallucinations and sometimes pleasant olfactory hallucinations may occur.

6. Cognitive function

There is decreased concentration. The patient is often very distractable and there is often a spurious hyper-amnesia.

7. Other associated symptoms

Of patients with mania, 10–20 per cent express schneiderian first rank symptoms, but these tend to be mood congruent and less persistent than those of schizophrenia. Insight is usually impaired.

8. Aetiology of affective disorders

There are many different theories and the detail is beyond the scope of this book. Most work has been done with depression.

1. *Genetic*—family and twin studies have revealed that the strongest genetic influence is with bipolar affective disorder (monozygous concordance of 79 per cent compared with a dizygous concordance of 19 per cent), followed by unipolar depressive disorders (monozygous concordance of 54 per cent; dizygous concordance of 20 per cent), whilst mild depressive disorders have little genetic basis (the concordance for both mono- and dizygous twins being approximately equal).

2. *Biochemical*—from the evidence of the action of drugs (drugs causing depression as a side-effect as well as those used to treat depressive illness), and the direct evidence of neurotransmitter status in post-mortem brains and estimated breakdown products of neuro-transmitters in urine and cerebrospinal fluid, a theory has been postulated that some deficit in the action of a neurotransmitter (possibly 5HT, noradrenaline, or, less likely, dopamine) could be the primary abnormality of depressive illness, or a closely related secondary effect. The evidence is intriguing, but as yet inconclusive.

3. *Psychological*—there have been many psychological theories put forward ranging from Freud's relating to loss, to the recent theory of negative cognition (Beck). There is some evidence to support the view that negative cognition is not secondary to a primary depressive disorder, but is the primary occurrence leading to depressive mood. A combination of negative thoughts, unrealistic expectations, and cognitive distortion (arbitrary inference, selective abstraction, over-generalization, minimalization of success, and magnification of errors) makes a person, programmed to think that way, more likely to suffer from a depressive episode when faced with a relatively minor worrying occurrence.

4. *Sociological*—'vulnerability factors' have been identified for depression in women, (a) over three children aged under 14 years in the family, (b) no work outside the home, (c) lack of confiding relationship in husband, and (d) death of own mother before the age of 11 years. These factors only apply to an urban setting and relate to low self-esteem.

5. *Life events*—stressful life events may obviously precipitate depression in someone so predisposed and there is an excess of life events (by a factor of six) before a depressive episode (there is an excess factor of seven before successful suicide and approximately four before an episode of schizophrenia). The type of episode is not related to the type of event (for example, not necessarily bereavement or loss in depression).

Differential diagnosis

Depression may mimic or be associated with a wide variety of physical illness, intoxication, or psychiatric illness. (See Section 4G (p. 197) for the differential diagnosis of depression and Section 4B (p. 130) for the differential diagnosis of mania.)

Treatment

As with treatment for any psychiatric illness, an initial assessment, confirmation of the diagnosis, and exploration of the differential diagnosis, should be made. This should also include an assessment of the patient's social resources, and also the effect that his illness is having on his family so that a rational decision can be made about where the patient should be treated, either at home or in hospital. This is also determined by his suicidal risk (p. 230). Physical treatment (including ECT) is discussed in Sections 5G (p. 412) and 5H (p. 417).

In addition to physical treatment, all depressed patients should have some form of simple psycho-therapeutic support. The choice of other forms of psychotherapy for depression is controversial, although most authors agree that it should take a problem-orientated form rather than a self-evaluating one whilst the patient is depressed. Currently popular is cognitive therapy, which aims to challenge negative thoughts and cognitive distortions. Social support is also often necessary (i.e., helping with financial or housing problems), particularly with regard to those problems that may facilitate relapse.

Prognosis

The average duration of a manic or depressed episode is said to be three months. The number of patients having their first affective episode who will eventually have other episodes is difficult to predict as quoted relapse rates vary widely. It is best to assume that perhaps half will relapse. Untreated, most episodes of either mania or depression will spontaneously remit, given time, although this may take several years. It may be helpful to keep this in mind when treating the more resistant depressions. Young patients are more likely to recover quickly than older ones.

Perhaps up to 17 per cent of all people with recurrent major depressive episodes will eventually commit suicide.

C Schizophrenia and other psychotic disorders

Definition

A mental disorder characterized by a persistent disturbance in the perception and evaluation of reality leading to characteristic changes in perception, thinking, affective response, and behaviour.

Epidemiology

The disease (for disease it probably is) has a prevalence rate of approximately 1 per cent in the general population. It is a major health problem (for example, the annual cost to the NHS is about £200 000 000 per year). It is equally common in men and women; the mean age of onset being 28 for men and 32 for women. The class structure and geographical location of people with initial schizophrenia approximates to that of the general population. Eventual social drift, however, distorts the picture. It occurs in all races and cultures; culture may alter prognosis and presentation.

Diagnostic criteria and clinical features

The diagnosis of schizophrenia is often difficult and not helped by the muddle and confusion of having different diagnostic criteria, even in the same country. The traditional British view, which you will most likely initially encounter, is to rely on '**first rank symptoms**.' Schneider first described what he called first rank symptoms, which are thought to be highly significant and diagnostic of schizophrenia in the absence of organic illness if they occur in a patient in clear consciousness and without a primary mood disorder. He also described second rank symptoms, which are associated with schizophrenia but are not diagnostic of it.

First rank symptoms

1. hearing one's own thoughts out loud;
2. voices conversing with one another about the patient ('third person');
3. voices keeping up a running commentary on the patient's behaviour;
4. somatic hallucinations with passivity experience;
5. thought insertion or withdrawal;
6. thought broadcasting;
7. feelings, impulses, or actions that are experienced as imposed on the person by outside agencies;
8. delusional perception.

Second rank symptoms

1. other hallucinations;
2. perplexity;
3. depressive and euphoric disorders of affect;
4. emotional blunting.

As a diagnostic concept, the importance attached to Schneider's first rank symptoms in the UK has tended to persist, although 20 per cent of patients diagnosed as having chronic schizophrenia have never had first rank symptoms, whilst 8 per cent of psychotic patients who eventually receive a diagnosis other than schizophrenia have had some of them (especially in hypomania). Schneider's symptoms are not good prognostic indicators, and schneiderian classification takes no account of how long the patient has had the symptoms.

Other classifications that have been tried include operational definition such as that in DSM III R (which includes length of time the patient has had the symptoms), and also a division into Type I and Type II schizophrenia. Type I is said to have an acute onset with positive symptoms, a good prognosis, and a good response to neuroleptics. Type II is characterized by a chronic state with predominantly negative symptoms. On CT scan of the brain an enlarged ventricular system is seen and there is a poor response to neuroleptics. The prognosis is poor. Type II is said to be associated with neuronal loss and organic brain damage.

Positive symptoms

1. hallucinations—usually auditory of the types defined in Schneider's first rank symptoms;
2. delusions—there are various types, but they must be *primary* delusions and not a secondary explanation of the patient's hallucinatory experience, for example, X-rays coming from the radio causing the auditory hallucinations;
3. formal schizophrenic thought disorder (see p. 79 and p. 84);
4. reduced contact with reality;
5. disturbed control of emotional response.

Negative symptoms

1. poverty of speech—this includes both amount and content of speech;
2. loss of volition, apathy, and reduced drive, energy, and interest;
3. slowed thinking and movement;
4. affective flattening;
5. attentional impairment.

Positive symptoms occur in acute schizophrenia and negative ones in chronic schizophrenia or in the defect state that follows an acute episode.

Classification

As with most things concerning schizophrenia, psychiatrists disagree on what classification should be adopted. Apart from the terms acute and chronic schizophrenia, and Type I and Type II, other terms you must be aware of and will come across in practice include:

1. *Catatonic schizophrenia*—positive symptoms of schizophrenia occur, as do episodes of catatonic stupor (negativism, elective mutism, and conscious stupor (cataplexy), plus waxy flexibility, echolalia or echopraxia, automatic obedience, stereotypy, manneristic behaviour, and perserveration (see Section 4P, p. 370)).

2. *Paranoid schizophrenia*—this presents with well systematized persecutory or grandiose delusions and hallucinations. Mood and thought processes are usually normal so that a victim can appear relatively intact until the delusional system is uncovered. This type becomes increasingly common with increasing age. If first rank symptoms of schizophrenia are absent, the condition is usually called a paranoid psychosis. It is uncertain whether this is a clinically useful or a merely arbitrary distinction.

3. *Hebephrenic schizophrenia* presents with silly, childish behaviours in association with affective symptoms and severe thought disorder. Delusions and hallucinations are common, but tend to be unsystematized and are not elaborate. An old term for this was 'buffoon state'. It needs to be correctly distinguished from mania and drug intoxication. It usually occurs in adolescents, and has a poor prognosis.

4. *Simple schizophrenia* implies an insidious development of psychosis with odd eccentric behaviour and declining social performance being prominent in the apparent absence of delusions, hallucinations, or thought disorder (although these are usually present,

but are concealed or develop later). This is also seen in the defect state that follows an acute episode. The prognosis is poor.

These are the classical categories of schizophrenia that you will still find widely used. There is however, little evidence to suggest that they actually exist as separate entities and the DSM III R classification ignores them completely.

Aetiology

The aetiology of schizophrenia has been much researched but little understood, probably because it is not a single entity. It almost certainly arises from a complex interaction between genetic, neurological, biochemical, psychological, and social factors, and does not have a single cause.

Differential diagnosis

There are several conditions that can mimic or be mistaken for schizophrenia, and these include physical illness, psychiatric illness, and intoxication. (For a full list see pp. 143–53 and p. 165.)

Management

Management must include care for both the patient and for relatives, and any plan must take account of psychosocial factors as well as medical ones. The first decision to make is where the patient should be treated. It is often said that admission for a first psychotic episode offers an asylum for the patient, rest for the relatives, and a clear space for observing and assessing the patient. Recent work has, however, shown that keeping patients in the community, even during their first episode, is equally, if not more, effective than hospitalization. The decision of where to treat the patient is an important one and must take into account the resources available to the patient (in terms of family support), and the resources available to the psychiatrist (in terms of home care teams, CPNs, etc.). An initial drug-free period of observation is said to be useful if the patient is not distressed by the symptoms he is experiencing, although not all psychiatrists accept this and prefer to treat psychotic symptoms swiftly to try to prevent increasing the length of the illness episode. It is also an advantage to observe the patient drug free for a short while in order to distinguish true and false side-effects of any antipsychotic medication.

Before an antipsychotic is chosen, a thorough medical history must be taken from the patient as well as the standard laboratory investigations mentioned earlier (p. 116). It is useful to run a checklist of possible side-effects before a drug is started. It is also useful to observe the patient's gait before commencing a drug to distinguish his pre-drug walking from his post-drug gait. Specific goals for the antipsychotic medication should be set such as:

1. eliminating hallucinations

2. improving socialization

3. decreasing hyperactivity

4. improving self-care

5. eliminating aggression.

It is easier to monitor drug effects if these goals are recorded beforehand. These goals should be explained to the patient as his compliance with the medication is vital. Simple supportive psychotherapy and counselling is required for the patient in the same way as any other acutely ill psychiatric patient. Explorative psychotherapy, however, is usually said to be contraindicated during acute psychosis. On discharge from hospital, a comprehensive plan should be made with the community team for out-patient follow-up. In the case of the patient treated at home, there should be a plan of continuing care. This should include both physical treatment, and social and rehabilitative work (for example, day-hospital placement if accommodation is a problem or there is family stress, and employment and financial help). Psychological care and counselling for both the patient and his family, and behavioural programmes (for example, social skills training) may well be required.

Outcome

About one-quarter of patients, after their first episode, will recover completely and will not relapse. A quarter will have no further problems after the first attack except for minor residual symptoms, but will have a possibility of relapse. A further quarter will make only a partial recovery and will continue to have marked post-psychosis dependency on others and social disablement with periodic relapses into acute illness. A quarter will have poor outcome with persistent symptomatology (especially negative symptoms) and severe social disablement. Perhaps 5 per cent of these will have chronic florid symptoms that will persist indefinitely despite all treatment.

Prognostic indicators

Good prognostic factors include an acute onset with positive symptoms, prominent affective symptoms, clear precipitating factors, old age at onset, and good premorbid psychosocial adjustment. Poor prognostic factors include a insidious onset of prominent negative symptoms (including flattening of affect and social isolation), the absence of affective or catatonic symptoms, a strong family history of schizophrenia, and previous poor social adjustment or previous personality disorder.

Paranoid psychosis

As indicated above, some patients, sometimes acutely and sometimes insidiously, develop a psychotic illness with delusions and hallucinations that do not have characteristic schizophrenic qualities and in which affective contact and emotional responsiveness is maintained. Such psychosis, more common in middle and old age, is usually considered to be a separate entity from schizophrenia. Because personality and social acceptability are better preserved, and patients are often non-cooperative, treatment is often difficult (and compliance difficult to obtain). The illness may often be hidden for long periods of time until some sudden act of violence or strange behaviour reveals it. Such paranoid states (for delusions are usually persecutory) may also occur in affective illness and in organic brain disease. They should be treated with neuroleptic drugs as in schizophrenia.

Delusional psychosis

Delusional psychoses, such as pathological jealousy ('Othello syndrome'), erotomania (de Clérambault's syndrome), and monosymptomatic hypochondriasis, are sometimes secondary to affective disorder, but sometimes appear to be primary disorders. Their classification is confused (i.e., DSM III R uses 'delusional psychosis', ICD 9 uses paranoid state), their aetiology obscure, and treatment difficult, although best results are probably gained by a combination of gentle and persistent confrontation and neuroleptic therapy.

D Organic brain disease

If its function is disrupted by toxic, inflammatory, infective, metabolic, or structural insult, the brain has only a limited repertoire of symptoms to indicate its distress. To some extent these symptoms depend on whether the whole or only part of the brain is affected, whether the insult is acute or insidious, and whether permanent or temporary damage has occurred. Very different conditions with completely different causes, natural history, and prognosis, may, however, cause very similar symptoms.

Likewise, very dissimilar symptoms may have the same physical cause. We have seen identical tumours in exactly the same part of the brain produce purely organic symptoms related to memory, predominantly schizophrenic symptoms, an apparent hysterical dissociation, a severe and intractable depression, and an aggressive behaviour disorder. All these different presenting syndromes were caused by left temporal tumours.

The reason that similar lesions in the same place may cause different symptoms is that the organic disturbance is taking place in brains that may have the same structure, physiological function, and chemistry, but which have different genetic inheritance, different memories, different experiences and upbringing, different cultures, and separate identities and personalities. The meaning of the insult to the functioning of the individual must also be taken into account, as well as what reserves the brain has to cope with the effects of the insult, and whether the integrity of the brain has already been breached (a small stroke in an individual with an intact brain may be hardly noticed but may be devastating in someone already brain damaged; alternatively, the same stroke, that critically but subtly interferes with language function and memory, may be hardly noticed in a manual worker but completely disable a teacher). In other words, when assessing a brain injury or an organic brain disorder one still has to consider the *person* whose brain function has changed.

The symptoms of brain insult or injury can be divided into four main classes:

1. delirium or confusional state (acute brain syndrome)
2. dementia (chronic brain syndrome)
3. focal symptoms (such as aphasia)
4. psychiatric syndromes.

The terminology of these states, at the moment, is a little muddled. A confusional state (which may be mild or severe) implies some degree of loss of awareness of surroundings, disorientation, and poor retentive memory. Delirium implies this state plus psychomotor excitement and usually hallucinations (this is probably an artifical distinction). Both conditions are also contained under the title of 'acute brain syndrome', which, although slightly ugly, is probably the better one to use. A chronic brain syndrome, or dementia, is more permanent, although sometimes reversible or arrestable, and there is progressive intellectual loss (sometimes static). Memory impairment is predominant, although secondary psychological, physical, and psychiatric sequelae may occur. There is no clear distinction between acute and chronic brain syndromes. An acute syndrome may gradually merge into a chronic one, and patients with a chronic brain syndrome are particularly liable to sudden episodes of confusion or delirium.

Delirium (acute brain syndrome)
Definition

Delirium is an acute, usually reversible (but potentially fatal) disorder of cerebral function in which there is an impairment (often fluctuating) of the person's ability to attend to, understand, and correctly perceive his environment. There is thus a degree of confusion (which may be profound or very slight), disorientation, an inability to retain new information, loss of attention and concentration, sometimes impaired consciousness, and characteristic perceptual disturbances. There may be misinterpretations, illusions, or hallucinations, which may occur in any modality, but are characteristically visual. There is characteristic wakefulness at night and drowsiness by day. The patient is often agitated with increased psychomotor activity (rarely there is stupor). The clinical features may develop suddenly, character-istically fluctuate, and are usually self-limiting, either because the patient spontaneously recovers or dies, or the condition is terminated by successful treatment.

Classification

Delirium is a *reaction* and can therefore only be clas-sified by cause. Although mild forms of delirium are often termed confusional states and severe forms en-cephalopathy, this is not an aetiological classification.

Epidemiology

This is uncertain, particularly as minor forms of de-lirium probably pass unrecognized or are accepted without comment. Some American studies have sug-gested that perhaps 15 per cent of patients in general hospitals have at least some degree of delirium. The commonest cause of delirium that you will encounter clinically is delirium tremens.

Clinical features of delirium

1. Appearance and behaviour

Initially the patient may look puzzled and sound queru-lous, but as the condition progresses he becomes wildly excited, irritable, and distractable (although quietness and stupor may also develop with the patient muttering and plucking at his bed clothes, 'I saw him fumble with the sheets and play with flowers and smile upon his fingers end . . . he babbled of green fields.'). Occupational delirium may occur, with the patient repeatedly carrying out some fragment of his former occupation, or the patient may be pursued by his own hallucinations.

2. Speech

Speech is often incoherent or related to distorted perceptions ('get them away—get off, get off'), or related to occupational delirium. It may be loud, may be muttering or whispering, or there may be shouting. Occasionally, the patient is mute.

3. Mood

The patient may be euphoric and excited, may appear depressed, or his mood may be normal. The patient may show a blunted affective response for a while.

4. Thoughts

The patient may be preoccupied with his inner experiences and may express delusional ideas (these are usually secondary to his altered perceptions). Paranoid delusions, particularly of being poisoned or interfered with by the nursing or medical staff, are common.

5. Perception

The illness is usually ushered in by misperceptions and illusions, which are then followed by hallucinations. Although auditory, olfactory, and occasionally tactile hallucinations can occur, the characteristic hallucinations of delirium are visual; they are often vivid (and may be lilliputian) and may have a threatening nature.

6. Cognitive function

This is always impaired, although sometimes subtly so that it is not immediately apparent. There is disorientation in time and place (occasionally in person), and impairment of attention and short-term memory, which may be profound (such patients require constant and repeated reassurance). At times there may be dysgraphia, dyslexia, dysphasia, and dyspraxia. Consciousness may be impaired.

7. Other associated symptoms

Sudden shifts in mood and changes in activity, consciousness, and perceptual experiences are very common. There is often a characteristic diurnal fluctuation in activity with wakefulness at night and sleepiness during the day, with worsening of behaviour in the early evening as darkness draws on. The patient may also complain of physical symptoms related to the underlying cause of the delirium. There may be tremor, sweating, circulatory collapse, tonic clonic seizures, vomiting, diarrhoea, the characteristic rash of pellagra or typhoid fever, or signs of meningism. There may be a flapping tremor (which should always be looked for). Occasionally, other movement disorders may be present.

Aetiology

For a full account of possible aetiology see Section 4F (p. 173) Most causes of delirium are systemic rather than cortical. It is never wise to assume that you are dealing with a single cause of the patient's condition, particularly in postoperative delirium and in patients with apparent delirium tremens (who, in addition to the alcohol-related component of the delirium, may also have pneumonia, pancreatitis, or severe electrolyte disturbance). In severe delirium, it is important to recognize hypoglycaemia, Wernicke's encephalopathy, and opiate poisoning quickly. If diagnostic facilities are not immediately to hand, it may be necessary to infuse intravenous glucose (not in severe liver disease), thiamine or B complex vitamins, and naloxone without waiting for laboratory results. Always check delirious patients for ataxia, nystagmus, and ophthalmoplegia, because failure to recognize Wernicke's encephalopathy quickly may lead to irreversible brain damage.

Differential diagnosis

Delirium may be confused with acute psychosis, mania, dementia, and other causes of excitement. For a full differential diagnosis consult Sections 4B (p. 130) and 4E (p. 165).

Treatment

Physiological and psychological support of the delirious patient is important, particularly good consistent nursing care with frequent reassurance, a quiet well lit environment, rehydration, and effective tranquillization (without undue sedation, which may be dangerous), whilst the underlying cause of delirium is recognized and treated. It is often best to avoid medication, particularly in severe anoxia or in acute liver failure (see p. 195 for details).

Prognosis

Delirium has a mortality rate. Although death in delirium is usually due to the underlying cause, occasionally a patient may die by accident, for example, stepping out of a window because he believes he can fly. Suicide may also occur. Patients may occasionally be dangerous to others. Morbidity may also be increased because patients may interfere with their treatment, may be so overactive that they interrupt their treatment, or may become so seriously exhausted that they die.

Dementia (chronic brain syndrome)
Definition

Dementia is a syndrome of intellectual loss, which is usually progressive. Other symptoms may appear, either related to the consequences of intellectual loss or to the patient's insight into his disability, or related to the specific cause of the intellectual loss. Thus in addition to memory loss, there may be specific distortions of language, perception, and motor skills, and there may be changes in personality with a loss of ability to cope with the environment. In the later stages of most dementias there is a merely vegetative existence with profound neurological signs.

Classification

Dementia may be classified according to its severity in terms of mild, moderate, or severe. In mild dementia, although there is some impairment of intellectual function, the patient can still live independently. In moderate dementia, the patient needs some degree of supervision, but can still live at home and may, under certain circumstances, be able to work. In severe dementia, continual supervision is required as the patient is unable to work, interact socially, or maintain his own hygiene.

Dementia is classified into cortical and subcortical dementia, and also into primary degenerative disorders and secondary degenerative disorders. Some authorities still divide dementia into presenile (occurring before the age of 65) and senile dementia (occurring over the age of 65), although the clinical utility of this type of classification may not be important and can be misleading. It is as important to investigate dementia in somebody of 85 as it is in somebody of 45, but the term senile dementia tends to be a 'write off' diagnosis, which is unfortunate because remediable causes of dementia exist even in advanced old age).

Epidemiology

The commonest form of dementia is Alzheimer's disease. Rare before the age of 65, it becomes increasingly common as age advances, so that by the age of 75 at least 5 per cent of the population will be significantly demented. This figure rises to perhaps 15–20 per cent by the age of 85.

Clinical features of dementia

1. Appearance and behaviour

In the early stages of dementia, little may be noticed wrong with the patient except that perhaps his language has lost its elasticity and rather empty stock phrases are being used. The patient complains of forgetfulness (or other people complain of it). Memory impairment eventually becomes socially important, and the patient may become lost whilst travelling, or forget important appointments, and may need to retire from work. Personal impairment occurs later. There may be significant speech difficulty and an obvious memory impairment, and the development of poor personal hygiene with incontinence. Eventually, very severe forgetfulness occurs, which is totally socially disabling and often accompanied by personality change and disruptive or disinhibited behaviour. Eventually, neurodegenerative changes occur so that the patient becomes bedridden and comatose.

Different forms of dementia will emphasize one or more of these features, and there are often secondary emotional and behavioural changes, occasionally accompanied by neurological symptoms or signs, like seizures, myoclonus, chorea, or cortical blindness. Poverty of ideation and disturbance of speech fluency become apparent as the dementia progresses, and there may be specific disorders of speech such as dysphasia.

2. Mood

Changes in mood often occur, usually producing transient sadness, euphoria, or irritability. There are occasional outbursts of explosive anger or catastrophic reactions. A sustained depressive mood should make one think very carefully about possible depressive pseudodementia. Sleep may be disrupted with night-time wakefulness and daytime drowsiness. In the later stages of dementia, there is often a loss of appetite with weight loss, whereas in the early stages there may be hyperphagia. Interest in sexual activity is usually lost, but occasionally, disinhibited sexual behaviour may occur.

3. Thoughts

Dementing patients may show preoccupations, over-valued ideas, ruminations, and delusional thinking, sometimes related to mood change and sometimes related to the patient's awareness of his failing powers. Delusions tend to be paranoid or hypochondriacal, and are usually fleeting. Occasionally, persistent delusional states may occur, very occasionally of a grandiose nature.

4. Perceptions

Misinterpretations and illusions are common and frank hallucinations may occur, either during transient delirium, which is common in dementia, during brief reactive psychosis, or occasionally, as part of the disease process itself.

5. Cognitive function

This is the primary disorder of dementia. Initially social memory is affected, but gradually retention of information and recent memory becomes progressively impaired until cognition can no longer be tested. Other associated symptoms, apart from transient psychiatric symptoms, are neurological symptoms and signs, such as myoclonus, chorea, tonic clonic seizures, dyspraxias, etc., which may occur as part of the condition that is causing the dementia. Hemiplegia may occur, and frontal lobe symptoms are common in dementias, as are neurological symptoms and signs indicating parietal lobe disturbance.

Aetiology

1. Cortical dementia
   (a) Primary degenerative dementia
      (i) Alzheimer's disease
      (ii) Pick's disease
   (b) Secondary dementias
      (i) vascular, particularly multi-infarct dementia;
      (ii) infections (neurosyphilis, Creutzfeldt–Jakob disease, AIDS and its associated cerebral infections);
      (iii) structural (normal pressure hydrocephalus);
      (iv) metabolic dementias (anoxic dementia, electrolyte abnormalities, hepatic and uraemic dementia);
      (v) dementias due to vitamin deficiency or alcohol abuse;
      (vi) thiamine deficiency, B12 deficiency;
      (vii) endocrine-related dementias (hypothyroidism, Cushing's disease, and Addison's disease);
      (viii) toxic dementias (drugs, heavy metals, solvents, etc.);
      (ix) cerebral tumours.
2. Subcortical dementias (Huntington's chorea, Parkinson's disease, Binswanger's disease, supranuclear palsy, Wilson's disease).

Differential diagnosis

See Section 4F (p. 173). Depression must be distinguished from dementia, but this is often not easy.

Treatment

It is important to recognize the potentially reversible or arrestable causes of dementia (see p. 190) and to treat these vigorously. For the progressive dementias that, at the moment, cannot be treated, good social support, good nursing care, retraining in social skills, and memory exercises are helpful and may aid in preventing deterioration.

Prognosis

The prognosis of dementia depends on the cause. It may be extremely rapid, as in Creutzfeldt–Jakob disease, stepwise, as in multi-infarct dementia, or a gradual but irreversible deterioration, as in Alzheimer's disease.

Alzheimer's disease

This is a slowly but inexorably progressive dementia that becomes increasingly common as age advances. Whether 'presenile' and 'senile' Alzheimer's patients are suffering from separate disorders, or whether age merely modifies the way the disease presents, has not been settled. In younger patients, the course is more rapid, the signs of parietal lobe damage are more obvious, and other neurological symptoms are more prominent, although perhaps in the elderly they are not looked for. Alzheimer's disease is characterized by initial memory disturbance, followed after one or two years by progressive signs of parietal lobe damage, and later by other neurological symptoms (partial seizures, extrapyramidal symptoms, etc.), followed eventually by neurovegetative degeneration.

The aetiology of Alzheimer's disease is as yet obscure, although there is a probable genetic factor (there is some recent compelling evidence to suggest that it may be a chronic reaction in the genetically predisposed to toxic substances in foodstuffs). Post-mortem characteristic histopathological changes (senile plaques and neurofibrillary tangles) are found widely distributed in the cortex, particularly in the frontal and temporal areas. There is a marked loss of cholinergic neurons, which may account for the memory defects, although whether this is the primary disorder in Alzheimer's disease or secondary to something else is uncertain. Much effort is being expended at the moment in trying to enhance cholinergic activity in the brains of patients with

Alzheimer's disease in the hope that this will improve memory function. Other neurotransmitter deficits, however, may be as important.

Alzheimer's disease remains a diagnosis of exclusion. A slowly progressive dementia is assumed to be Alzheimer's disease if other causes can be excluded. There is, as yet, no positive test for it in life apart from brain biopsy, which may be misleading. Characteristic changes in flash and pattern visual evoked responses may, however, prove to be useful, as may further developments in magnetic resonance imaging and position emission tomography.

Pick's disease

This is a rare form of dementia that affects women more often than men (2:1) and tends to occur in middle age. There is widespread involvement of the temporal and frontal lobes by degenerative atrophic changes that involve chromatolysis of the neurons with characteristic displacement of the nucleus to the periphery of the cell (balloon cell). The condition may be ushered in by focal symptoms (particularly related to speech and writing, or to dyspraxia) before much memory change is apparent. Personality change of a frontal lobe type is also common. The cause of this condition is unknown, although there is a genetic element. It tends to be a little more rapid than Alzheimer's disease in onset, and have a shorter course. There is no treatment apart from general supportive measures.

Multi-infarct dementia

It is uncertain how common this form of dementia is. Estimates of its prevalence vary widely, although it is not as common as Alzheimer's disease and is often over diagnosed. Multi-infarct dementia and Alzheimer's disease may, of course, exist side by side, since both are comparatively common conditions. Although patients who have had massive strokes (either embolic, thrombotic, or haemorrhagic) are often left with an intellectual deficit and may therefore dement, particularly if they have further strokes, multi-infarct dementia is usually taken to refer to patients who have multiple, small infarcts scattered widely over the brain (lacunae). The aetiology of these lacunae is thought to relate to hypertensive changes in small arterioles in the brain rather than to emboli. There seems to be a critical number of such lacunae below which little clinical impairment is apparent but above which even a small number of extra lesions seems to have a devastating effect. It is uncertain whether the lacunae themselves are the cause of the dementia or merely a by-product of the process that produces the dementia.

Multi-infarct dementia tends to have a stepwise deteriorating course with a patchy distribution of deficits in the early stages of the illness. Focal neurological signs are common. Many patients have evidence of vascular disease elsewhere or have hypertension or a history of having had a previous stroke. The course of the dementia is characteristically fluctuating with sudden episodes of worsening followed by periods of stability. Most patients die within five years from the onset of symptoms usually due, unless an intercurrent illness carries the patient off, to some vascular episode. Little can be done in the way of treatment. Some authorities advocate vasodilator drugs, but there is little evidence that they have more than a temporary effect. Occasionally, cautiously reducing hypertension may improve brain function for a while. Carotid surgery may be offered if carotid artery function is particularly impaired on one side, although it will not improve dementia that is already there. If the disorder is punctuated by transient ischaemic attacks, then aspirin may be offered. A subcortical arteriopathic dementia also occurs (Binswanger's disease).

Neurosyphilis

This condition (still known to many psychiatrists as general paralysis of the insane) is now rare, although it is still encountered. It relates to chronic brain invasion by *Treponema pallidum* and most commonly presents as a simple dementia in which occasional psychotic features, particularly paranoid and grandiose delusions, occur. Almost invariably some neurological features of tertiary syphilis will be present, particularly pupillary changes, which are seen in at least 80 per cent of patients with neurosyphilis, tabetic crises, or locomotor ataxia. It is diagnosed by testing for specific syphilitic serology, although some patients with cerebral syphilis have negative blood serology. Cerebrospinal fluid serology is therefore indicated if blood tests are negative but you retain a strong clinical suspicion that the patient may have cerebral syphilis. Get advice from the appropriate genitourinary department about what tests to use, particularly as false negative or positive results may occur or you may need to distinguish syphilis from yaws. The progress of the disease can be arrested by treatment with penicillin. Many physicians recommend a short course of steroids whilst penicillin is given to try to damp down the commonly occurring Herxheimer reaction (an acute toxic delirium following treatment with penicillin due to sudden release of toxic material from dead spirochaetes). Although neurosyphilis is rare nowadays, it is still important to keep a high index of suspicion for it. It is best to seek the advice of a colleague in genitourinary medicine before diagnosing and treating it or investigating the rest of the patient's family.

Creutzfeldt–Jakob disease

This is a fulminating dementia that is extremely rare, but of particular importance because there is little doubt that it is an infection probably transmitted by a slow virus. It often starts with symptoms of anxiety, depression, or emotional lability, that are swiftly followed by a rapidly developing dementia in which neurological symptoms (movement disorders like chorea, extra-pyramidal symptoms, myoclonus, muscle fasciculation, cortical blindness, or cerebellar symptoms) are common. The clinical course is extremely rapid and death will often occur within a year of the onset of symptoms. It should be assumed that the condition is infectious (particularly from transmission by blood or saliva) and appropriate precautions should be taken.

AIDS dementia

In about a tenth of patients with AIDS the presenting symptoms are a gradual memory loss with subsequent development of dementia, which often has features of a subcortical rather than a cortical dementia and may be associated with peripheral nerve involvement. There is little doubt that this relates to invasion of brain tissue with the AIDS virus (it will respond to AZT). AIDS is therefore part of the differential diagnosis of dementia, particularly in younger patients or those with an 'at risk' lifestyle. In addition to the AIDS virus directly causing a dementia-like syndrome, patients with AIDS may get other cerebral infections that may present either with focal neurological signs or with dementia or delirium. Particularly common in this country are toxo-plasmosis, cryptococcal meningitis, and tuberculomas. Lymphoma infiltration of the brain may also occur.

Normal pressure hydrocephalus

This is a rare but important dementing syndrome in which there is ataxia, urinary incontinence, and dementia accompanied by CT scan evidence of enlarged ventricles with usually normal cerebrospinal fluid pressure. In some cases the cause is unknown, but usually it is secondary to an obstructive hydrocephalus that may be the result of vascular or infective damage in the brain. Shunting procedures are usually very effective and the patient may recover completely, particularly if the condition is recognized in time.

Subcortical dementias

In these dementias most of the pathological change takes place in subcortical nuclear structures often with cortical sparing. Intellectual loss, although present, is often mild and not as severe as that seen in a cortical dementia. Extrapyramidal and movement disorders are prominent. There is relative preservation of language and parietal lobe function. The memory defect is often a difficulty in concentration and a slowing of memory processes rather than a failure to retain new information.

Huntington's chorea, although rare, is of particular importance because it is determined by an autosomal dominant gene on the short arm of chromosome 4. Genetic probe techniques (DNA probe G8) allows one to inform individuals (if sufficient family members can be tested and enough material is available from affected family members), with about a 95 per cent level of confidence, whether or not they are carrying the gene. The disorder is characterized by the development of generalized chorea, which gradually becomes more severe and eventually effects walking, manipulation, and swallowing (with potentially disastrous consequences). There is a slow intellectual loss that can be severe, although is often quite mild. Secondary emotional changes, particularly depression, are extremely common. Depression, paranoid psychosis, aggression, or personality disorder of frontal lobe type may precede the neurological symptoms.

The disease is due to neuronal degeneration, particularly in the striate cortex and globus pallidus, with some cortical loss, particularly in the frontal lobes. The condition usually manifests itself when the patient is in his thirties (the later the age of onset usually the slower the degeneration), but it may appear earlier, even in childhood, or may not occur until late middle age. There is no treatment, but intensive psychological support, treatment with antidepressants when necessary, and family therapy will prevent much suffering.

Wilson's disease is a rare autosomal recessive disorder causing both a brain and liver disorder due to retention of copper in the body because patients cannot excrete copper in the bowel. There is subsequent overloading of the liver with the metal, which results in liver failure. Eventual spillover of copper into the circulation with subsequent deposition of copper in the brain results in a subcortical dementia that produces an akinetic rigidity syndrome, dystonia, or cerebellar symptoms, and eventual dementia. Seizures occasionally occur. Almost invariably there is abnormality of liver function plus the presence of Kayser–Fleischer rings in the cornea. These are rings of greenish-brown pigmentation around the margin of the cornea that can usually only be seen with the aid of a slit-lamp. Deterioration can be stopped (and occasionally reversed) by treating the patient with penicillamine. Lifelong treatment is needed.

Focal symptoms

Focal neurological symptoms like dysphasia may sometimes be mistaken for a psychiatric illness, as may some parietal lobe syndromes. Symptoms like sensory inattention may be thought to be hysterical or functional unless the observer has a good knowledge of neurology and can recognize them for what they are. Severe damage to the frontal lobe may give rise to the frontal lobe syndrome, characterized by personality change involving loss of drive and volition, exaggeration of antisocial traits in the patient's character, a puerile sense of humour, and often a lack of attention to hygiene. Although this is classically a frontal lobe syndrome, it can be produced by lesions in other parts of the brain. Similarly, a temporal lobe syndrome is described that is related to bilateral temporal lobe damage. In addition to memory impairment, such a lesion may produce 'stickiness' of thinking, difficulty in shifting from one topic to another, a sensitive paranoid state, and a kind of oily religiosity.

Psychiatric syndromes

Brain damage, particularly in such areas as the corpus callosum or the frontal lobe, whether static or progressive, may release an apparent psychiatric syndrome such as a depressive illness or anxiety state, or a schizophrenia-like psychosis (particularly common in temporal lobe disorders) that is indistinguishable from the equivalent ordinary psychiatric syndrome except that, if looked for, subtle organic signs may be present. Such organically produced psychiatric syndromes are rare, but always need to be considered in the differential diagnosis of any patient presenting with a classical psychiatric illness. This is one of the reasons why a thorough physical and neurological assessment of any patient with a psychiatric disorder is necessary.

E Non-psychotic disorders (neuroses)

Many of your teachers and consultants will still be using a personal classification of psychiatric disorders that uses the terms 'psychotic' and 'neurotic'. Although modern classification avoids the terms because they are both relatively meaningless and pejorative, they are still in common usage. Psychotic disorder relates to the major mental illnesses like schizophrenia and manic depressive illness, in which insight is said to be lost and the patient's experience is outwith the normal range of human experience. Neurotic disorders (excluding organic brain disease, alcoholism, drug addiction, and personality disorder) include the rest of the customarily recognized psychiatric conditions, in which insight is said to be preserved and the patient's experience, although unpleasant and extreme, is within the normal range of human experience (in that most of us will have felt anxious or sad, will know what compulsive feelings are, or have had the desire to cut off from unpleasant events). Many 'neurotic' experiences are more understandable if we recall the way we thought and felt as children. Most 'neurotic' disorders can also be understood as reactions to stress.

How we respond to stress (and to what stresses we are particularly vulnerable) depends on our genetic make-up, on the example we have been set in terms of coping with stress, on our particular culture, on our previous life experiences (which render us vulnerable to particular stresses but not to others), and, to some extent, on our own pride in ourselves and our fighting spirit. Responses to stress may be adaptive or maladaptive. Adaptive responses are those that, even though they may make us feel uncomfortable, help us to deal with the situation that is causing the stress. Maladaptive responses fail to help us to deal with the situation, tend to reinforce the unpleasant symptoms caused by the stress, and therefore help them to become self-perpetuating.

It is important that you quickly learn to avoid 'medicalizing' normal and adaptive responses to stress and recognize that we cannot successfully respond to and deal with the normal stresses of life without, from time to time, feeling uncomfortable, and that these uncomfortable feelings are necessary. This is particularly so when considering anxiety. The problem is that you have a natural desire to help people and will find other people's distress unpleasant, and you will wish to alleviate it as quickly as possible. This desire may prevent you from seeing that often it is better to help the person to deal with the situation that is causing his symptoms, even though this may temporarily increase his distress, rather than by just treating him symptomatically. It is also better to help the person find resources within himself to cope with or deal with his symptoms than applying an external agent or remedy.

Reactive depression and grief

Mild depression is often accompanied by symptoms of anxiety, and deciding which is the predominant emotion can be difficult. Mild depression is also often reactive to life events, though out of keeping with what you judge the reaction of the patient should be—we have warned before of the treacherous nature of value judgements. For this reason, mild depression, particularly if contaminated with anxiety symptoms, is often called neurotic depression. Severe depression, however, can also be reactive. Many patients with what is clearly an endogenous depression will also have contaminating 'neurotic' symptoms (for example, prominent obsessional, hysterical, or anxiety symptoms). It is doubtful that any depression is completely reactive nor any depression completely endogenous. It is best to treat most depressions as though they were an aetiological mixture of both biological and psychological causes. The term neurotic depression is, however, still often widely used. The features of it are described in Section B (pp. 455–63) of this chapter.

Depression, whether mild or severe, should not be confused with grief, which is a psychological reaction to loss (usually, but not invariably, bereavement), or to loss of function or position. Grief takes a naturally long time to completely resolve, but it can become 'ossified' or 'stuck'. Naturally resolving grief needs support and counselling (although in the grief that accompanies terminal illness antidepressant therapy is sometimes indicated). Otherwise, chemical treatment for grief is indicated only in situations when the grief symptoms are seriously interfering with living. Stuck grief is usually treated with behavioural and cognitive therapy, although antidepressant therapy may have a place.

Anxiety disorders

Definition

Anxiety has both physical and psychological components (although it may be subjectively intense, but with little external objective evidence of its severity). The psychological feelings of anxiety are of dread, unpleasant anticipation, apprehension, or feelings of impending doom. This is associated with the physical symptoms of autonomic arousal with characteristic increase in muscle tension, breathing rate, and heart rate, sweating and piloerection, urinary frequency, and gut motility. There is poor sleep, often with early morning waking (sometimes there is hypersomnia), exhaustion, irritability, and difficulty with concentration. Pathological anxiety can be constant or fluctuate, may be reactive, occasionally appears to be endogenous, may come on gradually or occur suddenly, occur in association with specific stimuli or situations, or follow traumatic events.

Classification

A widely used classification is set out below:

1. generalized anxiety disorder
2. phobic disorder
3. panic disorder
4. obsessive–compulsive disorder
5. post-traumatic stress disorder.

Generalized anxiety disorder

Definition

This implies a sustained, prolonged increased level of anxiety that is out of keeping with the patient's circumstances, not part of a mood disorder or psychotic disorder, and accompanied by several of the psychological or physical symptoms of anxiety. Although the anxiety may fluctuate from day to day, it should be reasonably continuous and not merely occur as a phobic disorder.

Epidemiology

Generalized anxiety disorder is twice as common in women as it is in men and affects perhaps up to 4 per cent of the population at a time. It is also particularly common in chronic medical conditions, and may occur in patients with affective or psychotic illnesses, as a secondary phenomenon.

Clinical features of anxiety

1. Appearance and behaviour
Some patients can be very anxious without showing much evidence of this in their behaviour, but most anxious patients fidget, are restless, look inwardly preoccupied, cannot pay attention to tasks, may be pale or flushed, sweat, and chronically or acutely overbreathe, with resultant tingling in the limbs, chest pain, carpopedal spasms, and even attacks of unconsciousness.

2. Speech
Speech may be rapid or agitated and occasionally incoherent. It may be tremulous or interrupted by gasping or the effects of overbreathing.

3. Mood
The mood is one of tension and apprehension, with specific apprehensions about aspects of daily living that are out of proportion. Patients with chronic anxiety may be unhappy, but you cannot diagnose primary

generalized anxiety disorder in the presence of obvious mood disorder or a psychotic episode. The patient may be fatigued and also irritable. The patient may complain of initial insomnia, frequent waking with unpleasant dreams, or have early morning waking, and, as in depression, may ruminate anxiously whilst awake. Some patients retreat into hypersomnia as a defence against anxiety, as also happens in depression.

There is often loss of weight. A constant feeling of dread in the stomach or nausea may reduce appetite, although overeating occasionally occurs. Interest in sexual relations may be lost, and it may be difficult for people with high levels of anxiety to show much interest in work and their motivation may be lost.

4. Thoughts

These tend to be preoccupied with the events that are worrying the patient, and often are a preoccupation with the physical symptoms that accompany the anxiety. Self-reinforcement of the anxiety may occur, for example, palpitations occurring as part of the increased anxiety may make the patient think that he has heart disease, which therefore causes a further rise in his anxiety levels with a consequent increase in the number of his palpitations.

5. Perception

There are usually few perceptual changes in anxiety. Patients who are hyperaroused may have pseudo-hallucinations or suffer unpleasant derealization or depersonalization symptoms, and sometimes these may be the presenting and predominant symptoms. Some anxious patients may have olfactory or gustatory experiences, which may lead to the erroneous diagnosis of partial epilepsy.

6. Cognitive function

This may be impaired because of lack of concentration, although not to the degree seen in depression.

7. Other associated symptoms

The patient will complain of numerous physical symptoms including palpitations, breathlessness, air hunger, tingling in the extremities (due to hyperventilation), dizziness (often due to hyperventilation), non-cardiac chest pain, headache, backache, stomach ache, butterflies in the stomach, nausea, diarrhoea, fatigue, sweating, dry mouth, hot flushes, dysphagia, frequent swallowing, air swallowing, frequency of micturition, etc. All these need to be carefully assessed and physical disorders excluded.

Aetiology of generalized anxiety

The aetiology of this state is complex. Constitutional factors are important. Some people, due to their genetic structure and/or previous experiences, are more disposed to anxiety than others. It is also possible that a true endogenous anxiety state occurs. The combination of a constitution prone to anxiety coupled with unpleasant life events in people who have not learned how to cope with and deal with anxiety and who have had previous life experiences that predispose them to anxiety, is likely to cause a chronic anxiety state.

Differential diagnosis

It can be difficult to distinguish a severe anxiety state from a depressive illness, and sometimes patients who are anxious become so bizarre in their behaviour that they are mistakenly thought to be psychotic. This is particularly likely to happen in patients with obsessional behaviour or thinking or those who are so terrified that they appear to answer questions at random. There are many medical conditions that need to be excluded before making the diagnosis including endocrine disease, particularly hyperthyroidism, metabolic disorders, and cardiovascular disease. Anxiety may also occur as a component of delirium tremens, drug withdrawal, etc. Anxiety and physical illness commonly exist side by side.

Treatment

Although very short-term use of anxiolytic drugs like benzodiazepines, confined to a few days' treatment whilst the patient sorts out the life situation that is causing the anxiety, can be occasionally justified, the treatment of anxiety should be by behaviour therapy, cognitive therapy, counselling, and, if necessary, psychotherapy. Dependence on anxiolytic drugs must be studiously avoided.

Prognosis

Few formal studies have been done, but, the short-term prognosis for generalized anxiety is usually good, although in some patients relapses are frequent. Anxiety is often self-limiting.

Phobic disorder

Definition

Phobic anxiety only presents itself in certain circumscribed specific situations. There is a gradient of anxiety as the person approaches nearer to the feared situation, and anxiety remains as long as the person is exposed to it. He will usually terminate or avoid contact with the feared situation in order to avoid anxiety. Modern classification of phobias recognizes three subcategories: **agoraphobia** (literally fear of the market place, but better described as a fear of leaving one's secure base), **social phobia** (in which there is a specific fear related to embarrassment in front of other people, such as being unable to eat in the presence of others), and **simple phobia** (an **unreasonable** fear of insects, small mammals, heights, etc.). The anxiety generated by the situation and the patient's reaction to it must be outwith what is customarily considered to be the normal reaction to the particular stimulus, for example, uneasiness in the presence of an angry wasp is not a phobia.

Epidemiology

Simple phobias are very common (perhaps 16 per cent of the population have them) and are probably more common in women than in men. They need only be treated if they are severely disabling to the person involved. They tend to arise in childhood and persist into adult life. Sometimes a so-called 'one trial learning' will occur and the phobic reaction will be set up after a single traumatic incident in adult life. Social phobias are relatively uncommon and also tend to begin in childhood.

Agoraphobia is more serious and tends to start in early adult life, although it can occur for the first time at any age. It is commoner in women. Field studies have suggested that it may be, in its milder forms, quite prevalent, and up to 5 per cent of the female population may have a degree of it.

Clinical features

When not presented with the phobic stimulus the patient is normal (some patients will become anxious merely by thinking about or visualizing the feared stimulus), but when in the presence of the feared stimulus he shows all the clinical features of anxiety outlined on p. 493. The physical symptoms of both the anxiety itself, such as palpitations, and the secondary consequences of overbreathing will often increase the anxiety if the patient feels he is losing control (see below). Some patients, in the presence of the feared stimulus, will have an actual panic attack. Patients also show behaviours aimed at minimizing anxiety (for example, by embracing the trappings of religion or possessing lucky charms) or by avoiding the feared object, and such secondary behaviours may be very disabling, for instance, if they confine the patient to the house, and it is important to prevent such secondary handicaps from occurring by preventing other family members from overprotecting the patient. Some patients find themselves inextricably drawn to the feared stimulus (for example, children with fierce dogs) and seem almost to have a need to test out their feared behaviour. This is called counter phobic behaviour.

Aetiology

Many patients who develop phobic anxiety have a constitutionally high level of anxiety and are also more easily conditioned than most people so that a fear response develops to an often quite innocuous stimulus. Children often develop phobic symptoms if their parents have phobic anxiety; factors of modelling of behaviour are probably quite important.

Differential diagnosis

As with a generalized anxiety disorder, it can sometimes be very difficult to distinguish a phobic anxiety response, in which the person shows much preoccupation with the feared object, from an obsessional disorder. Patients with a phobic anxiety state who have panic attacks on presentation of the feared stimulus, should be distinguished from patients that have apparently spontaneous panic attacks that do not occur in association with a particular feared object, as their management may be different. People with frequent phobic responses develop secondary generalized anxiety and may become demoralized and unhappy, and the original phobic nature of the disorder may not be realized. Likewise, a depressive illness may activate previously controlled phobic responses that may be so prominent that the underlying depression is not recognized or is mistaken for a secondary depression. For the physical differential diagnosis of sudden attacks of anxiety see p. 502.

Treatment

Treatment for all phobic states should be with behavioural and cognitive therapy. Only very rarely should chemotherapy be used. Social and simple phobias are usually best helped by teaching the patient an individual method of relaxation that works for the patient (this may involve hypnosis or biofeedback) and then, following analysis of the various components of the phobia, desensitizing the patient to the feared stimulus by graded exposure from the least feared to the most feared component with the patient practising relaxation during the exposure. This can be done either in reality or in the patient's imagination. Occasionally, *flooding* the patient with the feared stimulus in a situation from which he cannot escape is effective, although it needs a willing patient and a supportive therapist. In agoraphobia, *operant conditioning* (whereby further and longer travels into the open air are rewarded by praise or other reinforcements) is also effective, particularly if combined with anxiety management. Occasionally, tricyclic antidepressants or monoamine oxidase inhibitors may be helpful when combined with behaviour therapy, particularly for agoraphobia. On no account should you prescribe benzodiazepines or other tranquillizing medication as the risk of dependence is too high.

Prognosis

The prognosis for agoraphobia depends on the enthusiasm and ingenuity of the therapist and on the resilience and motivation of the patient. It is particularly necessary to avoid secondary reinforcement of the agoraphobia (like a husband who is willing to go out and do all the shopping and leave his wife at home). The prognosis for both social and simple phobias is good.

Panic disorder

Definition

Patients with phobic disorders, particularly agora-phobia, may suffer panic attacks if suddenly or over-whelmingly exposed to their feared stimulus. The term panic disorder is used to describe a disorder in which panic attacks have no obvious precipitating reason and appear to occur spontaneously. Many people with panic attacks become phobic of the attacks themselves and become increasingly anxious about having an attack, which thus increases the likelihood that they will have one.

Panic attacks are sudden intense episodes of anxiety that are accompanied by a feeling of imminent dissolution, physical symptoms related to anxiety, and secondary physical symptoms related to the physiological effects of overbreathing (overbreathing is an important part of any panic attack).

Epidemiology

True panic disorder is equally common in men and women; it occurs in less than 1 per cent of the population, and commonly presents when patients are in their late twenties or early thirties.

Clinical features

1. Appearance and behaviour

There is a sudden onset of inner preoccupation with intense fear, particularly that the patient is about to die. In the middle of his panic the patient will often seek safety in flight, he will be shaking, have a high pulse rate, and, very characteristically, will be over-breathing. As a result he will often complain of tingling around the lips, in the hands and feet, may have stiffening of the hands, sometimes with true carpopedal spasm, and may occasionally become unconscious.

2. Speech

The patient will be difficult to communicate with because of his inner preoccupations, and speech may at times be incoherent.

3. Mood

The mood is one of intense anxiety and fear. Panic disorder may sometimes occur in the setting of a depressive illness and it is important to carefully exclude it. Panic episodes may last from a few minutes to several hours, and there will be a period of demoralization and unhappiness afterwards. At first, there will be little change in weight, though if secondary mood changes occur weight may be lost or occasionally gained. Work may be much impaired by the patient's fear of having an attack in public and making a fool of himself.

4. Thoughts

The patient is preoccupied with thoughts of death or insanity during the attack and will gradually become preoccupied with the fear of having the attack in between episodes. Hypochondriacal ideas may appear, particularly if the patient and his relatives feel that the attacks are organic in origin.

5. Perception

During a panic attack derealization and depersonalization are common and may well increase the patient's fear. Occasionally, pseudohallucinations occur.

6. Cognitive function

Because of the patient's intense preoccupation, concentration and attention span will be impaired during an attack.

7. Other associated symptoms

As mentioned above, patients may suffer from the secondary symptoms of hyperventilation. Patients often fail to recognize that they are hyperventilating, but will describe difficulty in getting their breath, not in terms of the characteristic expiratory difficulty of asthma, but more that they cannot get enough air into their lungs. They often have a feeling of suffocation, and their friends will report that they are gasping for breath. Chest pain is also common during hyperventilation, usually left-sided, and will often precede the attack.

Aetiology

The aetiology of panic disorder is uncertain. In the past, panic attacks have been thought to represent the sudden entry into consciousness of previously repressed thoughts (this may in fact be true for some patients with the disorder). Some panic attacks arise in the setting of a depressive illness. There is a growing belief that there may be some organic disorder present in some patients, possibly related to impaired lactate metabolism, or possibly even to some cortical lesion in the parahippocampal gyrus. Mitral valve prolapse was thought to be associated with this disorder at one time, but belief in this relationship is waning. Indeed, the pathological significance of mitral valve prolapse is in fact doubtful.

Differential diagnosis

Cardiovascular and cerebral disorders (particularly epilepsy) need to be excluded. In older patients, recurrent sudden left ventricular failure with angor animi needs to be distinguished. Occasionally, patients with recurrent small pulmonary emboli or pulmonary fibrosis may be misdiagnosed as having panic attacks. Hyperthyroidism, recurrent hypoglycaemia, phaechromocytoma, or the carcinoid syndrome may be mistaken for panic attacks, as may Ménière's syndrome (vertigo, nausea, and vomiting, that is often accompanied by sweating, pallor, an unpleasant subjective sensation, and occasionally other symptoms such as diarrhoea). In casualty, we have also seen acute drug intoxication and even early delirium tremens mistaken for panic attacks.

Treatment

If panic attacks are occurring in the setting of depression, the depression should be treated and then the panic attacks will often subside. Likewise, if, on analysing the patient's condition thoroughly, it is clear that you are actually dealing with agoraphobia in which panic attacks are occurring, then behavioural treatment is the therapy of choice. There is marked controversy about how pure panic attacks should best be treated. Some authorities hold, and there is some evidence for this, that even when depression is not present, antidepressant medication, either tricyclics or monoamine oxidase inhibitors, is the treatment of choice. It is possible that monoamine oxidase inhibitors are actually more beneficial than tricyclic antidepressants; a new generation of these drugs is being developed that does not have the unfortunate interactions with foodstuffs that the present drugs do.

Behaviour therapy, perhaps combined with cognitive therapy, also has its exponents. Behaviour therapy concentrates on teaching the patient intensive anxiety management and helping him to recognize the warning symptoms that an attack is coming on so that he can swiftly apply his new control skills. Once the patient is in the middle of a panic attack it becomes difficult for him to apply relaxation and so the aim is to teach him discrimination skills so that he can recognize the very beginnings of the attack before secondary reinforcement occurs. For many patients, a combination of an antidepressant and behaviour therapy is best. Although benzodiazepine tranquillizers have their exponents for this condition, because of problems of dependence it is better not to use them. Occasionally, beta-blocking drugs may be helpful in some patients, particularly those with prominent somatic symptoms. A non-cardioselective drug with beta-2-blocking properties is best, but use of these drugs should be combined with behaviour therapy.

Obsessive–compulsive disorder

Definition

In this condition there are characteristic obsessional patterns of thinking and ritualized compulsive behaviour. If the thoughts or the actions are interrupted, the patient becomes anxious. Some degree of ritual is, of course, common in human experience, particularly in childhood (it is not only primitive religions that use it), but when rituals take up most of the patient's waking life and totally alter his ability to work or to relate to other people then it becomes an illness. The patient will try to resist his obsessional thoughts or rituals but fail, and he retains full insight into the fact that they are pathological.

Epidemiology

The full syndrome is not common, occurring in less than 0.5 per cent of the population. It is equally common in men and women. Onset tends to be in the late twenties onwards. If the condition occurs in adolescence, it may be the precursor of schizophrenia. There is said to be an association between previous brain injury and the development of an obsessional illness.

Clinical features

1. Appearance and behaviour

The patient's behaviour will to some extent depend on what the ritualized behaviour is. When not engaged in his behaviour he may not appear to be anxious, but he will become extremely anxious if his behaviour is interrupted. Ritualized behaviour is prompted by an internal sense of compulsion that the patient finds difficult to resist. The patient may be compelled to repetitively check some domestic appliance (for example, a light switch), or may have cleaning rituals so that he spends two or three hours at the wash-basin repetitively scrubbing his hands to free them from imagined germs or contamination so that his hands become raw and bleeding. Touching rituals are common as well (analogous to the harmless touching rituals of childhood). Some patients have avoidance rituals.

2. Speech
Speech is usually unaffected, although occasionally may become part of a ritual. A variant of obsessive–compulsive disorder is **Gilles de la Tourette syndrome**, in which multiple tics and verbal ejaculations (often bleeping or grunting noises, which are disguised coprolalia) occur.

3. Mood
Mood is one of anxiety and tension. If rituals are interrupted or prevented, mood is often one of despondency and despair as the patient has full insight into the pathological nature of his condition. Sometimes a primary depressive illness will present as an obsessional disorder. The patient may be exhausted and fatigued by the necessity to carry out his rituals endlessly, and there is frequently sleep disturbance. Patients who have rituals that exhaust them or interfere with their eating may lose weight; sexual interest often declines, and concentration and motivation to work may be lost.

4. Thoughts
The patient's thinking may often be preoccupied with the need to carry out the rituals and many patients with obsessive–compulsive disorder have what has been called *folie de doute*. Whilst carrying out a ritual the patient repeatedly loses count or suddenly becomes doubtful about whether he carried out the ritual correctly and so has to stop and return to the beginning thus prolonging the ritualized behaviour, sometimes by many hours. Rituals may also involve thinking, and

the patient may be preoccupied with obsessional thoughts that he feels compelled to think about because if he does not he becomes anxious. Often obsessional thoughts are swear-words, scatological or blasphemous. The patient may also be struggling with the desire to speak them out loud, and, if compelled to do so, may disguise them as grunts or bleeps.

Although obsessional thinking often has a somewhat magical quality, it is not psychotic. The patient recognizes that the thinking arises from within his own mind and there is no suggestion that there is control from outside.

5. Perception
Very occasionally, if they have become acutely anxious during attempts at preventing their rituals, patients may depersonalize or develop derealization, but otherwise there are no perceptual distortions.

6. Cognitive function
This is usually not impaired unless the patient has become depressed, has developed a generalized anxiety, or is already brain damaged.

7. Other associated symptoms
Anxiety symptoms will be seen, particularly if the patient is prevented from carrying out his rituals, and occasionally depressive symptoms may be prominent, which indicate a better prognosis.

Aetiology
This is unknown, though there is growing evidence that it may relate to specific dysfunction in serotoninergic receptors, and there is a possible link with brain damage.

Differential diagnosis
Schizophrenia must be carefully distinguished, particularly in young patients. Always look carefully for evidence of an underlying depressive illness. Phobic

anxiety, especially fear of dirt and contamination, may occasionally be mistaken for an obsessive–compulsive disorder.

Treatment

Behaviour therapy, particularly response prevention (and thought-stopping techniques for obsessional thinking) is the treatment of choice. Some authorities recommend the use of clomipramine as an adjunct to behavioural treatment and there is some evidence that it may be helpful. If a patient's rituals are prevented there is an initial increase in anxiety, but if one can go on preventing the ritualized behaviour anxiety subsides and, after a while, the patient loses the need for the ritual. Such treatment can be carried out at home or in hospital, but requires the full cooperation of the relatives and a sufficient number of therapists to continually prevent the rituals being carried out.

Prognosis

Most patients do well. A few do badly and remain disabled by the symptoms. For such patients, leucotomy or other forms of psychosurgery are still occasionally indicated.

Post-traumatic stress disorder

Definition

Following a disaster or sudden traumatic event of a threatening nature (for example, earthquake, fire, transport accident, rape, or assault), victims show a characteristic emotional reaction, which also usually has a characteristic natural resolution and recovery (like grief). Some people, however, do not recover and continue to show signs of distress for a very long time after the traumatic incident.

The normal phases of response to a traumatic event have been classically described by Horowitz:

1. **Outcry** Although some people may appear un-ruffled by sudden disaster or trauma, most people show an immediate response ranging from acute fear and distress to being completely overwhelmed by the event so that the individual is dazed and stunned and appears to be totally unable to comprehend what has happened. Spectators of television coverage of natural or man-made disasters will have seen many examples of the stunned survivor.

2. **Denial phase** Following the outcry phase some survivors may show no emotional symptoms at all for a long time and only later develop emotional symptoms. Some people who use denial never develop emotional symptoms, and in the fighting services denial may be officially sanctioned ('why speak they not of comrades who went under'). Denial may be an effective coping mechanism and should not necessarily be punctured.

3. **Intrusive phase** After a period of denial, or immediately after the trauma, some victims do develop an anxiety state that is characterized by an exaggerated startle response, intrusive memories of the event, which are often intense and take the form of a 'flashback', and a morbid preoccupation with the events of the trauma (including obsessional concern with why the victim survived when others did not). There is a chronic, highly aroused state and sleep disturbance, with sleep often accompanied by vivid dreams of the event. If they are transient, such experiences are normal, usually respond to talking through the events, and natural resolution usually occurs. Sometimes, immediately after the event, hysterical symptoms may develop (usually symbolic of the trauma) and usually respond to immediate abreaction.

4. **Working-through phase** During this phase, which may need to be assisted by supportive psychotherapy, the victim works through the meaning of the disaster,

faces the memories of it, goes through a mourning phase, and begins to develop new plans for the future.

5. **Completion phase**   At the end of working through, the victim should have assimilated the meaning of the event (or come to terms with its meaninglessness), have realistic plans for the future, and resumed his normal activities.

The above describes a normal response to traumatic events. Pathological responses occur when symptoms do not resolve after a few weeks, or when symptoms are very severe and totally incapacitating, and the victim cannot redevelop his normal lifestyle or he shows marked maladaptive responses, such as total withdrawal, reliance on alcohol, chronic hysterical reactions, severe depression, or he develops a reactive psychosis.

Epidemiology
Pathological forms of traumatic stress disorder are likely to occur in people who are already predisposed to mental illness and who carry into the trauma ongoing personality or social conflicts, or those who have little social support, or who are young or very old. Men and women are equally affected. Pathological reactions are also more likely to occur in people who in some way feel responsible for the disaster, or who have been previously traumatized so that the disaster awakens previous memories of a similar event. *Esprit de corps* and a good fighting spirit will prevent pathological reactions, as will a strongly shared belief in a common purpose.

Clinical features
1. Appearance and behaviour
Except for those who use denial, people will initially show stunned shock-like behaviour and may appear confused, disorientated, and may well wander. Later they will have chronic symptoms of anxiety as outlined above, or have acute episodes of anxiety, particularly

if memories of the event arise unbidden into conscious-ness or if they are exposed to situations that remind them of the events of the trauma. They may show phobic avoidance of such situations. Victims may go to elaborate lengths to avoid anything that reminds them of their feelings about, or memories of, the traumatic incident. Children may show regressive behaviour, or the traumatic events may be reflected in their play.

2. Speech
Speech will be preoccupied with the event, and may have the signs of anxiety listed on p. 493.

3. Mood
Mood is one of tension, anxiety, and apprehension. It may be labile swinging between euphoria and depres-sion, and there is often chronic irritability and fatigue. Sleep disturbance, particularly initial insomnia and frequent waking during the night with nightmares, is commonly reported. Weight loss may occur, and there is usually a loss in sexual interest and difficulty in making deep relationships with other people. Interest in work and motivation is often lost for a long period of time.

4. Thoughts
Although denial may continue for a long period of time, there is often rumination about the events, particularly about why the individual has survived when others have not and, if the emotional symptoms are severe, a fear that the victim is going mad. Some victims show a morbid preoccupation with *not* thinking about the events that occurred and avoidance of any reminder of them.

5. Perception
Vivid pseudohallucinations may occur of the event (flashbacks), which are intense, very painful, and dis-turbing.

6. Cognitive function

There is often a loss of concentration and ability to attend to external cues, so that cognitive function may appear to be impaired.

7. Other associated symptoms

As in all anxiety states, the patient may complain of numerous physical symptoms, particularly breathlessness and palpitations, headaches, and other, muscular symptoms. A reactive psychosis, the awakening of a previous psychotic episode, or severe depression, may also occur.

Aetiology

As already indicated, the meaning of the trauma to the individual, his previous personality structure, life experiences (and any previous psychiatric illness), plus his own stoicism and reserves of psychological strength, will determine whether the condition occurs, how severe it is, and whether it becomes chronic and debilitating. It should once again be emphasized that many people exposed to trauma do not develop psychological sequelae afterwards, although in some the reaction is long delayed.

Differential diagnosis

Some victims will be carrying into the post-traumatic syndrome previous psychiatric illness or a disposition to it, and a number of the immediate victims of a disaster will already be psychiatrically ill. A few of them may also have been concussed or otherwise brain injured. Physical and neurological assessment is therefore essential, as well as a careful psychiatric evaluation of the victim so that other treatments, say for psychosis or severe depression, can be applied if necessary. Careful evaluation of alcohol and substance abuse is also necessary.

Treatment

Most victims of post-traumatic stress disorder need support, counselling, and reassurance that what has happened to them is normal and will resolve. Some need more intensive psychiatric treatment (including abreaction, particularly if they have hysterical disorders). Some who are psychotic or severely depressed may need medication, but otherwise medication should be kept to a minimum. Those who develop a chronic psychiatric disorder following trauma need intensive counselling, behavioural therapy, and cognitive therapy. Again medication should be avoided if at all possible, except in those who have a formal psychiatric illness.

There is a growing practice for sudden disaster to be attended by well-meaning, but often amateur counsellors who rush round the disaster site and its environs offering counselling to everyone and who, as a result, often become casualties themselves. Counselling of victims after a disaster should be done by professionals who can recognize that there are many people who do not need counselling at all because they have their own natural strengths and resources (or who merely need an explanation). It is important to avoid the trap of trying to help people avoid any mention of the disaster, because this reinforces sickness behaviour. People should be given the chance of talking through their experiences, and facing and dealing with their fears and anxieties, rather than running away from them. The human spirit has a natural resilience that should be supported and not medicalized.

Prognosis

For most victims of the post-traumatic syndrome, providing they are given the support that they need, the prognosis is good. A few victims remain psychologically disabled for long periods of time. Unfortunately, issues of litigation and compensation will often prevent such victims from getting the psychological help that they need, and may make the condition self-perpetuating.

Hysteria (conversion disorder)

Definition

Hysteria is being reclassified into part of the somatoform disorders (see p. 517), but we are including it before them because so often it can be seen as a particular kind of reaction to stress. In hysteria, psychological stress produces an apparent loss of (or alteration in) physical functioning, suggestive of a physical disorder. Often the change in function leads to a symbolic resolution of the stress. Hysteria may become self-perpetuating (i.e., primary gain becomes secondary gain), and the patient often shows a characteristic indifference to the symptoms. Hysteria is not the same thing as malingering, as to all intents and purposes the deliberate disability is unconsciously motivated.

Epidemiology

The condition is rare, is said to be commoner in women, and tends to occur in the young and in those perhaps already predisposed either by upbringing or by personality. Apparent hysterical behaviour can also be released by brain damage or by other mental illnesses, particularly depression.

Clinical features

1. Appearance and behaviour

The onset of the condition is usually sudden and the symptoms often brief, although, if not promptly treated, hysterical symptoms can become chronic. The underlying stress that has precipitated the disorder may not be immediately apparent. Usually the presented symptoms are neurological and take the form of paralysis or

sensory loss or both, sometimes of one limb, sometimes of both limbs on one side of the body, or a loss
of the ability to use or feel the lower limbs. There may
be hysterical blindness, deafness, ataxia, aphonia, or
seizures. The patient has a curious lack of the expected
emotional response to the sudden disability (*la belle
indifférence*).

2. Speech

Except in hysterical aphonia, speech is usually normal. 'Talking in tongues' may occur.

3. Mood

Mood is usually normal. Characteristically the patient,
although faced with what would normally be distressing physical symptoms, shows *la belle indifférence* to
them—do not mistake denial for this.

4. Thoughts

Except in the rare instances in which mental illness is
being unconsciously simulated, the patient's thoughts
are usually normal.

5. Perception

Even when perceptual disorder is being simulated, the
patient's perceptions are usually normal.

6. Cognitive function

Unless pseudodementia is being simulated or there is
a hysterical amnesia, cognitive function is usually not
impaired.

7. Other associated symptoms

In addition to neurological symptoms, mental illness,
dementia, or amnesia may be simulated. Other secondary changes may occur if the disability goes on for a
long time (for instance, the patient who has not moved
his limb for many months may develop some secondary atrophy; the patient who has been mute for a long

time will eventually find it difficult to speak again). If the patient's hysterical symptoms have been released by early schizophrenia, by depression, or by organic brain disease, then there will be some symptoms of the underlying disorder if they are looked for.

Aetiology

Almost invariably there is a history of some traumatic emotional event, which either may have been particularly important to the patient or was one that would be traumatic to most people (such as the stress of battle). Hysterical symptoms tend to occur in the predisposed and may become a learned pattern of behaviour. They are, of course, particularly common in childhood and if they are reinforced and rewarded in childhood may subsequently appear in adult life.

Differential diagnosis

Hysteria is rare. In many patients, genuine organic disorders, which perhaps start in an unusual way or with which the physician is unfamiliar, are erroneously labelled as hysterical. The problem is often that when a patient's illness first starts his symptoms are minimal and are more apparent subjectively than objectively so that, in order to be taken seriously by his physician, the patient actually exaggerates the degree of disability. This exaggeration is detected and hysteria therefore erroneously diagnosed. A thorough physical assessment both by history and by examination is essential and a *positive* diagnosis of hysteria made in terms of the symbolic nature of the disability, its lack of organic features, and *belle indifférence* (but do not confuse *belle indifférence* with denial or with stoicism). Hysterical symptoms are sometimes released in patients who are developing schizophrenia, depression, or organic brain disease, particularly in older patients. Hysteria, which is unconscious, must also be distinguished from straightforward malingering in which the deliberate disability is clearly consciously motivated. The distinction between the two is not always easy.

Treatment

Abreaction (see p. 411) is often helpful in discovering the underlying cause for the symptoms and often helps to relieve them. Hypnosis can also be used. It is important to prevent secondary gain and not allow the symptoms to be reinforced either by the patient or by the patient's relatives. The patient should also be engaged with supportive psychotherapy so that the underlying problems can be talked through and dealt with in the usual way, particularly if there has been an acute trauma. Hysterical symptoms are often easy to relieve if they have not been present for too long. If they have been present for a long time, then the patient must be helped not to lose face as he loses his symptoms, so that, for instance, a treatment programme involving physiotherapy, as well as psychotherapy and behaviour therapy, will be necessary. When the acute episode is over, psychotherapy is often indicated to help the patient recognize his propensity to develop hysterical symptoms under stress, and to find better ways of coping with stress. It is important that the patient is not stigmatized. Hysteria often leads to irritation and rejection (particularly by relatives and carers), and efforts should be made to prevent this by fostering a team approach.

Prognosis

Prognosis for the acute attack is usually good providing that secondary gain can be prevented, but in patients with histrionic personalities further attacks will occur if the patient is under stress (often the patient can be taught to recognize that the phenomena is occurring and to seek help). Hysteria that has become secondarily reinforced has a worse prognosis, and some kind of face-saving compromise may be needed. A sizeable proportion of patients with apparent hysteria eventually develop neurological or psychiatric illness.

Briquet's syndrome (somatization disorder)

Definition

This is not the same thing as hysteria, although it is often confused with it. It is not at all uncommon, although it often takes a long time for the penny to drop that one is dealing with this condition, particularly if the patient tends to present different symptoms to different doctors. The syndrome is one of multiple somatic complaints without a pathological foundation. In the DSM III R criteria, it is operationally defined as a patient who has a history of many physical complaints or a belief that he is sickly, beginning before the age of thirty, and persisting for several years. The patient must have at least 13 symptoms from the list below. A symptom is only counted as significant when it is not related to organic pathology, or to a pathophysiological mechanism, or, if there is underlying organic pathology, it is also only significant if it results in social or occupational impairment that is grossly in excess of what would be expected from the physical findings. The symptoms should not occur just during a panic attack and must cause the patient to seek frequent medical advice, alter his lifestyle, and take more than just 'over-the-counter' medication. The recognized symptoms are:

(a) Gastrointestinal symptoms:

1. vomiting, other than during pregnancy
2. abdominal pain, other than when menstruating
3. nausea, other than motion sickness
4. abdominal bloating
5. diarrhoea
6. intolerance of (get sick from) several different foods

(b) Pain symptoms:

    7. pain in extremities
    8. back pain
    9. joint pain
    10. pain during urination
    11. other pain (excluding headaches)

(c) Cardiopulmonary symptoms:

    12. shortness of breath when not exerting oneself
    13. palpitations
    14. chest pain
    15. dizziness

(d) Conversion or pseudoneurological symptoms:

    16. amnesia
    17. difficulty in swallowing
    18. loss of voice
    19. deafness
    20. double vision
    21. blurred vision
    22. blindness
    23. fainting or loss of consciousness
    24. seizure or convulsion
    25. difficulty walking
    26. paralysis or muscle weakness
    27. urinary retention or difficulty urinating

(e) Sexual symptoms (for major part of the person's life after opportunities for sexual activity):

    28. burning sensation in sexual organs or rectum other than during intercourse
    29. sexual indifference
    30. pain during intercourse
    31. impotence

(f) Female reproductive symptoms (judged by the person to occur more frequently or severely than in most women):

    32. painful menstruation
    33. irregular menstrual periods
    34. excessive menstrual bleeding
    35. vomiting throughout pregnancy.

Patients who have this disorder will almost certainly be referred after exhaustive (and often repeated) negative physical investigations often by a multitude of doctors. There may be evidence of a histrionic personality, with the patient showing a persistent tendency to form dependent relationships on others with childish, manipulative behaviour, alternating between seductive and rejecting behaviour that is directed towards the physician or psychiatrist, and an overly dramatic preoccupation with symptoms.

Epidemiology

This disorder is said to be commoner in women and may occur in up to one per cent of the female population.

Clinical features

1. Appearance and behaviour

These patients usually present at general hospitals or in general practice, and are usually referred from there in despair. They will therefore often be rather hostile initially, and bargaining may take place about the degree of psychological investigation that they are prepared to have, which they will often only allow if there is some trade-off for physical investigations that they feel they still need. They will be overly preoccupied with their symptoms.

2. Speech

Unless they have symptoms referrable to mechanisms of speech, this is usually normal, although it will be difficult to divert them from the topic of physical complaining.

3. Mood

In the pure syndrome, it is normal. Many of these patients pass through transient episodes of depression, and if there is a significant degree of depression the diagnosis may be in doubt.

4. Thoughts

There is a preoccupation with physical symptoms, although not to a delusional degree.

5. Perception

Perception is normally unchanged.

6. Cognitive function

Unless the patient is complaining of amnesia, this will usually be normal.

7. Other associated symptoms

They often have iatrogenic symptoms related to the medication they have been prescribed, and these need to be carefully distinguished from symptoms referable to the syndrome itself.

Aetiology

Although this is classified as a single syndrome, it is probably of multiple aetiology. There is evidence that some patients with this condition do have a personality disorder, and the number of other types of personality disorder is higher in first degree relatives than would be expected by chance. In some patients it is clear that most of the somatic complaints relate to tension and anxiety. In others it becomes apparent, as one gets to know them, that they have been 'taught' to present distress and unhappiness in a somatic form, and have perhaps become overly sensitized to those minor somatic complaints that occur in all of us all from time to time.

Differential diagnosis

Careful medical evaluation is necessary for all patients with this disorder because there are some medical ill-

nesses that often present initially with nebulous physical findings (such as collagen disorders), which may
be mistaken for this syndrome. Depressive illness with
hypochondriasis, somatoform pain disorder, hypochondriacal neurosis, and occasionally schizophrenia
(with somatic delusions), need to be carefully distinguished from this disorder.

Treatment

Treatment is possible but difficult, and initially one
has to develop, often very slowly, a therapeutic alliance with the patient and encourage him to develop
psychological awareness and to stop concentrating on
his physical symptoms. Initially some kind of bargain
may have to be struck about the extent of physical
investigation before he will accept that his symptoms
are psychologically based. This therapeutic alliance can
be developed with a tolerant therapist who is prepared
to use a mixture of psychotherapeutic, cognitive, and
behavioural techniques aimed at tension reduction,
stopping negative thinking and reinforcement of somatic symptoms, and helping the patient to develop
insight. Much can be achieved. This treatment programme unfortunately takes a long time, and many of
these patients opt out of treatment and seek physical
treatment elsewhere, or become so irritating to the
therapist that they are rejected.

Prognosis

This tends to be poor.

Hypochondriasis (hypochondriacal neurosis)

In this disorder the patient is preoccupied with the fear
of having (or the belief that he has) a serious disease,
based on the patient's misinterpretation of physical
sensations as evidence of physical illness. Appropriate
physical evaluation must have failed to reveal any

physical disorder, and the symptoms the patient describes must not just be symptoms of panic attacks. The fear or the belief persists despite reassurance. The duration of the disturbance must be at least six months. The patient retains some insight into the fact that his beliefs may be unfounded (i.e., they are not delusional). The symptoms usually relate to only one bodily symptom and do not have the characteristics of somatization disorder.

Epidemiology

It is not common in psychiatric practice (less than one per cent of the psychiatric population), but is more common in medical practice. It is probably equally common in men and women. The peak incidence is in early middle-age.

Clinical features

1. Appearance and behaviour

The presenting feature is worry about somatic health and preoccupation with the fear of having a serious disease (often, but not invariably, cancer). Physical symptoms are added to support the belief, but in this disorder it is the *fear* of physical disease that is predominant rather than complaining about symptoms.

2. Speech

May be preoccupied, but is otherwise normal.

3. Mood

Many of these patients have symptoms of some depression and anxiety, and anxiety symptoms, of course, tend to reinforce the patient's belief that something is wrong.

4. Thoughts

There are preoccupied with fears of physical disease and with the evidence that the patient believes supports his view that he is physically ill.

5. Perception

This is usually unchanged.

6. Cognitive function

This is usually unchanged.

7. Other associated symptoms

Transient depression and anxiety symptoms may occur. If they are prominent, reconsider the diagnosis.

Aetiology

As with somatization disorder, it is probably multi-factorial.

Differential diagnosis

Depressive disorder with multiple somatic complaints. Anxiety disorder, particularly panic disorder. Hypochondriasis may also be seen in prolonged or stuck grief, and it may then have the features of the physical illness from which the victim's relative died. Occasionally, in schizophrenia multiple somatic delusions may be the presenting feature.

It is important to rigorously exclude a physical disorder as a number of these patients do have an underlying physical disorder that only later will reveal itself. This is particularly true of patients with 'cancer phobia'.

Treatment

Making a therapeutic alliance is important in this syndrome, as it is in somatization disorder. Both behavioural and cognitive therapy may be important. Chemotherapy is useful in patients with associated depression, particularly antidepressants such as clomipramine. In some patients, even though their beliefs are not delusional, a neuroleptic such as pimozide may be helpful. Physical therapy in terms of exercise, physiotherapy, massage techniques, etc. may also be helpful.

Prognosis

In most patients with a marked degree of depression or phobic anxiety symptoms related to bodily function, the prognosis is usually good. In other patients it tends to be poor.

Other rarer somatoform disorders are **dysmorphophobia**, in which the patient is preoccupied with imagined bodily defects (for example, the shape of the nose, ears, or other part of the body). There may be frequent requests for surgery to correct these imagined disorders (preoccupation with real and important disorders, such as bat ears, may also occur). In some of these patients the preoccupation becomes delusional, and some of these patients eventually become psychotic. Corrective surgery does not help and should not be recommended. Chemotherapy for those who are depressed or psychotic may be appropriate, but otherwise long-term cognitive therapy probably offers the best help for a disorder that is often intractable.

Some patients have the **somatoform pain disorder**. To qualify for this diagnosis they must have been preoccupied with a pain for at least six months, and the pain must have no organic background, or there must only be minor organic pathology present, and the complaining must be grossly in excess of what would be expected. Such patients are rare in psychiatric practice, but common in pain clinics and medical practice. Patients often become habituated and even addicted to analgesics. Pain can be a withdrawal symptom following the abuse of analgesics. The condition is common in compensation cases in which the patient readily adotps the role of an invalid. Many become depressed. The differential diagnosis includes patients with severe depression in whom pain may be the presenting symptom. Even if a severe depression is not present, patients often respond to antidepressant medication combined with cognitive and behavioural therapy, providing that they are prepared to accept treatment.

Anorexia nervosa

Definition

The patient cannot or will not maintain a normal body weight (weight is usually at least 20 per cent below that expected for the patient's age and height). In juvenile anorexia, expected weight gain is not seen during adolescence. There is a phobia of becoming fat with a perceptual distortion of body image so that the patient both feels and sees herself as fat even though she is emaciated. There is amenorrhoea.

Epidemiology

The prevalence is uncertain. Most people with established anorexia nervosa are female. Perhaps five per cent of the young female population are sufficiently underweight to have amenorrhoea, but not all of these people will have the full-blown syndrome. It occurs in all social classes, but may be more prominent in the middle classes. Contrary to popular belief, there is no real evidence that it is increasing in prevalence.

Clinical features

1. Appearance and behaviour

The patient is emaciated, but will usually try to hide this with baggy clothes. Some patients achieve weight loss purely by eating minimally, some use laxatives and diuretics, some induce vomiting, and some have episodes of binge eating followed by vomiting (this is called bulimia nervosa). The patient's perception of herself is as fat, even when she is painfully thin, and the thinner she gets often the fatter she sees herself. There are often feelings of guilt after eating. There is often a preoccupation with feeding others and with cooking; excessive exercise is taken and the patient is often hyperactive; and there may be some sleep disturbance with early morning waking. Bizarre vegetarian diets, particularly involving fresh vegetables, are common and many patients have carotinaemia.

Physically, patients may have characteristic parotid gland swelling; there is preservation of secondary sexual characteristics even though the body is emaciated; there is fine downy hair on the back and cheeks; and in extreme cases there is peripheral cyanosis. In those who vomit there may be pitted dental enamel and chronic sinusitis. Mild obsessional rituals are also common.

2. Speech

This is usually unaffected, except the patient is preoccupied with a desire to be thin.

3. Mood

There is sometimes a secondary depression. Often, however, there is a rather brittle cheerfulness. Broken sleep with early morning waking occurs, even in the absence of depression.

4. Thoughts

These include a preoccupation with body shape, fatness, food, and diet. The patient will often lie about her eating behaviour.

5. Perception

There is a distorted bodily perception as outlined above, although this is not of psychotic intensity. It is a kind of dysmorphophobia.

6. Cognitive function

This is usually preserved, except in extreme starvation when concentration and then memory become impaired.

7. Other associated symptoms

There is often, but not invariably, a loss of sexual interest, loss of libido, and difficulty in making relationships with others. Severe starvation may lead to peripheral oedema, hypoalbuminaemia, renal failure, hypocalcaemia, cardiomyopathy, neuropathy, and anaemia.

Aetiology

The aetiology is uncertain. There is probably an underlying physical predisposition that is possibly related to disturbed hypothalamic function (it is difficult to tell which is the chicken and which is the egg). Psychological factors related, for example, to difficult relationships with parents, response to stress, etc., interplay with the presumed physical disorder. Social factors, particularly society's evaluation of thinness as an ideal, may also play a part and in some patients there may be an unconscious denial of sexuality.

Differential diagnosis

Anorexia nervosa is not the same thing as being excessively thin and does not usually follow starvation. Occasionally, central nervous system lesions of the hypothalamic pituitary axis or in the midbrain may cause a syndrome resembling anorexia nervosa. Malabsorption, Addison's disease, and juvenile diabetes mellitus, may all be mistaken for it. In pituitary and hypothalamic disease there is extreme pallor and loss of the secondary sexual characteristics. In Addison's disease, there is deep pigmentation. These conditions can be distinguished by measuring hormone levels and by failure to respond to appropriate hormone stimulation tests. The patient does not have the positive psychological features of anorexia nervosa (including preoccupation with weight and fear of fatness), and has a normal perception of her weight loss.

Depressive illness can present with anorexia and

weight loss, but the patient does not have the other symptoms that go with anorexia nervosa. Some schizophrenic patients can lose a great deal of weight, but again do not have the characteristic features of anorexia nervosa.

Treatment

If the patient is severely ill so that her physical health is threatened, (for example, by hypokalaemia or by a very low serum albumin), admission to hospital is mandatory. This should initially be to a medical ward where lifesaving measures can be carried out (most psychiatrists in this country would feel that this can be on a compulsory basis if necessary). The aim should then be to achieve a slow rate of weight gain that is acceptable to the patient. Gradually extending targets can then be negotiated with the patient. Initially it is often better to compromise and just help the patient to stabilize her weight. When she is used to being a certain weight, increase the target weight very slowly with the goal of eventually helping her to achieve a weight at which she will menstruate. Try to establish a regular three meals a day regimen with supplements at other times (which can be withdrawn when enough weight gain has been achieved). Too rapid a weight gain merely increases any fatness phobia and makes the patient more resistant to treatment. Likewise, treatment regimens, although very popular, that put the patient into a childlike dependent state so that she is kept in bed and only allowed out as she gains weight, are to be avoided if possible. Do not weigh the patient too often; once a week is usually sufficient. Make sure weighing takes place under standard conditions on the same machine and try to persuade the patient not to weigh herself in between. Too frequent weighing leads to eating behaviour becoming contingent on weight, which is the very condition that you are trying to treat!

It is better to try to develop a therapeutic alliance with the patient, using both cognitive and behavioural means, to help her to gradually increase her weight and come to terms with and conquer the unpleasant feelings that such weight gain initially induces. This can often be done on an out-patient basis. Anorexia nervosa raises great anxiety in parents and other carers, and often family therapy is necessary to overcome this. As treatment progresses one can usually begin to get to know the patient as a person and begin to understand the particular psychological pressures that have helped to produce her behaviour. Occasionally, antidepressant medication may help to increase weight and also to relieve any secondary depression. Appetite-enhancing drugs such as cyproheptadine have a limited place.

Prognosis

In uncomplicated anorexia nervosa the prognosis is often good and most patients achieve a reasonable compromise, although menstruation often does not occur for some months after regaining normal weight. The patient will be vulnerable to developing anorexic symptoms in the future during any stressful periods in her life. Patients with severe personality difficulties have a poorer prognosis, as do those that have bulimic behaviour in addition to anorexia. Despite everything that can be done, some patients die of anorexia. There is particular difficulty in deciding when, and if, to coerce and force treatment. Laxative and diuretic abuse increases the risk of death.

Bulimia nervosa

Definition

In this condition there are recurrent episodes of binge eating that are outwith the patient's control, usually followed by self-induced vomiting. The behaviour should be persistent, with at least two binge-eating episodes per week for at least three months. Anorexic behaviours are common, such as the use of laxatives, diuretics, episodes of dieting or fasting, vigorous exercise, and an overconcern with body shape and weight.

Epidemiology

Occasional binge eating ('pigging out') is common, and mild degrees of bulimia are also common, particularly in the young female population (perhaps five per cent or even higher). Bulimia nervosa, as an established disorder with serious social and physical consequences, is not common. It is sometimes difficult to decide if one is dealing with anorexia nervosa in which bulimic features are prominent, or vice versa. There is some argument about whether they are variants of a single disorder or are distinct diagnostic categories. Bulimia is rare in men.

Clinical features

1. Appearance and behaviour

Some patients are underweight, many are of normal weight, and a few are overweight. Rapid alterations in weight are also common (for example, two stone in a month). Most bulimics get recurrent urges to overeat and binge, some of which they can control, some of which they cannot. Patients often describe developing a dream-like state before the bingeing occurs (some report a sweet taste in the mouth at this time). Bingeing is usually done in secret, and very large amounts of (usually sweetish) carbohydrate-containing food are eaten. Some patients steal in order to binge, others root for food in pig bins, and find themselves compelled to eat almost anything. Most vomit after an episode (those that do not tend to gain weight). Vomiting may become reflex and is often both preceded and followed by intense feelings of guilt and despair. The frequency of bingeing varies enormously as does the time of day at which bingeing is done, particularly since it has to be done in secret. Patients severely affected by the disorder will often binge at least once a day.

2. Speech

This is usually unchanged.

3. Mood

Secondary depression seems common, as in anorexia nervosa, and there may also be sleep difficulties.

4. Thoughts

Thinking tends to be preoccupied with the problem and with guilty thoughts, particularly after a bingeing episode.

5. Perception

This is usually little changed, although some patients that have strong anorexic features will have the typical anorexic perceptual distortion of body image.

6. Cognitive function

This is unchanged.

7. Other associated symptoms

Anxiety and depression are common, and alcoholism and occasionally drug abuse are probably commoner in bulimics than in the general population. Severe bingeing and vomiting leads to metabolic disorders, particularly hypokalaemia and metabolic acidosis. Occasionally, gastric rupture or oesophageal tears occur (Mallory–Weiss syndrome). Dental changes, including characteristic pitting of the enamel, are common, as is chronic sinusitis. Salivary gland swelling is also common.

Aetiology

As with anorexia nervosa, it is uncertain. There may be an underlying organic predisposition that is triggered into life by environmental stress or by the development of comfort eating that gets out of control. Personality disturbance is said to be more common in the siblings of patients with this disorder than in the general population. Other addictive behaviour is also seen.

Differential diagnosis

A distinction, which is not always possible, should be made between primary bulimia and primary anorexia nervosa. Depressive illness may sometimes present with bulimia, and occasionally the behaviour may occur for the first time in somebody facing a major life crisis or acute situational reaction. Organic syndromes causing a similar condition are rare. Epilepsy is often blamed, though in our experience never causes this condition. Rarely, organic disease of the brain, particularly bilateral hippocampal damage, gives rise to the Kluver–Bucy syndrome (characterized by cognitive difficulty, tendency to examine the environment with the mouth, hyperphagia, and hypersexuality). The Kleine–Levin syndrome, episodic hyperphagia and hypersomnia, originally thought to only to occur in males, has now been described in females.

Treatment

If there is a strong anorexic element, it may be better to treat for anorexia nervosa, but if behaviour is more clearly bulimic then behavioural and cognitive therapy aimed at teaching the patient control skills to prevent bingeing and to eat more regularly are indicated, as well as exploring the underlying reasons for the bulimia. Occasionally, as in anorexia nervosa, medical treatment is necessary first. Bulimia is often well treated by group therapy. Some patients respond well to physical therapy such as massage. Fluoxetine may have a place, particularly in the overweight, but should not be used in the underweight.

Prognosis

This is often a difficult condition to treat (both for the therapist and the patient). Relapses are common during periods of life stress. The recent development of group therapy techniques has undoubtedly improved prognosis.

F Personality disorders

The classification of personality is a problem of relative shades of grey rather than differentiation between black and white. This is reflected in the many different systems and categories suggested at various times for the description and delineation of personality. Another problem is that the term personality disorder is often used as a pejorative label, as a dustbin, and as a refuge for the cynical or incompetent.

Much confirmatory evidence is required to make a hard and fast diagnosis of personality disorder, and much more than the day-to-day assessment of personality that we all carry out instinctively is needed. A generally accepted definition is that of the World Health Organization (1978).

Deeply ingrained maladaptive behaviour generally recognized by the time of adolescence or earlier and continuing throughout most of adult life, although often becoming less obvious in middle to old age. Because of his deviation of psychopathology, the patient suffers or others have to suffer, and there is an adverse effect on individuals or society.

Epidemiology

This obviously depends both on the definition of personality disorder employed and how it was measured, and the population studied. One recent study in the USA suggested a 2.1 to 3.3 per cent lifetime risk of antisocial personality disorder.

Classification

There are two accepted classifications used in current practice—the ICD 9 (shortly to be ICD 10) and DSM III R. The DSM system is more operationally defined and so is cumbersome to present in a short textbook. ICD 9 is descriptive and we have felt it useful to include it to give a quick overview. The following descriptions imply a persistent lifelong and prominent trait that makes the individual collide with other individuals or with society.

Paranoid   Either consistently oversensitive and blaming others, or aggressively occupied with personal rights and having an excessive tendency to self-reference and to entertain overvalued ideas.

Affective   Persistent abnormality of mood, depressed or euphoric, or alternating between them, but not amounting to manic depressive disorder.

Schizoid   Extreme reserve, shyness, and aloofness. May be persistently eccentric in behaviour.

Explosive   Hostile to approaches, explosive instability of mood, liable to sudden irritability and impulsive aggression, but is normal at other times.

Anakastic 'obsessional'   Extremely cautious, rigid, perfectionist, doubting, prone to anxiety, may have obsessional traits such as repeated checking.

Hysterical   Shallow, labile moods, very dependent on responses from others, erratic relationships, histrionic, and may dramatize physical symptoms to excess.

Asthenic Passive dependence, lacking resilience and mental vigour.

Sociopath Persistent antisocial behaviour with lack of sympathetic feeling or remorse. May be abnormally aggressive.

ICD 9 recommends avoidance of the terms 'immature' and 'inadequate' personality as these have been used as pejorative labels in the past and have no real definition in the ICD system, and it also allows the category of 'other' and 'unspecified'.

Aetiology

Little is known for certain of the factors involved in the aetiology of personality disorder. Research is scanty and incomplete, reflecting particularly the obvious difficulty in recognizing early life events that *may* shape a personality that is to be classified many years later. Aetiology is a complex interaction between genetic endowment, childhood upbringing, influence and environment, and the morals of the society in which the individual lives, some societies welcoming personality traits that other societies abhor.

Assessment

The assessment of a personality disorder is a long process if it is done thoroughly. It must include not only prolonged interviews with the patient, on more than one occasion, but also interviews with other professionals, such as social workers or probation officers. It must also include interviews with the patient's employer, others who have come into contact with the patient, and the family and friends of the patient (not only to corroborate what the patient says but also to gain a good idea of the problems that the particular personality presents to the patient and those around him). Standard personality questionnaires (for example, the Personality Assessment Schedule by Tyrer and Alexander) have been devised to aid a more consistent diagnosis of personality disorder. With all the confusion of terminology and the use of different personality assessment scales, it is often better in practice to describe briefly the main features of a patient's character rather than to try to attach a single diagnostic label to them.

Treatment

The treatment of problem personalities is notoriously difficult. Aims should be modest and a considerable amount of time must be allowed to achieve them. Since the personality disordered are often difficult and unrewarding to work with, if long-term therapy is indicated, care should be taken to ensure that the patient is not rejected by the medical or nursing staff, and that the patient's personality is not taken as a reason for disengagement and disenchantment. It is also important to discourage the patient from adopting a passive sick role, with an expectation that there is a treatment that can be given to him to 'cure' his problems. The truth is that a change will only come with a lot of hard work by the patient, who must enter into a therapeutic contract based on shared responsibility.

Drug treatment

Drugs have almost no part to play in the management of these disorders. Anxiolytics or major tranquillizers may occasionally be given for short periods at times of extreme stress, but are not indicated for long-term treatment, particularly because of the problems of addiction.

Psychotherapy, behaviour and cognitive therapy

Such therapies are indicated to help the patient to understand the way his behaviour both affects other people and causes him problems, leading to a gradual understanding and change in, or tolerance of, his personality. A supportive approach is especially needed as changes will occur over years rather than weeks or months. A true therapeutic community will be especially valuable, but difficult to find.

Prognosis

Although personality disorders are difficult to treat or change rapidly, evidence suggests that they tend to become less of a problem with increasing age.

G Alcohol/drug abuse and dependence

Various models have been used to describe dependent syndromes, including both medical models and behavioural models, but these are simplistic and it is better to adopt a multifaceted approach to the problem. The World Health Organization said that 'the view that dependence is a clustering phenomenon (cognitive, behavioural, and physiological) implies that multiple criteria are necessary for its assessment'. The psychosocial as well as the physical aspects of dependence are equally important.

Dependence implies subjective awareness of a compulsion to use a drug or drugs, usually during attempts to stop or to moderate use, a desire to stop drug use in the face of continued use, a relatively stereotyped drug taking habit, i.e., a narrowing in the repertoire of drug taking behaviour, evidence of neuroadaptation (tolerance and withdrawal symptoms), use of the drug to relieve or avoid withdrawal symptoms, the prominence of drug seeking behaviour relative to other important priorities, and rapid reinstatement of the syndrome after a period of abstinence.

A useful source book is the Royal College of Psychiatrists' report *Drug scene* published in 1988, which gives a good historical perspective as well as details of current drug use.

Epidemiology

About a tenth of admissions to psychiatric care are for alcohol-related problems: perhaps 3–5 per cent of the population have problem drinking. Alcohol also accounts for a significant proportion of general medical admissions. Alcoholism is commonest in young adult males, but there are disturbing increases in the female proportion. Most alcohol *dependence* begins in the late teens or early twenties.

Alcoholism is said to be commoner in the high and low social classes; its prevalence is lowest in the middle classes. It is more common in the divorced or separated, but is often the cause of marital disharmony. There are some occupational risks, for example, those who work in the brewing trade or in pubs, and business men and journalists who use alcohol as social lubricants, and in occupations in which work stress is high, for example, doctors.

Clinical features

These can be divided into acute intoxication phenomena, acute withdrawal phenomena, chronic effects, associated psychiatric syndromes, and harmful social effects. The **acute intoxicating effects** of alcohol are easy to recognize—fatuous euphoria, unsteadiness, and slurred speech ('Marry, sir, nose painting, sleep, and urine. Lechery, sir, it provokes, and unprovokes')—but you should already know that they often are a misleading cover for other disorders (such as hypoglycaemia or head injury). Drunkenness may be too readily diagnosed when the patient is actually suffering from something else—not all unconscious patients smelling of drink are actually drunk. In psychiatry in particular, apparent intoxication may mask a physical illness, a psychosis, or a drug overdose. Intravenous naloxone, which temporarily 'wakes up' the alcohol-intoxicated, can be very helpful. A consequence of repeated intoxication (or a single severe intoxication) are **memory blackouts**, or failure to recall the events of the night before. They should be taken as a warning that brain damage is starting to occur.

Pathological drunkenness (*mania àpotu*) also occurs when a very small amount of alcohol triggers off an acute behaviour disturbance. It may occur in the brain damaged or in the psychotic. Occasionally, it occurs as an alcohol-withdrawal phenomenon.

Delirium tremens (see p. 473) may occur as a withdrawal phenomenon, may occur in the face of continued drinking, or in response to intercurrent illness or infection in the alcoholic.

Although it is often thought to be the hallmark of alcoholism, only approximately five per cent of alcoholics attending clinics have experienced delirium tremens. The syndrome is characterized by tremor, restlessness, loss of contact with reality, disorientation, and illusions that may progress to terrifying hallucinations (commonly visual, but may be auditory or tactile, and often accompanied by paranoid delusions). If associated with withdrawal, the onset is usually about 72 hours after cessation of drinking. Tonic clonic seizures may accompany the syndrome at any time from the first day to two weeks after the last alcoholic drink. The syndrome carries a mortality of approximately 10 per cent.

Chronic disorders include those of thiamine deficiency; the acute form is termed Wernicke's encephalopathy, which has four main characteristics. There is an acute onset of global confusion, nystagmus, ataxia, and occular paralysis (of conjugate gaze). It is more common in those who drink over a number of years with concomitant poor nutrition, and is often preceded by prodromal symptoms of anorexia, nausea, and vomiting, which deteriorate over a few days into the full picture. It carries a mortality of approximately 15 per cent, and about 80 per cent of cases go on to develop Korsakoff's psychosis. It is a medical emergency, like delirium tremens, and should be recognized and treated as soon as possible with parenteral vitamin supplements containing thiamine.

An important part of the differential diagnosis of confusion in alcoholics, is a subdural haematoma, which is often sustained after a drunken fall.

Korsakoff's psychosis may occur with Wernicke's encephalopathy or may follow it. It shares the same pathology and aetiology and is due to thiamine deficiency. The main clinical feature of Korsakoff's syndrome is a marked memory disorder with preservation of other cognitive functions. It may require subtle cognitive testing to establish the diagnosis. Gross cases of it have severe recent memory impairment, confabulation, disorientation in time and place, and lack of insight, often accompanied by a disorder of the sense of the timing of events in relation to each other. It is important to differentiate this syndrome prognostically from alcoholic dementia (in which the cognitive deterioration is more global), and from a reversible alcoholic cognitive deterioration that clears quickly if the patient 'dries out'. Treatment is with thiamine. The prognosis, in terms of eventual social recovery, is probably better than most textbooks imply, although recovery may take two to three years.

Some alcoholics develop *a dementia of a more global kind* resembling Alzheimer's disease, which is progressive and which does not remit even if the patient remains dry. This is usually termed alcoholic dementia. It should be remembered that some permanently intoxicated people can appear quite brain impaired, but will gradually recover their wits during the drying out period if it extends for several weeks. The diagnosis of alcoholic dementia can therefore only be made if the patient has been known to be dry for some time.

In addition to cognitive changes, alcoholics may suffer from acute or permanent damage to the cerebellum and the peripheral nervous system, the gastrointestinal tract, the liver, and the heart. Certain cancers are are more common in alcoholics, particularly if they smoke. A very careful physical assessment is therefore mandatory for anyone with alcoholism.

Related psychiatric symptoms

1. Alcoholic hallucinosis

These are auditory hallucinations occurring in clear consciousness, often carrying on from hallucinations first experienced during alcohol withdrawl, although occasionally they may occur *de novo*. They often start as elementary hallucinations, but usually progress to formed words and sentences, usually of a derogatory nature. They may be accompanied by secondary persecutory delusions. Studies show that all but a few (5–10 per cent) will resolve spontaneously within 6–12 months if the patient dries out, although a return to drinking often brings a recurrence of the hallucinosis. If troublesome, it will respond to treatment with phenothiazines.

2. Affective disorder

Many alcoholics have some degree of depression, not just because of their chaotic lifestyle and relationships. Perhaps a fifth have recurrent affective illness (some writers suggest that alcoholics have depressive personalities and therefore lose themselves in the comfort of drink). Alcoholics are over-represented in both attempted and successful suicide statistics. Completed suicide is fifty times commoner in alcoholics than in the general population, and suicide risk therefore needs careful assessment. Completed suicide is commoner due to both impulsivity and the tendency to depression.

3. Pathological jealousy (Othello syndrome)

This is a firmly held delusion of a partner's infidelity. It is potentially very dangerous to the partner's well-being and so should always be taken seriously.

4. Psychosexual problems

These are common in alcoholism, particularly impotence and decreased sexual drive. Impotence is usually due to a combination of physical (neurogenic) and psychological factors. Potency often returns if the victim can stay dry.

Alcohol-related social problems

1. Family problems

Alcohol is said to contribute to approximately one third of divorces: 52 out of 100 battered wives report that their husbands are heavy drinkers. There may also be an increase in the occurrence of minor depressive disorders in the families of alcoholics as a direct result of coping with the illness. Children of alcoholics are at increased risk from an alcohol-related disorder at a later date.

2. Employment

Alcoholics are said to lose over twice the number of working days as other people. This is coupled with poor time-keeping and productivity. There is a three times greater risk of accidents in people who have blood levels of alcohol above the 80 mg% level than in those who are sober. Over a third of drivers involved in fatal road traffic accidents are intoxicated at the time of the accident.

3. Crime

Of prison inmates, 40–60 per cent have previous significant alcohol problems. There is also a group of problem drinkers who drift into crime to sustain their drinking habit. It is important to note that the above factors are interdependent and may lead into a slow spiral downwards of homelessness, vagrancy, and petty crime.

Aetiology

It is likely that the aetiology is multifactorial. Twin studies indicate a minor genetic effect, and biochemical factors may be involved. It has also been shown, however, that the rate of alcohol dependency is related to the general level of alcohol consumption within society. Children follow their parents' drinking habits and so it may be that these are also behaviourally mediated. Certain personality types have also been linked with excess alcohol consumption, although such findings are not consistent. An important group of patients are those with a pre-existing psychiatric disorder (especially an affective disorder, but including the neuroses and schizophrenia), who tend to 'self-medicate' with alcohol. This fact should be kept in mind when assessing someone with an alcohol problem.

Treatment

For *acute withdrawal*, it is necessary to sedate the patient with a decreasing course of either chlormethiazole or a benzodiazepine, which should be tailed to zero over seven to ten days. It is also essential that high potency multivitamin preparations are given to avoid the possible complications of Wernicke's and Korsakoff's syndromes. Thorough investigation and examination of other complicating factors (for example, liver or heart disease, concurrent infection, or dehydration) should always be made.

Maintenance after initial withdrawal is more of a problem. The warmth and enthusiasm of the therapist has been found to be an important factor in eventual success. Goals must be set after negotiation, and they must be realistic and, when possible, involve the family. Supportive psychotherapy should be used both to enhance the patient's self-esteem and to identify possible pitfalls (for instance, cues of habitual drinking). There are many other agencies, for example, Alcoholics Anonymous, that must be considered when working out a programme for the reformed alcoholic.

There are often many practical problems (housing, employment, etc.) that will need to be tackled at some point during the rehabilitation programme. Many find group therapy useful and some find security in the use of drugs such as disulfiram (Antabuse), although obviously this is totally dependent on the patient's choice as he will need to comply with the drug. Although controlled drinking has its advocates, the initial aim should be to keep the patient dry; for most patients, forever.

Prognosis

Untreated this is poor with only a tenth stopping spontaneously and a tenth regaining some control. Over half will continue to have a drinking problem. Whether treatment has any real effect is uncertain; it only works in those who have recognized that they have a problem and have the motivation to stop drinking.

Drug dependency

The concepts of substance abuse and dependency have already been covered in the section on alcohol abuse.

Treatment of drug dependency is specialized and so we will just touch on the clincal features of addiction and the effects of withdrawal from common drugs. It should be borne in mind that drugs of abuse do not only include illegal drugs, but also many psychoactive drugs available freely on prescription.

Opiates (heroin, morphine, codeine, DF 118)

Methods of drug taking include oral, by inhalation, and by injection (intramuscularly, subcutaneously, or intravenously). Acute effects include a detached dream-like state, the user becoming unconcerned with his usual cares, relaxation, and an initial increase of libido.

Rapid physical dependence and tolerance develops. Acute withdrawal symptoms include restlessness and fear, nausea, diarrhoea, sweating, sleeplessness, and abdominal and muscle pain. There may be a rebound autonomic excitability including tachycardia, involuntary movements, and hypertension. Mortality and morbidity of drug abuse is mainly due to the method of use. Infections (hepatitis B, AIDS, and endocarditis) are common with intravenous use. Other complications are accidental overdose, respiratory depression, and suicide. Treatment is similar to that for alcoholism, and is dependent on the patient's desire to give up as well as the ability to make practical changes in his lifestyle. This is often a problem as their social life for people from 'drug subcultures' may revolve around the people they take the drug with, giving abstinence a very high price. Specialized units are empowered, within the law, to maintain heroin addicts on (hopefully decreasing) doses of oral methadone.

Amphetamine

Amphetamine is the main abused stimulant drug. It is taken orally (occasionally intravenously). The initial effect is one of euphoria, excitement, increased drive and concentration, reduced appetite, and fatigue. This is followed the next day by dysphoria, fatigue, headache, etc. This pattern of response is particularly dangerous as it encourages quick dependence. If taken in high doses, amphetamines may produce a 'symptomatic schizophrenia', with prominent persecutory delusions that may be accompanied by visual and tactile hallucinations. Occasionally, a symptomatic mania is seen. These psychotic states tend to resolve within a week of drug withdrawal, although may require treating with phenothiazines.

Cocaine

This is another stimulant, which is sometimes used in conjunction with heroin. It is usually inhaled, although may be used orally or intravenously. It causes intense euphoria and excitement with increased energy of short duration. Prolonged use causes a hypervigilant syndrome, often with paranoid ideation. Withdrawal causes craving and depression, tremor, and discomfort. Occasionally, it has the side-effect of causing visual or tactile hallucinations (formication). Increasingly, especially in the USA, cocaine is converted to a base substance (crack cocaine) that is a highly addictive drug when smoked (this habit is known as free basing). It has the features of cocaine but with increased intensity, which increases the addictive potential as the patient craves the crack-induced highs and wishes to avoid the deep depression that follows them.

Hallucinogenic substances (LSD or acid)

This is taken orally. Even very low doses can cause an acute state with multiple hallucinations (usually visual) with perceptual distortions and intense emotions. The experience may be intensely pleasant leaving the user feeling that he has gained insight, or may be a terrifying and unpleasant experience of depression or paranoia.

There is a real risk of suicidal behaviour during such experiences. Insight may be retained or thinking may become delusional (for example, developing the false belief that one can fly with disastrous consequences). After-effects include unpleasant flashback phenomena (the exact prevalence of this disorder is unknown). Occasionally, an LSD-induced schizophreniform psychosis may develop, which may be persistent (it is uncertain whether LSD is the primary cause or simply releases a psychosis in predisposed individuals).

Cannabis

Cannabis is widely used by a variety of social groups and is similar to alcohol in its effect on mood. It is usually taken for a feeling of relaxation, well-being, and tranquillity. It induces some psychological dependence. Occasionally, a short-term affective psychosis may develop. Chronic use is said to cause an 'amotivational syndrome' of lethargy, apathy, and dullness.

Sedatives

These include benzodiazpines and barbiturates, often initially supplied on a prescription. They are sometimes used in conjunction with other drugs. Barbiturate abusers become rapidly dependent with a withdrawal syndrome of disturbed sleep, restlessness, irritability, and possible seizures. Chronic abuse gives rise to slurred speech, nystagmus, and a drowsy feeling. Overdose causes respiratory failure. Although usually taken orally, these drugs can be injected intravenously. Benzodiazepines also rapidly cause physical dependence. Acute withdrawal mimics the insomnia or anxiety state for which the drugs were first prescribed. Abrupt withdrawal may also precipitate seizures or confusional states. Benzodiazepines, often those obtained illicitly, can be crushed and injected. When taken in this way they tend to cause acute inflammatory reactions, which may bring the addict to the notice of the medical services.

Solvent abuse

The solvents used include those used for cleaning, aerosols, glues, modelling cement, paints, and lacquers. Abuse is said to be prevalent in preadolescent and adolescent boys, usually as a group activity, although there are persistent lone users. They are inhaled, often from plastic bags including empty crisp packets. There is an initial euphoria followed by drowsiness or stupor. Occasionally, perceptual disturbances occur. Psychological addiction occurs, although solvents are said not to be physically addictive. Deaths have been reported for a variety of reasons (for example, respiratory failure following inhalation or smothering by the plastic bags used to create the solvent environment, or death due to cardiac arrhythmias). There are a variety of other direct toxic effects on the liver, kidneys, peripheral and central nervous systems, and bone marrow.

Summary

When taking a drug history from a drug addict, you will find that he is often more knowledgeable than yourself about drugs, and it can be fascinating to listen and learn from him about the drug scene. Until, however, you have gained a great deal of experience and have built up a good therapeutic alliance with the individual patient, do not trust what you are told and always seek independent verification. The addict's lifestyle and constant need to secure supplies makes him manipulative and untrustworthy. Unless you are part of a specialist team with a clear prescribing policy *never* prescribe drugs of addiction to an addict (cover acute withdrawal with phenothiazines).

Reading list

We include here texts that you will find useful in your first few months in psychiatry. For a comprehensive list consult your tutor and the reading lists published by the Royal College of Psychiatrists. Check with your book seller about prospective new editions before purchasing.

General texts

Clare, A. (1988). *Psychiatry in dissent*, (2nd edn). Routledge, London.
Well worth reading during those lonely evenings on call, puts psychiatry into a necessary perspective.

Gelder, M., Gath, D., and Mayou, R. (1989). *Oxford textbook of psychiatry*, (2nd edn). Oxford University Press, Oxford.
A good general text, well referenced.

Hill, P., Murray, R., and Thorley, A. (1986). *Essentials of post-graduate psychiatry*, (2nd edn). Grune and Stratton, London.

Kendall, R. and Zeally, A. (1988). *Companion to psychiatric studies*. Churchill Livingstone, Edinburgh.

Weller, M. and Eysenck, M. (1991). *Scientific basis of psychiatry*. Saunders, London.

Special texts

Bebbington, P.E. and McGuffin, P. (1988). *Schizophrenia: the major issues*. Heinemann, London.

Birchwood, M. et al. (1988). *Schizophrenia: an integrated approach to research and treatment*. Longman, Harlow, Essex.

Bloch, S. (1986). *Introduction to psychiatry*, (2nd edn). Oxford University Press, Oxford.

Bluglass, R. (1984). *A guide to the Mental Health Act.* Churchill Livingstone, Edinburgh.
Another 'bible' you will consult often.

Cassem, N. (1991). *Handbook of general hospital psychiatry*, (3rd edn). Mosby Year Book, Massachusetts General Hospital, Boston.
A brilliant outline of liaison psychiatry.

Faulk, M. (1987). *Basic forensic psychiatry.* Blackwell, Oxford.

Graham, P. (1991). *Child psychiatry: a developmental approach.* Oxford University Press, Oxford.

Hawton, K. and Catalan, J. (1990). *Attempted suicide.* Oxford University Press, Oxford.

Hawton, K., Salkovskis, P.M., Kirk, J., and Clark, D.M. (1989). *Cognitive behaviour therapy for psychiatric problems.* Oxford University Press, Oxford.
A brilliant book that will greatly influence your practice.

Lader, M. and Herrington, R. (1991). *Biological treatments in psychiatry.* Oxford University Press, Oxford.

Lishman, W.A. (1987). *Organic psychiatry: psychological consequences of cerebral disorder*, (2nd edn). Blackwell, Oxford.
The 'bible' of neuropsychiatry: you will consult this book again and again.

Silverstone, T. and Turner, P. (1991). *Drug treatment in psychiatry*, (4th edn). Routledge, London.

Snaith, P. (1991). *Clinical neurosis.* Oxford University Press, Oxford.

Worden, J.W. (1991). *Grief counselling and grief therapy*, (2nd edn). Tavistock, Routledge, London.

Index